Hepatology and Transplant Hepatology Board Review

Hepatology and Transplant Hepatology Board Review

Jawad Ahmad, MD, FRCP, FAASLD
Icahn School of Medicine at Mount Sinai
New York, NY, USA

Shahid M. Malik, MD
University of Pittsburgh Medical Center
Pittsburgh, PA, USA

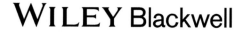

Registered Offices
John Wiley & Sons, Inc., 111 River Street, Hoboken, NJ 07030, USA
John Wiley & Sons Ltd, The Atrium, Southern Gate, Chichester, West Sussex, PO19 8SQ, UK

For details of our global editorial offices, customer services, and more information about Wiley products visit us at www.wiley.com.

Wiley also publishes its books in a variety of electronic formats and by print-on-demand. Some content that appears in standard print versions of this book may not be available in other formats.

Library of Congress Cataloging-in-Publication Data applied for
ISBN: 9781119853510 (paperback)

Cover Design: Wiley
Cover Images: © natali_mis/Adobe Stock Photos

Set in 10/12pt WarnockPro by Straive, Chennai, India
Printed and bound by CPI Group (UK) Ltd, Croydon, CR0 4YY

C9781119853510_040123

Contents

Preface

Like several other specialties in medicine, historically, hepatology was always an interesting field with diagnostic conundrums that required getting a good history, a whole slew of eponymous physical exam findings, interpretation of multiple blood tests, and the "easy access to the liver" to get a biopsy that you could spend many hours reviewing. And then provide the patient with supportive care and observe!

This changed in the last 30–40 years ago with advancements in our understanding of viral hepatitis that led to initially effective and then highly effective therapies and vaccines and most importantly the development of immunosuppressive drugs that allowed liver transplantation to become the definitive treatment for patients with end-stage liver disease.

As a result, hepatology and transplant hepatology have emerged as individual disciplines, separate from gastroenterology, and this has been recognized by the American Board of Internal Medicine (ABIM) who have offered a transplant hepatology board exam since 2006.

Since taking the exam in 2006 (and then recertifying in 2016), I have been frustrated at the lack of study guides or board review material in hepatology as there are in gastroenterology (including an annual course that I co-direct at the Icahn School of Medicine at Mount Sinai in New York). There are many seminal textbooks of liver disease, but they are not the place to turn to when studying for the board exam. Hence, the idea for this book.

The ABIM website for transplant hepatology (https://www.abim.org/Media/lo0jcigs/transplant-hepatology.pdf) gives quite a lot of information about the content of the examination. In 2021, the examination was divided into pre-transplant (45%), peri-operative (20%), post-transplant (25%), transplant immunology (5%), and miscellaneous (5%) categories.

Shahid and I have tried to cover all the main topics that could make an appearance in the board examination, but in a more concise format, so it can be read at leisure or while you have a few spare minutes between seeing patients or on rounds. To keep things interesting, we have added cases that display an interesting image or teaching point and an occasional zebra.

To mimic the examination, we have assembled 257 multiple-choice questions, but we have deliberately not divided them into chapters. All the questions involving patients are based on real cases we have seen (with some changes to protect patient confidentiality) and the images, pathology slides, cholangiograms are all original. The bulk of the actual examination is case based. We have used the most current management guidelines from the main liver societies, but as with most of medicine, there is room for individual comments. After each question, there is a brief overview of the topic and "pearls" are scattered throughout the book for points that we felt needed to be emphasized and are likely to come up on the board examination.

The fact of the matter is, the ABIM board examination is very well written (it's written by people like us!). The questions are clinically relevant and based on scenarios you will encounter in your hepatology practice. Very few of the questions are "out of left field." There may be a handful of terms that you may not be familiar with (such as prope tolerance, Tregs, SF-36 questionnaire), but we hope we've covered most of these terms in this text. The questions on the exam are not meant to trick you. The questions are meant to test your medical knowledge, clinical acumen, and management skills. The test writers they are not going to try to trip you up you with a technical point, for example the genetic defect for BRIC is ATP8B1 (and not ATP7B which is seen in Wilson disease).

With that being said, the boards are the boards and there will be questions that are "board answers" but are not necessarily what we do in clinical practice. Three examples that jump to mind:

1. Deferring treating for autoimmune hepatitis (AIH) unless the enzyme elevation is more than 2–3× upper limits of normal. Most hepatologists would end up treating in the setting of even mild enzyme elevation, assuming other parameters (serologies and biopsy) are consistent with AIH.
2. Obtaining a liver biopsy in a patient with hemochromatosis with a ferritin >1000 ng/mL to rule out cirrhosis. Today, most of us would obtain a noninvasive imaging study (FibroScan, Shear-Wave Elastography, or MRE) to assess the degree of fibrosis as opposed to a liver biopsy.
3. The role of ursodeoxycholic acid (UDCA) in patients with primary sclerosing cholangitis (PSC). Most hepatologists are still trialing patients on a course of UDCA, but for the boards, UDCA is always the wrong choice when it comes to PSC.

When in doubt, answer the question based on guideline recommendations.

Our main objective in writing this review was to have it be the only source you will need to (comfortably) pass the transplant hepatology examination. We have included key references in case you wanted to delve deeper into a subject, but we are hopeful that everything you need for the examination will be in this book. Until now there were no MCQ/review books specifically designed for the transplant hepatology boards. There are gastroenterology board reviews with liver questions, but nothing covering the full range of topics outlined by the ABIM.

From 2016–2020, there were 265 transplant hepatology test-takers. The past rate has consistently been over 95%. Why such a high pass rate? Well, it goes without saying that hepatologists in general are quite smart. However, the fact of the matter is to pass the examination you only need to get at least 70% of the questions correct (this will change slightly from year to year). Based on the overall high pass rates, we can surmise that test-takers take these exams very seriously. Not surprising given the cost of the ABIM examinations (seriously, how they justify the $3000 price tag is beyond me!). The overall pass rate of the 56,420 test takers for the 19 specialty board examinations over the last 5 years is 91%. So maybe hepatologists aren't as special as we thought, or doctors make sure they get their money's worth.

Board examination questions should be clear and unambiguous. The board will avoid questions with a lead-in containing "all of the following EXCEPT." We also tried to avoid questions like these, but ultimately included a handful as they are a nice means of solidifying factual points and there are a couple of trick questions (to keep you on your toes). The board questions also typically lag 1–2 years from clinical practice. Therefore, although we included the new hepatocellular carcinoma (HCC) therapies in our review, these agents are unlikely to be tested on for a few years. The boards also include some "throw away" or "litmus" questions used to gauge answers for future examinations. Remember a vast majority of test-takers should answer most examination questions correctly. The boards like to use questions where the correct answers are agreed upon by most. You, of course, will assume that every test question on your examination will be counted toward your grade.

The questions in this book are meant as a springboard to the clinical pearls which are the real "meat" of this review. We designed each "pearl" to be a potentially testable point. Therefore, in essence, this book has well over 1500 potential testable points.

The day of the examination will go by relatively quickly, but it is easy to get burned out while studying for the examination. Pacing yourself is key. Studying can be a tedious process. We've included some personal anecdotes to help break the monotony of studying. Our recommendation is to start this review about 12 weeks before your examination. We suggest doing about 25 questions a week with a concentration on learning the clinical pearls. About 10 days before the examination, I would suggest re-doing the questions to bolster your confidence.

All right, enough stalling. Let's get to studying and smash these boards!

Remember: save livers…save lives.

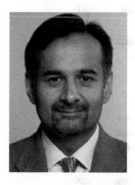

Jawad Ahmad

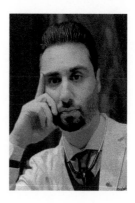

Shahid M. Malik

Acknowledgments

"The fool doth think he is wise, but the wise man knows himself to be a fool"
As You Like It

William Shakespeare

From your first day of medical school, it becomes quickly apparent that despite being the smartest kid in school, you know very little. This is especially so in the British system of medical school training where an 18 year-old adolescent is given a short white coat and becomes a medical student, just 5 short years away from reciting the Hippocratic coat, donning a long white coat, and prefixing Dr. to their name. However, those 5 years are just the start of your medical education, the start of a journey where there is no destination but the route you take during that journey will define how wise you become.

Becoming a doctor is hard. Teaching others how to practice medicine is even harder. Neither happens without the influence of many individuals – other doctors, nurses, physician extenders, fellows, coordinators, endoscopy technicians, students, and staff, but most of all patients. We go into medicine for many different reasons but earning the trust of another human being, putting their health and life in your hands, remains the integral part of your journey.

I was privileged to spend my 5 years of medical school in London at the Royal Free Hospital School of Medicine. It was there that I first developed an appreciation for liver disease through sometimes fun, sometimes intimidating, but always rewarding interaction with giants in the field of hepatology including Dame Sheila Sherlock, Professor Peter Scheuer, Professor Andrew Burroughs, and all the others who worked on the Liver Unit.

One of the most gratifying aspects of medicine is the interaction with colleagues within your specialty and in different disciplines during weekly conferences, on rounds, or just in the hallway. Throughout the last 20 plus years, there have been hundreds of individuals ranging from eminent professors to first year medical students, who I am indebted to for teaching, stimulating and continually appraising what I think I know and the decisions that I make. At the University of Pittsburgh, it was my honor to be taught by and work with Drs. Obaid Shaikh, Mordechai Rabinovitz, Adam Slivka, John Martin, and Kathy Downey. At the Icahn School of Medicine at Mount Sinai, it has been a privilege to work with some of the smartest people I know and the epitome of a multi-disciplinary team.

I would like to acknowledge the production team at Wiley for their incredible professionalism and patience in putting this book together during an unprecedented pandemic.

I would not be here without love and stability that family brings. I have been blessed with three beautiful children, Leila, Noor, and Aryia, who remind me, that for all my mistakes, at least three times I did something right. Finally, I dedicate this book to my loving parents, Iftikhar and Gulzar, who remain the wisest people I know.

January 2022   Jawad Ahmad, MD, FRCP, FAASLD
New York, NY

All good things begin
In the name of God, the Most Beneficent, the Most Merciful

I can't help but roll my eyes when I hear doctors being described as or having developed a God complex. Any doctor who does hold him or herself in such high regard either has not worked long enough or is delusional. Medicine is the most humbling of professions. Patients remind us of that on a daily basis.

Writing a book of this breadth is also a humbling experience. Being an educator to medical trainees is a great responsibility. Please accept my apologies for any errors, oversights, or omissions.

I want to thank all those who helped educate and train me over the years, in particular, Doctors: Kevin McGrath, Adam Slivka, Rocky Schoen, Abhinav Humar, David Whitcomb, and of course Jawad. Of all my mentors, I am most appreciative to Dr. Mordechai Rabinovitz, whose passion and "love for all things liver" was one of the main reasons I pursued a career in hepatology. To this day, discussing (some may perceive it as arguing) challenging cases with the Professor (in the hallways of Montefiore Hospital) is one of the joys that keep me in academic medicine.

Thank you to all my trainees, nurses, and mid-level providers. A special thanks to Cathy Freehling for always looking out for me. Thanks, are also due to my patients (and families) who have entrusted their health in my hands.

I want to thank my three brothers, all accomplished physicians in their own right: Salman, Shehzad, and Sajjad Malik.

I want to thank my wife Rafia for her loyalty, patience and devotion, but most of all for giving me my three most precious gifts, Safa, Summer and Ejaz.

I have been given so much, very little of which is the result of my own efforts. I am forever in debt to the unwavering support of my parents. I am blessed with the constant prayers of my Mother, Abida Malik, and the beautiful example of my Father, Dr. Maqsood A. Malik, a great cardiologist and an even better person.

Finally, I want to acknowledge the four Pennsylvania cities that have played an integral role in my medical journey: Pottsville, Erie, Philadelphia, and Pittsburgh!

Pittsburgh, PA
January 2022

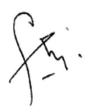

Shahid M. Malik, MD

Exam Blueprint

The entire exam is on computer and lasts one day. It is divided into four 2-hour sessions containing up to 60 multiple-choice questions. Test takers are allotted up to 100 minutes of break time. Breaks can only be taken in between the 60 block sessions (not during). There is a 30-minute optional tutorial session, an honesty pledge which is up to 10 minutes, and an optional 10-minute survey; the total test duration could be up to $4 \times 120 = 480 + 100$ minutes break $+ 50$ minutes (tutorial, pledge, and survey) $= 730$ minutes or up to **10.5 hours.**

Medical content category % of transplant hepatology board exam

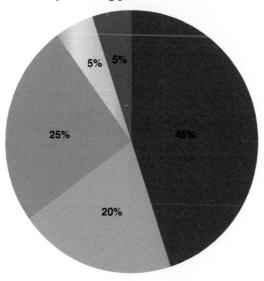

■ Pretransplant ■ Perioperative ■ Post-transplant ▨ Transplant Immunology ■ Miscellaneous

The blueprint below from the ABIM expands additional detail on the five broad exam content categories.

Pretransplant	108 questions
Biliary atresia (Pediatrics)	4–5 questions
Genetic liver diseases	9–10 questions
Alpha1-antitrypsin deficiency	
Cholestatic syndromes (PFIC, BRIC)	
Cystic fibrosis	
Fibrocystic diseases (caroli and choledochal cysts)	
Familial amyloid polyneuropathy	
Hereditary hemorrhagic telangiectasia	
Iron overload syndromes	
Mitochondrial defect	
Urea cycle defects	
Wilson	
Autoimmune disorders	7–8 questions
Primary biliary cholangitis	
Autoimmune hepatitis	
Overlap syndromes	
Primary sclerosing cholangitis	
IgG4 cholangiopathy	
Sarcoidosis	
Celiac disease	
Viral hepatitis	16–18 questions
A-E	
Other viruses (EBV, CVM, HSV)	
Outflow diseases (Budd Chiari, VOD)	3–4 questions
Growth failure (pediatrics)	4–5 questions
Portal hypertension	4–5 questions
Varices	
Ascites	
Hepatic hydrothorax	
SBP	
Encephalopathy	
HRS	
HPS	
PPHTN	
Noncirrhotic PHTN	
Liver tumors	9–10 questions
HCC	
Hepatoblastoma	
Cholangiocarcinoma	
Hemangioendothelioma	
NET	
Benign tumors (adenoma, FNH, hemangioma)	

Pretransplant	108 questions
Selection and evaluation for transplantation	21–23 questions
PELD and MELD scoring systems including exceptions	
Contraindications to liver transplantation	
Live donor selection	
Impact of infection, malignancy and malnutrition on outcomes	
Co-morbidities including HIV	
Acute liver failure	12 questions
Epidemiology	
Etiology	
Pathophysiology	
Assessment	
Prognostic indicators	
Treatment	
Indications for liver transplantation	
Outcomes based on age and diagnosis	
Alcoholic liver disease	4–5 questions
Transfer of care	3–4 questions
DILI	3–4 questions

Perioperative	48 questions
Donor Selection	7–8 questions
Extended criteria donors	
Steatosis	
Viral infection	
Domino liver transplant	
Surgical options, complications to graft and donor types (including ABO blood type)	7–8 questions
Perioperative complications	14–15 questions
PNF	
Vascular complications	
Infections (bacterial, viral, fungal)	
HBV and HCV therapy	
Biliary complications	
Allograft rejection	
Metabolic complications (including neuro and nephrotoxicity)	
Drug hepatotoxicity	4–5 questions
Nutritional support	4–5 questions
Living donor	2–3 questions
Small for size	
Donor complications	
Recipient complications	
Donor transmission of disease	2–3 questions
Donation after cardiac death	2–3 questions
Split graft transplantation	2–3 questions

Post-transplant	60 questions
Immune complications	9–10 questions
Rejection	
GVHD	
Alloimmune and autoimmune diseases (De novo)	
Nonimmune complications	12 questions
Diabetes	
Renal	
Bone	
Growth and development (pediatrics)	
Cardiovascular complications	
Vascular complications	
Infectious Complications	12 questions
Viral infections (CMV, EBV, HSV)	
Bacterial infections	
Fungal infections	
Recurrence Disease Post Transplant (HCV, PBC, AIH, malignancy)	7–8 questions
Post-Transplant Malignancy	4–5 questions
PTLD	
Surveillance	
Indications for Retransplantation	4–5 questions
Adherence	4–5 questions
QOL	4–5 questions

Transplant immunology	12 questions
Basic immunology	4–5 questions
Innate and adaptive immune system	
Immune response	
Tolerance	
Mechanism of action and pharmokinetics of IS meds	4–5 questions
Cyclosporine and tacrolimus	
MMF and azathioprine	
Sirolimus and everolimus	
Antibody therapy	
Drug–drug interactions	
Corticosteroids	
Short-term immune and nonimmune toxicity of IS medications	2–3 questions

Miscellaneous	12 questions
Statistics	4–5 questions
Kaplan–Meier	
Cox proportional hazards	
Relative risk	
Odds ratio	
Receiver operating characteristic curves	
Ethics	4–5 questions
Psychosocial evaluation	
Living donor transplantation	
Transplant tourism	
Clinical trial participation	
Managed care and reimbursement	2–3 questions
Regulatory issues	2–3 questions
Policy implication of organ shortage regulation	

Table of Abbreviations Used and Units for Laboratory Tests

	Abbreviation	Units
Total bilirubin	Tbili	g/dL
Aspartate aminotransferase	AST	U/L
Alanine aminotransferase	ALT	U/L
Alkaline phosphatase	ALP	U/L
Gamma glutamyl transferase	GGT/GGTP	U/L
Albumin		g/dL
Total protein		g/dL
International normalized ratio	INR	
Creatinine	Cr	mg/dL
Hepatitis B surface antigen	HBsAg	
Hepatitis B surface antibody	Anti-HBs	
Hepatitis B e antigen	HBeAg	
Hepatitis B e antibody	Anti-HBe	
Hepatitis B core antibody total	Anti-HBc	
Hepatitis B core antibody IgM	Anti-HBcIgM	
Hepatitis B virus	HBV	
Hepatitis C virus	HCV	
Hepatitis A virus	HAV	
Hepatitis E virus	HEV	
Hepatitis D virus	HDV	
Human immunodeficiency virus	HIV	
Hepatitis A antibody	Anti-HAV	
Hepatitis D antibody	Anti-HDV	
Hepatitis C antibody	Anti-HCV	
Anti-nuclear antibody	ANA	
Smooth muscle antibody	SMA	
Anti-mitochondrial antibody	AMA	
Immunoglobulin	IGG	mg/dL
Alfa-fetoprotein	AFP	ng/mL

	Abbreviation	Units
Carbohydrate antigen 19-9	CA19-9	U/mL
Ultrasound	US	
Computed tomography	CT	
Magnetic resonance image	MRI	
Positron emission tomography	PET	
Endoscopic retrograde cholangiopancreatography	ERCP	
Endoscopic ultrasound	EUS	
Percutaneous transhepatic cholangiogram	PTC	
Hepatocellular carcinoma	HCC	
Cholangiocarcinoma	CCA	
Upper limit of normal	ULN	
Ursodeoxycholic acid	UDCA	
Primary biliary cholangitis	PBC	
Primary sclerosing cholangitis	PSC	
Hemoglobin	Hb	g/dL
White blood cell count	WBC	$\times 10^3/\mu L$
Platelet count	Plts	$\times 10^3/\mu L$
Electrocardiogram	EKG	
Chest X-ray	CXR	
Hepatopulmonary syndrome	HPS	
Portopulmonary hypertension	PPHTN	
Liver transplant	LT	
Orthotopic liver transplant	OLT	
Live donor liver transplant	LDLT	
Calcineurin inhibitor	CNI	
Cytomegalovirus	CMV	
Epstein Barr virus	EBV	
Herpes simplex virus	HSV	
Polymerase chain reaction	PCR	
Post-transplant lymphoproliferative disorder	PTLD	
Gastric antral vascular ectasia	GAVE	
Argon plasma coagulation	APC	
Trans-jugular intra-hepatic porto-systemic shunt	TIPS	
Balloon retrograde transvenous obliteration	BRTO	
Kaposi sarcoma	KS	
Human herpes virus	HHV	
Mammalian (mechanistic) target of rapamycin	mTOR	
Donation after cardiac/circulatory death	DCD	

	Abbreviation	Units
Extended criteria donor	ECD	
Hepatic artery stenosis/thrombosis	HAS/HAT	
Primary non-function	PNF	
Non-alcoholic steatohepatitis	NASH	
Esophagogastroduodenoscopy	EGD	
Liver function tests	LFTs	
Tacrolimus	Tacro/FK	ng/mL
Cyclosporine	Cyclo	ng/mL
Mycophenolate mofetil	MMF	
Sirolimus/everolimus		ng/mL
Inflammatory bowel disease	IBD	
Mycobacterium avium-intracellulare	MAI	
Acquired immunodeficiency syndrome	AIDS	
Fluorescent in situ hybridization	FISH	
Next-generation sequencing	NGS	
Neuroendocrine tumor	NET	
Yttrium 90	Y90	
Transarterial chemoembolization	TACE	
Radiofrequency ablation	RFA	
Nonsteroidal anti-inflammatory drug	NSAID	
Model for end-stage liver disease	MELD	
Pediatric model for end-stage liver disease	PELD	
Body mass index	BMI	kg/m^2
Lactate		mmol/L
Ammonia	NH3	µmol/L
Emergency room	ER	
Resistive index	RI	
Focal nodular hyperplasia	FNH	
Nodular regenerative hyperplasia	NRH	
Recurrent pyogenic cholangitis	RPC	
Major histocompatibility complex	MHC	
Interleukin	IL	
Antigen presenting cell	APC	
T cell receptor	TCR	
Interferon gamma	IFN-g	
Delayed type hypersensitivity	DTH	
Ferritin		ng/mL
Hemophagocytic lymphohistiocytosis	HLH	

	Abbreviation	Units
Acute cellular rejection	ACR	
Rejection activity index	RAI	
Autoimmune hepatitis	AIH	
Serum ascites albumin gradient	SAAG	mg/dL
Drug-induced liver injury	DILI	
Biliary atresia	BA	
Alpha-1-antitrypsin (deficiency)	A1AT, AATD	
Graft to recipient weight ratio	GRWR	
Anti-thymocyte globulin	ATG	
Hepatorenal syndrome	HRS	
Glomerular filtration rate	GFR	
Organ procurement and transplantation network	OPTN	
Progressive familial intrahepatic cholestasis	PFIC	
Hepatitis B immune globulin	HBIG	
Tuberculosis	TB	
Ceruloplasmin		mg/dL
Nonselective beta-blocker	NSBB	
Benign intrahepatic cholestasis	BRIC	
N-acetyl-L-cysteine	NAC	
Mean corpuscular volume	MCV	FL
Triglyceride	TG	mg/dL
Direct acting anti-virals	DAA	
Hemolytic uremic syndrome	HUS	
Right upper quadrant	RUQ	
Intravenous drug use/abuse	IVDU/IVDA	
Kilo-pascal	kPa	
Tenofovir disoproxil fumarate	TDF	
Tenofovir alafenamide	TAF	
Acute fatty liver of pregnancy	AFLP	
Hemolysis, elevated liver tests and low platelets	HELLP	
Sinusoidal obstruction syndrome	SOS	
Food and drug administration	FDA	
Spontaneous bacterial peritonitis	SBP	
Portal hypertension	PHTN	
Sodium	Na	
Potassium	K	
Cold ischemia/ischemic time	CIT	
Warm ischemia/ischemic time	WIT	

	Abbreviation	Units
Antibody mediated rejection	AMR	
Donor specific antibody	DSA	
Hereditary hemorrhagic telangiectasia	HHT	
Arterial-vascular-malformations	AVM	
Posterior reversible encephalopathy syndrome	PRES	
Portosystemic encephalopathy	PSE	
Acetaminophen	APAP	
Pulmonary artery systolic pressure	PASP	
Small for size syndrome	SFSS	
Spontaneous splenorenal shunt	SSRS	
Thromboelastographic	TEG	
Graft-versus-host disease	GVHD	
Donor risk index	DRI	

Questions and Answers

Question 1

A 31-year-old lawyer presents with a 2-week history of pruritus and dark urine. He finally came to the emergency room when his wife noted his eyes were yellow. His symptoms started following an upper respiratory infection. Review of systems is notable for an 8-pound weight loss. The patient recalls one prior episode of self-remitting jaundice and pruritus 10 years prior that was attributed to an infectious hepatitis.

On physical exam, the patient has marked scleral icterus and diffuse excoriations. His abdominal exam is benign. Mentation and neurological exam are normal.

Laboratory studies:

Total bilirubin of 14.6 with a direct component of 11; AST 112, ALT 118, ALP 333, and GGT of 32; INR is 1.

An extensive acute liver workup including serologies for viral and autoimmune hepatitis are negative; ceruloplasmin is 32. An ultrasound reveals gallstones but is otherwise normal.

Symptomatic management is recommended. The patient's symptoms resolve, and labs return to normal in 10 weeks. The diagnosis is established based on genetic testing.

▶ Question

Which of the following is FALSE regarding this disease?

A Liver pathology would be mostly benign.
B A cholangiogram would be normal.
C Corticosteroids are the treatment of choice.
D The most commonly associated genetic abnormality is in ATP8B1.
E Total serum bile acids would be expected to be increased.

Hepatology and Transplant Hepatology Board Review, First Edition. Jawad Ahmad and Shahid M. Malik.
© 2023 John Wiley & Sons Ltd. Published 2023 by John Wiley & Sons Ltd.

C is the correct answer.

Commentary – BRIC

Clinical Pearls: Benign Recurrent Intrahepatic Cholestasis (BRIC)

1. Recurrence of an episode of jaundice is required for the diagnosis of benign recurrent intrahepatic cholestasis (BRIC).
2. For the boards gamma glutamyl transferase (GGT) will be normal.
3. Total serum bile acids are typically markedly elevated.
4. BRIC is an autosomal recessive disease.
5. Defects are associated with ATP8B1 (caution with the gene for Wilson: ATP7B); the more severe defects in this gene are associated with progressive familial intrahepatic cholestasis (PFIC); this gene is likely also responsible for intrahepatic cholestasis of pregnancy (ICP).
6. Episodes usually appears after an upper respiratory infection (>50% of cases), followed by drugs (namely hormonal).
7. Mean duration of episodes is six months.
8. A total of 80% of individuals will present within the first two decades of life. The mean age of first episode is 15 years.
9. ATP8B1 is also expressed in pancreas and small intestine (hence, pancreatitis and diarrhea as potential clinical clues).
10. Treatment is supportive; rifampin, ursodeoxycholic acid (UDCA) and in extreme cases plasmapheresis.
11. Proposed diagnostic criteria:
    a. At least two episodes of jaundice separated by symptom-free interval lasting months to years
    b. Elevated alkaline phosphatase (ALP) (typically GGT low to mildly elevated)
    c. Severe pruritus
    d. Liver histology relatively benign other than centrilobular cholestasis
    e. Normal cholangiogram
    f. Absence of other causes of cholestasis (namely drug and pregnancy)

Notes

BRIC is one of my favorite diseases. Making a diagnosis can make you look quite smart! The disproportionately low GGT is a hallmark of BRIC and should raise high suspicion. The presentation can be dramatic, but ultimately everyone is relieved when the diagnosis is established. To fulfill diagnostic criteria, a "recurrent" attack is necessary. Given the severity of the itching episodes, patients (and spouses) may describe this disorder as anything but "benign."

Reference

Triggers of benign recurrent intrahepatic cholestasis and its pathophysiology: a review of literature. PMID: 34599573.

Question 2

Review the following liver biopsy slide.

▶ Question

Which statement regarding this disease is FALSE?

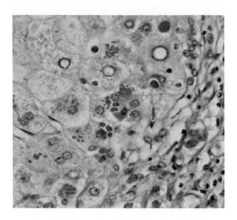

A A deficiency of the protein alpha-1 antitrypsin within the liver leads to hepatic damage.
B Mutation in the *SERPINAI* gene causes deficiency of alpha-1 antitrypsin.
C Alpha-1 antitrypsin protects the body from neutrophil elastase.
D Patient's with ZZ phenotype are at the highest risk of developing progressive liver disease.
E PAS globules are not specific for alpha-1-antitrypsin deficiency (A-1ATD).

A is the correct answer.

Commentary – A-1ATD

Clinical Pearls: Alpha-1-Antitrypsin Deficiency (A-1ATD)

1. A-1ATD is an autosomal recessive disease.
2. Alpha-1 Antitrypsin is a protease inhibitor of the proteolytic enzyme elastase.
3. Mutation in the **ser**ine **p**rotease **i**nhibitor gene: *SERPINAI* gene causes deficiency of alpha-1 antitrypsin.
4. Liver disease results from the accumulation within hepatocytes of unsecreted variant alpha-1 antitrypsin protein.
5. Alpha-1 antitrypsin protects the body (specifically the lung) from neutrophil elastase, an enzyme released from white cells to fight infection but can also attack normal (lung) tissue.
6. Pulling this all together: A-1ATD is a genetic disease that leads to a mutation in *SERPINA1* which leads to deficiency/defective A-1ATD. Variants of alpha-1 accumulate in the liver and causes damage. Less alpha-1 in the circulation leads to less destruction of neutrophil elastase. More neutrophil elastase leads to lung damage.
7. Carotid artery dissection and ulcerative neutrophilic panniculitis are associated manifestations.
8. The most clinically significant phenotype is : ZZ, followed by SZ and MZ:
   a. Prevalence of liver disease in ZZ patients is ~10%:
      i. Of which half can progress to cirrhosis.
      ii. Lung disease estimated to be ~25% in patients with ZZ phenotype.
9. In infants, it can present as prolonged jaundice after birth.
10. Intravenous alpha-1 augmentation is given to ZZ individuals who have reduction in FEV1.

Notes

A representative slide of a patient with A-1ATD. The Periodic acid Schiff (PAS)-positive stain demonstrating the striking fuchsia-colored diastase-resistant globules within hepatocytes.

Reference

Alpha-1 antitrypsin deficiency. PMID: 20301692.

Question 3

A 44-year-old male presents to his primary care physician with complaints of bilateral joint pain in his hands. Review of systems is notable for loss of libido and erectile dysfunction. Bloodwork reveals an iron saturation of 73% and ferritin of 690.

▶ Question

Treatment of this underlying condition would be expected to lead to improvement in all of the following EXCEPT:

A Improved cardiac function
B Improvement in arthropathy
C Improved control of diabetes
D Improvement in liver enzymes
E Improvement in skin pigmentation

B is the correct answer.

Commentary – Hemochromatosis

Clinical Pearls: Hemochromatosis

1. Response to phlebotomy in patients with hereditary hemochromatosis:
   a. does not reverse testicular atrophy
   b. leads to minimal improvement in arthropathy
   c. does not reverse established cirrhosis
   d. does not reduce risk of HCC in patients with established cirrhosis
2. The second and third metacarpophalangeal (MCP) joints are the classic rheumatologic manifestation (illustrated below):

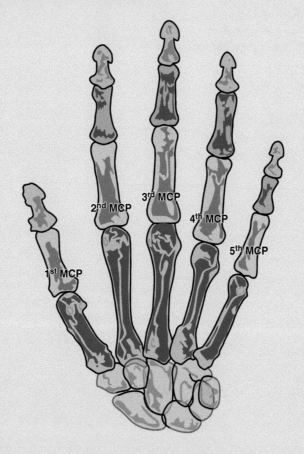

3. Other extrahepatic manifestations include congestive heart failure, porphyria cutanea tarda, testicular atrophy, chondrocalcinosis, impotence, and diabetes.

Question 4

▶ Question

Which of the following regarding hepcidin is FALSE?

A Hepcidin is a 25 amino acid peptide produced in the liver that downregulates iron absorption.

B When hepcidin binds to ferroportin, the ferroportin is internalized and degraded.

C Hereditary hemochromatosis leads to increased levels of hepcidin.

D Hepcidin is expressed predominantly in hepatocytes.

E HCV infection may lead to an increased iron deposition in the liver through inhibition of hepatic hepcidin transcription.

C is the correct answer.

Commentary – Iron Homeostasis

Clinical Pearls: Hepcidin, Ferroportin, and Hemochromatosis

1. The interaction of hepcidin with ferroportin constitutes the key control step in systemic iron homeostasis.
2. Hepcidin is produced predominantly in the liver and is secreted into the circulation. It binds to ferroportin which is found in macrophages and on the basolateral surface of enterocytes:
   a. Ferroportin is a trans-membrane protein that transports iron from the inside of a cell to the outside of the cell; it is the only known iron exporter.
3. When hepcidin binds to ferroportin, the ferroportin is internalized and degraded, and thus iron export is inhibited.
4. Hepcidin downregulates iron absorption.
5. Hereditary hemochromatosis (HH) leads to a reduction in hepcidin which leads to an overexpression of cell membrane ferroportin and, hence, an increased excretion of iron into the circulation.
6. In summary: HH is a mutation in *HFE* gene which leads to: reduced hepcidin – increased ferroportin – increased iron into circulation leading to systemic iron overload.

Question 5

A 41-year-old male is referred to you for elevated iron studies. He has a history obesity and hypertension. He is of Irish descent. His father died at age 62 of heart failure. His mother is 78 years old and alive.

The patient feels well other than mild fatigue. Exam is relatively unremarkable other than a BMI is 34 kg/m².

Laboratory studies:

WBC 7, Hb 16, Platelets 222; Normal renal function and electrolytes. TBili 0.8, AST 28, ALT 40, ALP 118.

Iron % saturation is 72 with a ferritin of 628 ng/mL. HFE testing: C282Y +/+.

Ultrasound is normal. Viral serologies are negative.

▶ Question

What do you recommend now?

A MRI with iron quantification
B Percutaneous US-guided liver biopsy with iron quantification
C Phlebotomy
D Repeat iron studies after 12 hours fast
E Dietary reduction in iron and then monitor iron studies

C is the correct answer.

Commentary – Iron Studies

> ### Clinical Pearls: Clinical Hemochromatosis
>
> 1. A ferritin of >1000 should prompt liver biopsy to rule out cirrhosis; on the other hand, if homozygous for C282Y and ferritin less than a 1000 – guidelines recommend against liver biopsy, i.e. go straight to phlebotomy:
>   a. Ferritin >1000 = liver biopsy is a favorite board question, although in practice most are obtaining some form of liver stiffness measurement (LSM).
> 2. Pearls' Prussian blue stain (see histology image) is used for evaluating the degree of cellular iron distribution within hepatocytes: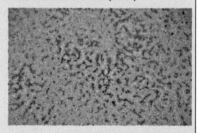
> 3. In secondary iron overload, iron deposition is usually mild (1–2+) and generally occurs in Kupffer cells (as opposed to hereditary hemochromatosis in which iron deposition is concentrated with hepatocytes).
> 4. As in most other forms of chronic liver disease, HCC surveillance in patients with hemochromatosis is only recommended when a patient has cirrhosis.
> 5. Cirrhosis + Hemochromatosis? This combination has the highest incidence of HCC.
> 6. *Vibrio vulnificus* have been associated in HH patients who eat raw shellfish.
> 7. Dietary adjustments in iron are not necessary.
> 8. Avoid vitamin C supplementation.
> 9. With phlebotomy, you are aiming to reduce ferritin to less than 50–100.
> 10. Phlebotomy is recommended initially 1–2×/week; ferritin can be repeated after 10–12 phlebotomies.
> 11. Chelating agents (deferoxamine, deferiprone) have many side effects and are only reserved for patients who can't tolerate phlebotomy (anemia, poor venous access, etc.).
> 12. Homozygous C282Y accounts for 85% of HH (less so C282Y/H63D; C282Y/S65C)

> ### Notes
>
> Of all the diseases that I get consulted for, genetic hemochromatosis is the most "overly" and "mis"-diagnosed. Remember, iron studies are commonly elevated in many forms of hepatic injury. For the boards you must be familiar with the algorithm for diagnosis. I anticipate the rule of "ferritin >1000 should prompt liver biopsy to rule out cirrhosis" will be phased out soon (with the increasing use of LSM), but until then, that is the board answer. The roles of hepcidin and ferroportin are also commonly tested.

Reference

ACG clinical guideline: hereditary hemochromatosis. PMID: 31335359.

Question 6

A 27-year-old first-time pregnant female presents to her OB-GYN with complaints of itching. She is 32 weeks pregnant.

Laboratory studies:

TBili 0.8, AST 48, ALT 63, ALP 216, GGT 23.
Total bile acids: 48 micromol/L (normal <11).

▶ Question

All of the following should be recommended EXCEPT:

A Viral serologies for HBV and HCV.
B Ursodeoxycholic acid should be prescribed at 10–15 mg/kg.
C Delivery should be arranged at 34 weeks, given the increased risk of fetal distress.
D The patient should be advised that the recurrence rate for the condition with subsequent pregnancies is up to 70%.
E Symptomatic management for pruritus can include hydroxyzine.

C is the correct answer.

Commentary – ICP

Clinical Pearls: Intrahepatic Cholestasis of Pregnancy (ICP)

1. The highest incidence of ICP occurs in patients of Bolivian and Chilean descents.
2. There appears to be a higher incidence in twin pregnancy.
3. ICP occurs in second and third trimester; symptoms can take up to 6 weeks to resolve postdelivery.
4. Mutations have been associated with several genes, but for the boards: ABCB4.
5. The diagnosis typically requires bile acids >10; bile acids >40 is associated with worse fetal outcomes:
   a. preterm, meconium, bradycardia, fetal distress; fetal loss is rare.
6. Ratio of bile acids: cholic acid >chenodeoxycholic acid.
7. Delivery is recommended at 37–38 weeks.
8. ICP recurs 45–70% in subsequent pregnancies.
9. Patients can develop vit-K deficiency from malabsorption.
10. As in BRIC, GGT is usually normal or low.
11. There is data to suggest an increased risk of ICP in women infected with HCV.

Reference

Intrahepatic cholestasis in pregnancy: review of the literature. PMID: 32384779.

Question 7

An 18-month-old child presents to your office with pruritus, jaundice, diarrhea, and failure to thrive.

Laboratory studies:

TBili 14 (direct 10) AST, 124, ALT 110, ALP 480, GGTP 18.
After establishing a diagnosis, you recommend partial external biliary diversion (PEBD).

▶ Question

All of the following are true regarding PEBD EXCEPT?

A PEBD is a procedure in which bile is diverted from the gallbladder through a loop of jejunum connecting the dome of the gallbladder to the skin.
B The procedure interrupts the enterohepatic circulation of bile salts.
C It can alleviate intractable pruritus.
D It can improve liver histology, but seldom improves liver function tests.
E It can preclude the need for liver transplant in up to 75% of children.

D is the correct answer.

Commentary – PFIC

Clinical Pearls: Progressive Familial Intrahepatic Cholestasis (PFIC)

1. PFIC is an autosomal recessive condition.
2. It is associated with defects in ATP8B1 (the same gene linked to BRIC).
3. Defects in ATP8B1 lead to an overload in bile acids in hepatocytes due to reduced bile salt secretion and increased bile salt reabsorption.
4. This leads to downregulation of farnesoid X receptor (FXR): a receptor related to regulation of metabolism of bile acids:
   a. Relevant link: Obeticholic acid is an agonist against the FXR.
5. AT8B1 is also expressed in the membrane of cells of the small intestine, kidney, and pancreas.
6. Byler disease (as opposed to Byler syndrome) has been associated with extrahepatic diseases (pancreatitis, hearing loss, and diarrhea), this is classified as **PFIC1.**
7. **PFIC2 or** Byler syndrome is a mutation in ABCB11 which results in more severe hepatobiliary disease than PFIC 1:
   a. transaminase elevation is higher than PFIC 1
   b. higher risk of liver tumors
   c. giant cells on histology
8. **PFIC3:** ABCB4: high GGT and cholesterol stones (ABCB4 genetic defect is associated with ICP).
9. Biliary diversion procedures: partial external biliary diversion (PEBD): 70–80% of patients with PFIC respond both biochemically and histologically.

Notes

The phenotypic spectrum of ATP8B1 deficiency manifests anywhere from mild, "benign" disease (BRIC) to severe life-threatening disease (PFIC).

Reference

Progressive familial intrahepatic cholestasis: diagnosis, management, and treatment. PMID: 30237746.

Question 8

A 19-year-old female is evaluated in the neurology clinic for a progressively worsening movement disorder. Ceruloplasmin returns at 12 mg/dL. The patient is referred to you. You obtain the following tests:

Repeat ceruloplasmin 10 mg/dL
Albumin 3.7
24-hour urine copper 88 mcg
Ophthalmology consult is negative for Kayser–Fleisher (KF) rings

▶ Question

Which of the following do you recommend next?

A Total serum copper
B Liver biopsy with copper quantification
C Molecular testing
D EGD with small bowel biopsies for copper staining
E Serum zinc

B is the correct answer.

Commentary – Copper Metabolism

> ### Clinical Pearls: Wilson Disease and Copper Metabolism
>
> 1. Wilson disease is an autosomal recessive disease.
> 2. Mutation is in the ATP7B gene.
> 3. Copper is absorbed by enterocytes, mainly in the duodenum (absorption of dietary iron is also at the level of the duodenum). Copper is then transported into the circulation and associated with albumin and the amino acid histidine and then taken to the liver.
> 4. The liver secretes the copper containing protein: ceruloplasmin and excretes excess copper into bile.
>   Ceruloplasmin carries 90% of copper in the blood:
>   a. A ceruloplasmin of less than 20 in the right clinical scenario should prompt further investigation.
>   b. It is not uncommon to have borderline ceruloplasmin in patients with cirrhosis (i.e. 15–20).
> 5. Processes that impair biliary copper excretion can lead to increases in hepatic copper content (most notably cholestatic diseases such as PSC).
> 6. Total serum copper is usually decreased in proportion to reduced ceruloplasmin in circulation.
>   a. Nonceruloplasmin bound copper is elevated.
>   b. Nonceruloplasmin bound copper can be estimated by: total serum copper concentration minus ceruloplasmin bound copper.
> 7. Absent or reduced function of ATP7B leads to decreased hepatocellular excretion of copper into bile and results in hepatic copper accumulation.
> 8. Hepatic parenchymal copper concentration is the gold standard for the diagnosis of Wilson; >250 mcg/dry weight.
> 9. Failure to incorporate copper into ceruloplasmin is an additional consequence of the loss of functional ATP7B protein; a defect in ATP7B in essence causes a decrease in ceruloplasmin.
> 10. A 24-hour urinary excretion of copper reflects the amount of nonceruloplasmin bound copper in circulation:
>   a. The cut off value for 24-hour urine copper is >40 mcg.
> 11. A combination of KF rings, ceruloplasmin, and 24-hour urine copper collection are used to arrive at a diagnosis or need for further testing (i.e. liver biopsy or molecular testing).
>
> **In Summary:** Wilson disease: a defect in ATP7B – leads to a decrease in excretion of copper into bile – which then causes an increase in hepatic copper accumulation.
> A defect in ATP7B also leads to a decrease in ceruloplasmin which leads to decrease in TOTAL serum copper (less is able to be bound as there is little ceruloplasmin), but an elevation in nonceruloplasmin bound copper (usually above 25) and an increase in 24-hour urinary excretion of copper.

Reference

Wilson's disease: a comprehensive review of the molecular mechanisms. PMID: 25803104.

Question 9

A 23-year-old college student is brought to her local community hospital by her room-mate with a rapid decline in mental status. In the emergency room, the patient's vitals are the following: temperature: 37.6, pulse 110, BP 94/48, RR 8, 95% on room air. She cannot be aroused even to deep sternal rub and is immediately intubated. Exam is notable for marked jaundice.

STAT labs are notable for a Hemoglobin of 6.
TBili 42 (unconjugated 31), AST 108, ALT 98, ALP is undetectable:

   Cr 3.4
   INR is 7.2
   Serum ammonia level is 343 micromol/L

▶ Question

Which of the following should be done immediately?

A Trial of corticosteroids
B Penicillamine-D
C *N*-acetyl-L-cysteine (NAC)
D Transfer to a liver transplant center
E Transjugular liver biopsy

D is the correct answer.

Commentary – Wilson Disease

Clinical Pearls: Wilson Disease

1. Hemolysis is seen in 10% of patients with acute Wilson disease:
   a. Coombs negative hemolytic anemia (predominantly unconjugated hyperbilirubinemia).
2. KF rings are present in 50% of patients:
   a. KF rings are present in nearly 100% of neurological Wilson.
3. Up to 30% of patients will have psychiatric manifestations.
4. Uric acid is decreased because of associated renal tubular dysfunction (Fanconi's syndrome).
5. There is rapid progression to renal failure.
6. Alkaline phosphatase is typically low, sometimes undetectable; ALP/TBili ratio <4 is highly sensitive and specific for Wilson.
7. Extrahepatic manifestations include the following: aminoaciduria, kidney stones, osteoporosis, arthritis, cardiomyopathy, pancreatitis, hypoparathyroidism, infertility.
8. First degree relatives with Wilson must be screened.

Notes

Chronic Wilson is a tricky diagnosis to make. Wilson disease rarely presents in a straightforward manner and more often than not requires piecing together the results of multiple tests. Acute Wilsonian crisis on the other hand is dramatic, with some of the most striking labs in all of liver disease. Clinical clues may include the uniquely low (and sometimes undetectable) alkaline phosphatase and the marked elevation in total bilirubin, largely from hemolysis.

Reference

Screening for Wilson disease in acute liver failure: a comparison of currently available diagnostic tests. PMID: 18798336.

Question 10

Zinc is most commonly used as maintenance therapy in patients with Wilson disease.

▶ Question

What is the mechanism of action of zinc?

A Promotes urinary excretion of copper.
B Promotes copper excretion by the kidneys.
C Downregulates ATP7B.
D Induces enterocyte metallothionein and interferes with copper uptake from the GI tract.
E It downregulates metallothionein and interferes with copper uptake from the GI tract.

D is the correct answer.

Commentary – Wilson Disease Therapy

Clinical Pearls: Treatment of Wilson Disease

1. D-penicillamine promotes urinary excretion of copper. 30% of patients develop adverse reactions including proteinuria and lupus-like syndrome. D-penicillamine should be taken without food.
   Urinary copper should increase and nonceruloplasmin copper should normalize. Should not be taken while breastfeeding.
2. Trientene is a chelator. It promotes copper excretion by the kidneys; it can be used even in decompensated disease.
3. Adequacy of treatment is monitored by measuring 24-hour urine copper excretion. Levels should run between 200 and 500.
4. In those with nonadherence to therapy, nonceruloplasmin bound copper is elevated, whereas overtreatment values will be low.
5. Zinc interferes with the uptake of copper from the GI tract. It induces enterocyte metallothionein. Metallothionein has a greater affinity for copper than zinc and binds copper and inhibits its entry into the circulation. The nonabsorbed copper is defecated.
6. Foods high in copper include shellfish, nuts, chocolate, mushroom, and organ meat.
7. Treatment of Wilson should continue in pregnant females. Mothers should not breast feed on penicillamine.
8. KF rings can improve on treatment.
9. After hepatic manifestations, neurologic symptoms are the most frequent. Dysarthria is the most frequent neurological symptoms, reported in nearly 97% of patients. Drooling is a classic symptom and is seen in nearly 70% of patients:
   a. *Risus sardonicus* (uncontrollable grinning) ☺ may be a clinical clue.
10. Classic imaging findings: symmetric hyperintense changes of the basal ganglia.
11. Neurological manifestations for the most part improve post-LT, but severe neurological impairment may not and may contraindicate LT.

Reference

Wilson disease. PMID: 30190489.

Question 11

A 38-year-old female presents with jaundice and severe fatigue. Exam is notable for marked scleral icterus, asterixis, spider angiomata, parotid gland enlargement, and conjunctival pallor. A flow murmur is appreciated on cardiac exam and a bruit is audible in her right upper quadrant (RUQ).

Laboratory studies are notable for a Hb of 6, platelets of 47 TBili of 22 (unconjugated 17), AST 98, ALT 47. and ALP of 112.
A blood smear is shown below.

▶ Question

Which of the following would NOT be consistent with this presentation?

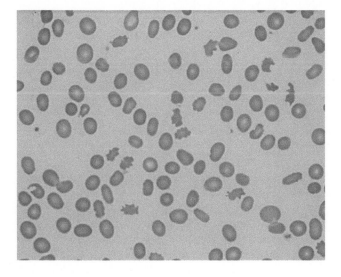

A MCV 114
B GTP 740
C Unconjugated bilirubin 17
D Triglyceride level 92
E INR 2.7

D is the correct answer.

Commentary – Cirrhosis and Anemia

Clinical Pearls: Anemia and Cirrhosis

1. Massive GI hemorrhage think variceal bleed or peptic ulcer.
2. Slow, chronic bleeding requiring intermittent transfusion, think gastric antral vascular ectasia (GAVE):
   a. Tranexamic acid has been used for GAVE in patients who fail argon plasma coagulation (APC), but it has been associated with an increased risk of thrombotic events.
3. Hypersplenism is secondary to portal hypertension that can lead to a drop in all cell lines, but most notably platelets.
4. Aplastic anemia is characterized by pancytopenia and hypocellular bone marrow following viral hepatitis (namely HBV, HCV, EBV, parvovirus 19).
5. Complications of HCV therapy (namely interferon-inducing bone marrow suppression and ribavirin-induced hemolysis, although these are now more historical, given DAA therapy).
6. Alcohol, Zieve's syndrome, may also be exacerbated by folic acid and/or B12 deficiency; inadequate dietary intake or malabsorption: Hemolytic anemia (spur cells and acanthocytes displayed in smear above), hyperlipoproteinemia, jaundice, and abdominal pain. Clinical clue may be elevated TG.
7. Hemolytic anemia: rarely as a result of destruction secondary to transjugular intrahepatic portosystemic shunt (TIPS).
8. Rapidly growing vascular tumor (usually giant hemangioma), thrombocytopenia, microangiopathic hemolytic anemia, and consumptive coagulopathy. More commonly seen in infants: Kasbach–Merritt syndrome.
9. Acute Wilsonian crisis can present with spherocytic severe acute hemolytic anemia (Coomb's negative) with marked elevation in total bilirubin which is predominantly unconjugated.
10. DIC: It may be difficult to distinguish DIC from liver disease related hemostatic abnormalities. Factor VIII activity levels are generally increased or normal in liver disease, as opposed to DIC, where consumption causes decreased factor VIII levels. DIC and liver disease may coexist especially in the setting of infection and sepsis.
11. Iron deficiency anemia and mild elevation in LFTs? Think celiac
12. It is not uncommon to see elevated liver enzymes in thrombotic microangiopathy (thrombotic thrombocytopenic purpura and hemolytic uremic syndrome):
    a. Calcineurin inhibitor (CNI)-induced HUS has been described posttransplant.
13. Liver is affected by multiple complications related to sickle cell disease:
    a. Multiple transfusions and risk of viral hepatitis, iron overload.
    b. Pigmented gallstones related to chronic hemolysis.

  c. Acute sickle cell hepatitis crisis occurs in about 10% of patients. RUQ pain, low-grade fever, and tender HM; jaundice; enzyme elevations can be as high 1000; likely related to ischemia and sinusoidal obstruction.

  d. Sickle cell intrahepatic cholestasis due to disseminated vaso-occlusion in the sinusoids can present with marked jaundice.

  e. Acute hepatic sequestration defined as sudden increase in liver size associated with RUQ pain and an acute decrease in Hb >2, thrombocytopenia, jaundice, and liver failure.

14. Leptospirosis: Zoonotic disease usually acquired from animal urine, infected animal tissue, or contaminated water. Hawaii reports the greatest number of cases in the United States. Presents with fever, headache, conjunctival redness. May be complicated by jaundice (can be markedly elevated) and renal failure (Weil's disease). DIC is not uncommon. Most cases are self-limiting. Severe cases will require antibiotics (doxycycline or azithromycin).

15. Adult-onset Still's disease (AOSD) is an inflammatory disorder characterized by quotidian (occurring daily) fevers, arthritis, and an evanescent salmon-colored rash typically found on the trunk. It is a diagnosis of exclusion. In addition to marked serum ferritin, hematological findings such as hemolytic anemia and DIC are not uncommon. Elevated LFTs are seen in 75% of patients.

16. Cytopenia is related to hemophagocytic lymphohistiocytosis (HLH).

Notes

Liver disease often presents with anemia. In these clinical pearls, we have included 15 scenarios to be aware of, including a smear from a patient with Zieve's; a syndrome which carries a very high mortality.

Reference

Zieve's syndrome: an under-reported cause of anemia in alcoholics. PMID: 31037235.

Question 12

A 47-year-old male from the United States is admitted to the hospital with complaints of fatigue and dark urine. The patient says he began to feel unwell about 4 days ago. He returned from an overseas trip about 4 weeks ago, where he admits being involved in high-risk sexual activity.

Exam is notable for normal vital signs. The patient is icteric, his mentation is normal, and he has no asterixis. He is slightly tender in the RUQ but has no ascites.

Laboratory studies:

TBili 6.4, AST 1345, ALT 987, ALP 181
INR 1.3
Serum venous ammonia level is 34 micromol/L.
A right upper quadrant ultrasound is normal.
Viral serologies reveal: HBsAg positive, HBeAg positive, anti-HBe negative, anti-HBc IgM positive, anti-HBs negative; HBV DNA pending.
HAV IgM negative; HCV PCR negative.
HIV negative.

▶ Question

Which of the following do you recommend?

A Lamivudine 100 mg daily
B Tenofovir 300 mg daily
C Entecavir 0.5 mg daily
D Supportive care and close monitoring
E Referral for liver transplantation

D is the correct answer.

Commentary – Acute HBV

Clinical Pearls: Acute HBV

1. Acute HBV can be either de novo or reactivation; the hallmark for acute HBV is a positive anti-HBc IgM (although it may only be positive in up to 70% of cases of reactivation). Acute vs. de novo infection can be very difficult to distinguish without past serologies.
2. 95% of acute de novo HBV in adults resolves spontaneously and does not require treatment.
3. Some experts advocate treating acute "severe" de novo HBV defined as a protracted, protracted or severe course as indicated by TBili of >3 and INR >1.5, encephalopathy or ascites.
   a. High risk of lactic acidosis in decompensated patients placed on HBV therapy, especially when MELD >20.
4. ALF from acute HBV warrants liver transplant consideration.
5. Because of resistance, Lamivudine and Adefovir are unlikely to be answer choices on the boards.
6. Window phase: anti-HBc IgM may be the only marker of infection: HBsAg and anti-HBs are not detected. This is an immunologically mediated phenomenon caused by precipitation of antigen–antibody complexes in their zone of equivalent concentrations and thereby, their removal from circulation. A favorite exam question.
7. Traditionally, HBV in adults is via sexual transmission, but, more recently, IVDU transmission is an equally common risk factor.

Notes

Hepatitis B used to drive me crazy as a medical student, but once you get your bearings, it's a fascinating disease. HBV can present in many different ways, lending itself to multiple test questions. Remember for the boards de novo HBV never needs to be treated, reactivation must be treated, and ALF should be referred for liver transplant.

Reference

Management of acute hepatitis B and reactivation of hepatitis B. PMID: 23286861.

Question 13

A 26-year-old graduate student originally from China with chronic HBV presents to your clinic regarding lowering the chances of HBV transmission to her child.

▶ Question

All of the following increase the risk of vertical transmission from HBV EXCEPT?

A Coinfection with HIV
B HBeAg positive status
C High maternal DNA (i.e. >200K)
D Baby receiving less than three doses of the HBV vaccine
E C-section

E is the correct answer.

Commentary – HBV and Pregnancy

Clinical Pearls: HBV and Pregnancy

1. HBIG x 1 dose and first dose of HBV vaccine series should be administered to newborns of infected mothers less than 12 hours after deliver; vaccine series is completed at 6 months (0-, 1-, and 6-month schedule).
2. For the boards: HBV DNA >200,000 should warrant anti-viral therapy to decrease risk of vertical transmission. Anti-viral therapy should be given in third trimester (initiate at 28–32 weeks). Anti-viral can be discontinued at 4 weeks postpartum.
3. Risk of transmission is associated with HBeAg-positive status (70–90% versus 5–40% in HBeAg negative; assuming no HBIG/vaccine and no anti-viral).
4. Amniocentesis may increase risk of transmission in mothers with HBV DNA $>10^7$.
5. Tenofovir (TDF) is drug of choice in pregnant females (telbivudine may also be used).
6. Infants born to HBV mothers should undergo testing for HBsAg and anti-HBs at ~12 months of age.

Reference

Hepatitis B – Vertical transmission and the prevention of mother-to-child transmission. PMID: 32249130.

Question 14

A 24-year-old male from Beijing, China, establishes care in the liver clinic. He is very concerned about his high HBV DNA level. Other than some mild anxiety, he feels well. His exam is normal.

Laboratory studies:

TBili 0.8, AST 14, ALT 14, ALP 89.
HBsAg positive, HBeAg positive, anti-HBe negative, HBV DNA 28,000,000 IU/mL; anti-HBs negative.
An ultrasound with elastography reveals a normal-appearing liver; elastography shows a kPa of 3.2 with an IQR of 8%.

▶ Question

What do you recommend?

A Liver biopsy
B MRI with elastography
C Reassurance and monitoring
D Interferon alpha-2a
E Tenofovir 300 mg daily

C is the correct answer.

Commentary – HBV Therapy

Clinical Pearls: HBV Therapy

1. Immunotolerant HBV: most commonly seen in younger patients, characterized by normal LFTs, HBeAg positive, and marked elevation in DNA; biopsy usually not indicated, but would typically show minimal inflammation/fibrosis. Treatment is not recommended.
2. Three medications approved for chronic HBV:
   Tenofovir (TAF or TDF)
   Entecavir
   Interferon alpha-2a
   a. Anti-retrovirals approved to treat HIV that are also active against HBV include the following: emtricitabine, lamivudine, and tenofovir.
3. Factors associated with HBV response to Interferon alpha-2a: HBeAg positive, older age, female, higher ALT, lower DNA (less than 2K), genotypes A and B.
4. Decision on HBV therapy depends on a combination of: LFTs, HBeAg status, DNA, and liver biopsy findings (there is a shift for biopsy to be replaced by elastography).
   Exception is HBV *cirrhotic* patients in which treatment is generally recommended regardless of DNA and LFTs. Dose of entecavir increases from 0.5 mg to 1 mg in decompensated cirrhosis.
   Regarding treatment of chronic HBV
   HBeAg positive:
     If ALT is normal, no need to treat (regardless of DNA).
     If ALT is between 1 and 2×, ULN recommendations are to make treatment decision based on biopsy findings.
     If DNA >20K and LFTs >2× ULN, then treat.
     If HBeAg negative and DNA is less than 2K and normal LFTS, then no treatment.
     If ALT is 2× ULN and DNA less than 2K, then liver biopsy.
     If ALT 2× ULN and DNA >2K, then treat.
5. Hepatitis e antigen (HBeAg) is a secretory protein that is processed from the pre-core protein. It is generally considered to be a marker of HBV replication and infectivity. HBeAg is usually associated with high DNA levels and higher rates of transmission:
   a. HBeAg loss occurs early in patients with acute infection.
   b. However, HBeAg seroconversion may be delayed in patients with chronic HBV. In such patients, it is usually associated with high DNA and active liver disease (the exception to this is immunotolerant phase who are HBeAg positive with very high DNA but typically minimal to no liver injury).
   c. Seroconversion (loss of HBeAg, development of anti-HBe) is usually associated with remission in liver disease; however, some patients continue to have

---

active liver disease after HBeAg seroconversion. Such individuals may have wild-type HBV or variants that prevent or decrease production of HBeAg: pre-core mutants. (Hence, why the DNA threshold level is lower in HBeAg negative patients).

6. Entecavir resistance is 1% at 5 years in naive patients. The development of tenofovir resistance at this time has been limited to case reports.
   Entecavir and Tenofovir are both highly effective in lowering DNA levels to undetectable levels and have been shown in long-term studies to lead to fibrosis regression.

7. Lamivudine resistance is reported >50% at 5 years.

8. High risk of lactic acidosis in decompensated patients placed on HBV therapy especially when MELD is >20; liver transplant should be considered in appropriate patients.

9. Tenofovir Disoproxil Fumarate (TDF) versus Tenofovir Alafenamide (TAF):
   a. TAF is prodrug and is absorbed more quickly. Given in smaller doses than TDF (25 versus 300) and so less kidney and bone toxicity.

10. Healthcare workers should not perform high-risk procedures if their HBV DNA is >1000 IU/ml.

Reference

Management of chronic hepatitis B infection: current treatment guidelines, challenges, and new developments. PMID: 24876747.

Question 15

A 37-year-old male from Peru with HBV is seen in your clinic. He has established cirrhosis, but is well compensated. His LFTs are normal. He is HBeAg negative, anti-HBe positive, HBV DNA is undetectable on entecavir 0.5 mg daily.

Delta Antigen positive

An EGD reveals grade I esophageal varices.

▶ Question

What do you recommend?

A Ultrasound +/– AFP for HCC surveillance
B Nonselective beta-blockade
C Increase entecavir to 1 mg daily
D DEXA scan
E HBV DNA-resistance panel

A is the correct answer.

Commentary – HBV, HDV, HCC

Clinical Pearls: HBV and HCC and DELTA

1. HBV has genotypes A–J:
   a. C and D have been associated with a comparably higher incidence of HCC.
2. HCC surveillance (US +/− AFP) for the most part is only recommended for cirrhotic patients (assuming they can tolerate therapy if HCC is found), the exceptions are: HCV with progressive fibrosis (F3 or F4) and chronic HBV in the following patients. Asian or Black MEN ≥40; Asian women ≥50
   Persons with first-degree family members with HCC or those with HDV regardless of fibrosis.
3. The incidence of HCC is highest in those with advanced fibrosis and elevated DNA levels.
4. Delta screening is recommended in patients from high-risk areas: Africa, Asia, Pacific Islanders, Middle East, Eastern Europe, South America, Greenland; persons who have sex with IVDU; MSM, co-infected HIV/HCV, multiple sexual partners. Some guidelines are now recommending testing for Delta in all HBsAg positive patients.
5. Make sure to check for Delta in persistently elevated ALT despite low HBV DNA levels.
6. In a patient who is Delta Ag positive, current recommendations are to check for HDV RNA, and if positive consider PEG-IFN alpha for at least 48 weeks (if HBV DNA >2000 IU/mL treat with combination nucleos ((tide)) analogues). Treatment results in HDV RNA negative in 25–40% of cases.

Notes

Awareness of hepatitis Delta is expanding. It is likely under-recognized with up to 10% of patients with HBV coinfected. Many experts are now recommending screening all patients with HBV. Patients with Delta progress more rapidly and have a higher incidence of HCC.

Reference

Hepatitis B/D-related hepatocellular carcinoma. A clinical literature review. PMID: 34611832.

Question 16

A 57-year-old African American male is referred to the liver clinic for "clearance" prekidney transplant. The patient is receiving a kidney from his 24-year-old nephew. Recipient and donor HBV serologies are noted below.

Laboratory studies:

Recipient: HBsAg positive, anti-HBc total positive, anti-HBs negative, HBeAg negative, anti-HBe positive, HBV DNA undetectable.
Donor: HBsAg negative, anti-HBc negative, anti-HBs >1000.
Immunosuppression induction consists of rabbit anti-thymocyte globulin (rATG) and maintenance for the first year is a combination of low-dose prednisone, tacrolimus, and mycophenolate.

▶ Question

Which of the following do you recommend?

A HBIG and HBV vaccination posttransplant
B Tenofovir 300 mg daily indefinitely
C No steroids as part of induction immunosuppression
D HBIG alone
E No prophylaxis is necessary; monitor LFTs and DNA q4–6 months

B is the correct answer.

Commentary – HBV Reactivation

Clinical Pearls: HBV Reactivation and Prophylaxis

1. Reactivation in: HBsAg positive, anti-HBc positive patients, is defined as follows:
   a. ≥2 log increase in HBV DNA compared to baseline
   b. HBV DNA ≥3 log in a patient with previously undetectable DNA
   c. HBV DNA ≥4 log if baseline is not known

Reactivation in HBsAg negative, anti-HBc positive is defined as follows:

1. HBV DNA detectable
2. HBsAg reappearance

A hepatitis flare is defined as ALT ≥3× baseline level.
Reactivation and a hepatitis flare are termed: *HBV-associated hepatitis*

Liver

1. All HBsAg-positive patients undergoing LT should receive prophylaxis with nucleotide analogues with or without HBIG posttransplant.
2. All HBsAg-negative patients who receive an anti-HBc positive organ should receive lifelong anti-viral therapy.

Nonliver

1. All HBsAg-positive organ transplant recipients should receive lifelong anti-viral therapy to prevent reactivation. Tenofovir (TAF, TDF) or entecavir are preferred drugs.
2. Those that are isolated anti-HBc total positive should be monitored for reactivation or alternatively anti-viral therapy for the first 6–12 months (period of maximal immunosuppression) may be considered.
3. HBsAg negative and anti-HBc total negative recipients who RECEIVE an anti-HBc positive organ should be monitored without prophylactic therapy.

Cytotoxic and Immunosuppressive Drugs

1. HBsAg-positive patients should initiate prophylaxis before therapy.
2. Isolated anti-HBc positive patients should be carefully monitored with ALT, HBV DNA, and HBsAg every 1–3 months during therapy and up to 12 months after cessation.
3. If a patient is anti-HBc positive, recommendations are to use prophylaxis if using CD20 therapies (rituximab is what the boards will test on) AND patients undergoing stem cell transplantation.
4. Anti-viral prophylaxis should start before immunosuppressive (IS) therapy, continue during IS therapy and for at least 6–12 months after IS therapy is completed.

Notes

Which patients to recommend prophylaxis against reactivation HBV causes confusion in many trainees. Identifying reactivation HBV is of critical importance as it can lead to severe injury and even death. We provide a concise review of the most commonly tested scenarios.

Reference

Prevention of hepatitis B reactivation in patients requiring chemotherapy and immunosuppressive therapy. PMID: 34368296.

Question 17

A deficiency in the enzyme that catalyzes the step-in beta-oxidation of mitochondrial fatty acid that forms 2-ketoacyl-CoA from 2-hydroxyacyl-CoA is responsible which of the following pregnancy related liver diseases:

A Acute fatty liver of pregnancy
B HELLP
C Hyperemesis gravidarum
D Intrahepatic cholestasis of pregnancy
E Preeclampsia with hepatic involvement

A is the correct answer.

Commentary – Pregnancy and Liver Disease

Clinical Pearls: Pregnancy and Liver Disease

1. Hyperemesis gravidarum: First trimester
2. Intrahepatic cholestasis of pregnancy (ICP) typically late second or third trimester
3. HELLP is a complication of severe pre-eclampsia. **H**emolysis, **E**levated **L**iver Tests and **L**ow **P**latelets. Clinical clues include schistocytes, normal INR, elevated LDH, edema; fetal mortality in up to one-third of cases. Most occur in third trimester.
4. Acute fatty liver of pregnancy (AFLP) results from mitochondrial dysfunction. Inherited mutations with deficiency in long-chain L-3 hydroxyacyl-CoA dehydrogenase (LCHAD). Mother is heterozygote, fetus is homozygous: fatty acids of fetus spill into mother. Early detection and treatment of LCHAD deficiency improves prognosis of newborn.
   a. AFLP: elevated INR, ammonia, pancreatitis, renal failure, DIC, GIB, elevated WBC. Liver biopsy shows MICROvesicular steatosis:
      i. Other causes of microvesicular steatosis: Reye syndrome (usually occurring after viral infection; 90% associated with aspirin use), valproic acid, lysosomal acid lipase deficiency and tetracycline.
   b. Both HELLP and AFLP can occur postpartum.
5. Herpes simplex virus (HSV): Genital or oral vesicular lesions only seen in 50% of cases. ALF from HSV on boards likely will be either immunocompromised host or pregnant female (typically, third trimester). Marked elevation in transaminases, but underwhelming bilirubin (although seems to be higher in pregnant females) with fever and abdominal pain. Can check HSV DNA (HSV IgM can be falsely positive). Rare cause of ALF, but very high mortality and in pregnant females, risk of transmission in up to 50% of cases:
   a. If there is any clinical suspicion for HSV as cause of ALF, administer IV acyclovir 10 mg/kg TID.
6. Most common cause of jaundice in pregnancy remains viral hepatitis:
   a. Vertical transmission of HAV is limited to case reports.
   b. HBV vertical transmission as high as 90% without prophylaxis.
   c. HCV vertical transmission in up to 5% of cases.
   d. HEV as a cause of ALF in pregnant females in second and third trimester. A total of 25–50% rate of vertical transmission.
7. Pregnancy promotes bile lithogenicity and sludge. Estrogen increases cholesterol synthesis. Progesterone impairs gallbladder motility. A total of 10% of pregnant women have gallstones. Cholecystectomy is best done in second trimester.
8. If varices are present in pregnant females, risk of bleeding is as high as 75%. Band-ligate in second trimester or early third. Propranolol preferred over nadolol.
9. Splenic artery aneurysm seen in 2.5% of pregnant women with PHTN; consider IR embolization if >2 cm.

Clinical clues to help differentiate AFLP versus HELLP.

	HELLP	AFLP
Incidence	0.5%	0.005%
Pre-eclampsia	Yes	50%
LFTs	++	+++ (usually higher)
Platelets	Low	Usually >120
INR	Normal	Elevated
Fibrinogen	Normal to increased	Low
Anti-thrombin activity	Any AT activity	<65%
Glucose	Normal	Low
Renal failure	+/−	+

Notes

Differentiating between HELLP and ALFP can be challenging. This table provides some of the most notable contrasts between the two diseases.

Reference

Liver disease in pregnancy. PMID: 18265410.

Question 18

A 23-year-old first-year medical student undergoes a routine physical exam. He is asymptomatic and has no complaints. The patient reports that he does notice a slightly yellow tint to the whites of his eyes during periods of fasting and when he does not get enough sleep. Exam is normal.

Laboratory studies:

TBili 2.6 (conjugated: 0.3), AST 22, ALT 23, ALP 109.

Which of the following is FALSE?

A A majority of bilirubin is derived from the breakdown of senescent red blood cells.
B Gilbert syndrome is the most common cause of conjugated hyperbilirubinemia.
C The enzyme defect in Gilbert syndrome and Criggler Najjar is with UDP-glucuronyl transferase.
D Males are affected more than females in Gilbert syndrome.
E IV nicotinic acid may raise bilirubin levels in patients with Gilbert syndrome.

B is the correct answer.

Commentary – Bilirubin Metabolism

Clinical Pearls: Bilirubin Metabolism

1. Bilirubin is derived from the breakdown of senescent (old) red blood cells. Heme portion is oxidized into unconjugated bilirubin.
2. Unconjugated bilirubin is NOT water soluble. It is attached to albumin and taken to the liver.
3. Unconjugated bilirubin is conjugated by the enzyme uridine diphosphonate glucuronyl transferase (UDPGT or UDP-glucuronyl transferase). Conjugated bilirubin is water soluble and can be excreted in urine.
4. This conjugated bilirubin is then excreted through the biliary system into the small bowel.
5. In the bowel conjugated bilirubin is converted to urobilinogen, which is what gives stool it's "brown" color.
6. Obstructive jaundice (stone, mass, stricture, etc.) prevents the excretion of conjugated bilirubin from the liver. Conjugated bilirubin is water soluble and is excreted in the urine – leading to the classic, "dark urine."
7. Less-conjugated bilirubin in the bowel leads to less urobilinogen and lack of "pigment" in stool, i.e.: pale/white stool or "acholic."
8. Gilbert syndrome/disease (pronounced: zheel-BARYS)
   a. Mainly autosomal recessive
   b. More common than people think, seen in 3–7% of the population
   c. 2 : 1 male to female ratio
   d. Higher bilirubin with illness, fasting, low fat meal, nicotinic acid infusion
   e. Not necessarily for test purposes, but more so for rounds, phenobarbital an inducer of UDPGT can lower bilirubin levels in patients with Gilbert's

Notes

Why does every board exam present Gilbert syndrome in a medical student? We decided to follow the tradition. Gilbert syndrome runs in my family. No doubt, the whites of the eyes do get a tad yellow during "call nights."

Question 19

The disorder which leads to an inability of conjugated bilirubin to leave the liver is known as:

A Crigler Najjar type I
B Crigler Najjar type II
C Rotor syndrome
D Gilbert's disease
E Dubin Johnson

E is the correct answer.

Commentary – Bilirubin Defects

Clinical Pearls: Bilirubin Defects

1. Hemolysis: Increase in breakdown of RBCs leads to increase in unconjugated bilirubinemia.
2. Defects in UDPGT lead to less conjugated and so an increase in unconjugated bilirubin: Gilbert syndrome.
3. Crigler Najjar type 1 is severe and is a result of no enzyme UDPGT activity.
4. Crigler Najjar type II is a decrease in enzyme activity and is not nearly as severe in clinical consequence.
5. Less UDPGT is why many newborns are initially jaundiced.
6. Inability of conjugated bilirubin to leave the liver: Dubin Johnson; clinical clue: "black liver."
7. Defects with storage of conjugated bilirubin: Rotor syndrome.

Reference

Inherited disorders of bilirubin clearance. PMCID: PMC4821713.

Question 20

Which of the following is generally considered a contraindication to liver transplantation for metastatic neuroendocrine tumor (NET)?

A Functional liver parenchymal involvement of 30%.
B G3 tumor with Ki-67 index >20%.
C Resection of primary tumor outside of the liver.
D Stable disease on imaging for 9 months.
E Age 55 years.

B is the correct answer.

Commentary – Neuroendocrine Tumor and Liver Transplant

> **Clinical Pearls: Liver Transplantation for Metastatic Neuroendocrine Tumor (NET)**
>
> 1. Neuroendocrine tumors are rare neoplasms with generally indolent growth behavior. Two major categories:
>   a. Well differentiated. Traditionally referred to as carcinoid tumor and pancreatic NET (islet cell tumors).
>   b. Poorly differentiated.
> 2. The hallmark of neuroendocrine cells is the production of abundant neurosecretory granules, as reflected in the strong and diffuse immunohistochemical expression of neuroendocrine markers such as synaptophysin and chromogranin.
> 3. The liver is the most common site of NET metastasis. Primary tumor site:
>   a. Small intestine 45%
>   b. Pancreas 42%
>   c. Colon 40%
>   d. Stomach 15%
>   e. Rectum 6%
>   f. Appendix 3%
>   g. In 10% of cases, the primary tumor is not identified
> 4. Liver transplantation is a viable treatment option for patients with unresectable isolated liver metastases from NET with 5-year survival approaching 70% in select patients. 5-year disease survival is only ~25% without transplant.
> 5. Criteria for liver transplantation:
>   a. Less than 50% of the liver should be involved.
>   b. Primary tumor should be resected.
>   c. Metastatic disease must be limited to the liver (negative PET scan).
>   d. Age less than 60 years.
>   e. Stable disease for at least six months.
>   f. Histological grade G1 or G2 with Ki-67 index <10%.

Reference

Liver transplantation in the treatment of unresectable hepatic metastasis from neuroendocrine tumors. PMID: 32655939.

Question 21

A 27-year-old female is referred to your clinic by her OB-GYN when a pelvic ultrasound noted an incidental lesion in the liver. The patient is healthy and has no medical history. She is planning on starting a family. She was previously on oral contraception (OCP) since the age of 16. Liver tests and tumor markers are normal.

You obtain an MRI of the abdomen with eovist. A representative image is shown below. The official read is a 8.6 × 5.4 cm lesion in the left lobe that is T2 iso-to slightly hyperintense, T1 hypointense, moderately hyperenhancing on arterial phase with washout on portal venous and delayed phases. In addition, it demonstrates loss of signal on out-of-phase imaging, indicative of microscopic fat. Findings are compatible with HNF-1 alpha-mutated lesion.

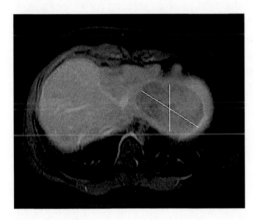

What do you recommend?

A Surgical resection of the lesion
B Radiofrequency ablation
C Referral for liver transplantation
D Advise the patient that she should not get pregnant
E Subcutaneous octreotide

A is the correct answer.

Commentary – Hepatic Adenoma

Clinical Pearls: Hepatic Adenoma

1. Hepatic adenomas are typically seen in females aged 20–44; predominantly in the right lobe.
2. Associated with OCPs, anabolic steroids, glycogen storage disease.
3. As opposed to hemangioma and FNH, OCP should be discontinued in females with hepatic adenoma.
4. Three major groups. Will require liver biopsy to differentiate (although radiographic features may be discernible).
   a. Mutations in hepatocyte factor 1 alpha (HNF1alpha): account for 46% of adenomas histologically: marked steatosis. Good prognosis, least aggressive.
   b. Mutations in beta-catenin. 14% increased risk of malignant transformation; more frequent in male patients.
   c. Inflammatory type, usually small; risk of malignancy is reported ∼10%.
5. Bleeding is an established complication of adenomas; risk increases when the lesion is >3.5 cm, especially prepregnancy.
6. Hepatic adenomas >5 cm should be considered for surgical resection given the high risk of bleeding.
7. Consider resection in all male patients.
8. Histologically: dilated sinusoids.
9. Adenomatosis is a distinct pathological entity. Diagnosis is made when there are >10 lesions.
10. CT scan: adenomas are isodense on noncontrast phase and show peripheral enhancement during early phase and subsequent centripetal (inward) flow during portal venous.
11. Adenomas appear hypervascular, but less so than FNH.
12. Centripetal filling: fills inward (as opposed to FNH which has centrifugal filling: inward to outward).
13. Lesions are well circumscribed and nonlobulated.
14. High lipid content.
15. Because adenomas are nonfunctional, most do not take up technetium Tc-99m sulfur colloid; scintigram shows a "cold spot" (as opposed to hemangiomas).

Notes

Some experienced abdominal radiologists are able to surmise on the subtypes of adenomas based on radiographic features. At the moment however, subtyping adenomas is based on histological findings.

Reference

Benign liver tumors. PMID: 33005655.

Question 22

A 37-year-old female with worsening nausea and nonbloody emesis is taken to the emergency room by her 19-year-old daughter. On arrival, the patient is somnolent but arousable. She is oriented only to person. She has asterixis. Exam is also notable for jaundice and an enlarged tender liver with an audible bruit. The patient has spider angiomata, palmar erythema, and parotid gland enlargement. The patient's temperature is 99.8, HR 102, BP 100 systolic; 96% RA, RR 14; BMI 28.

Laboratory studies:

WBC 18, Hb 12, Platelets 76K; 92% neutrophils; MCV 112
Sodium 131, Cr 1.1
TBili 9.8, AST 88, ALT 34, ALP 116, GGT 788; Albumin 3.3
INR 2.2
NH3: 88
Beta-HCG negative
Chest-X-Ray: negative, Bcx negative, UA: 2+ urobilinogen.
Ultrasound: enlarged, steatotic liver with trace perihepatic ascites; gallbladder with mild wall thickening; CBD 3 mm.
Serum alcohol and urine alcoholic metabolites: negative.
Anti-HAV IgM negative, HBsAg, anti-HBc total positive, anti-HBc IgM negative, anti-HBs 500, HBV DNA negative; anti-HCV negative.
IgG 1900, IgM 200, IgA 480; ANA 1 : 40, smooth muscle negative.
Ceruloplasmin 33.

On day 3 of admission, the patient looks slightly better and is more awake. WBC remains elevated without obvious infection. Total bilirubin is now 13. A transjugular liver biopsy is obtained with a hepatic venous pressure gradient of 16 mmHg. Representative images are shown below.

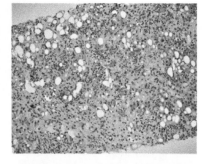

You recommend
A Empiric antibiotics
B MRCP to rule out biliary obstruction
C Trial of prednisolone
D Pentoxifylline 400 mg po TID
E Trientene 500 mg po TID

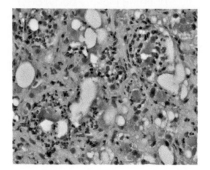

C is the correct answer.

Commentary – Acute Alcoholic Hepatitis

Clinical Pearls: Acute Alcoholic Hepatitis

1. AST/ALT ratio 2 : 1, but if AST >350 is very unlikely to be alcohol (especially on the boards).
2. Relatively normal alkaline phosphatase, but marked elevation in GGT can be a clue. Marked elevation in GGT with normal ALP is almost always alcohol.
3. Disproportionate TBili and INR; elevated MCV; low platelet count
4. Elevated WBC and low-grade fever.
5. Enlarged, tender liver; hepatic bruit is pathognomonic.
6. Steatotic liver on imaging; +/− cirrhotic features.
7. A majority of patients with acute severe alcoholic hepatitis will have underlying advanced fibrosis/cirrhosis:
   a. Up to 85–90% based on biopsy studies.
8. Severe disease is defined as follows:
   a. Maddrey discriminant function (MDF) ≥32:
      i. Know how to calculate MDF (patient PT − control PT (12 is a safe number to use for control) × 4.6 + TBili.
   b. MELD score ≥21 can also be used to define "severe" alcoholic hepatitis.
9. For the boards, severe disease warrants strong consideration of corticosteroids assuming no contraindications, namely active GI bleeding, severe kidney injury and sepsis.
   a. Prednisolone (better bioavailability then prednisone) 40 mg daily × 28 days, then taper to off ~2 weeks. (IV methylprednisolone 32 mg daily IV if patient can't take oral).
   b. Some small studies using granulocyte colony stimulating factor (G-CSF) show promise for acute severe alcoholic hepatitis (and ACLF), but further studies are needed before they can be widely recommended.
10. The histological image above reveals active steatohepatitis with Mallory–Denk bodies; cytoplasmic hyaline inclusions of hepatocytes with classic "twisted rope appearance" (see image to the right with blue arrow pointing Mallory body) often seen in alcoholic liver disease, but not necessarily specific or sensitive for.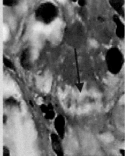
11. Alcohol metabolites in urine: Ethyl glucuronide (EtG) and ethyl sulfate (EtS) can remain detectable in urine for several days. Phosphatidylethanol (PEth) can be detected for up to 12 days.

Notes

Unfortunately, we see too many cases of alcoholic hepatitis and the prevalence seems to be rising. In a bold move, EASL guidelines call for the banning of all alcoholic advertising and marketing! Will the AASLD follow suit? The presentation of alcoholic hepatitis can be dramatic and the outcomes dismal. A huge clinical clue? A marked elevation in GGT in the setting of a relatively normal ALP; a ratio missed by too many!

Reference

Diagnosis and treatment of alcohol-associated liver disease: a review. PMID: 34255003.

Question 23

You are reconsulted on a 51-year-old male admitted to the hospital 9 days ago for acute alcoholic hepatitis. Your team recommended a trial of steroids for acute severe alcoholic hepatitis (DF 92, MELD 31). The patient has remained infection-free. His day 7 Lille score calculates at 0.65. This is the patient's first hospitalization. He has no other significant medical history. He seems to have good insight and is willing to attend formal rehabilitation.

On exam he is awake and oriented. He has mild asterixis and moderate ascites. His family has been supportive and has been at his bedside daily.

You recommend

A Continue steroids
B Add pentoxifylline
C Transjugular liver biopsy
D Consideration for early transplantation for acute severe alcoholic hepatitis
E Transjugular intrahepatic portosystemic shunt

D is the correct answer.

Commentary – Treatment of Acute Alcoholic Hepatitis

Clinical Pearls: Treatment for Alcoholic Hepatitis

1. Despite corticosteroids being called into question for acute alcoholic hepatitis, it will be the answer of choice as first line treatment on the boards.
2. Recommendations are to calculate the patient's 7-day Lille score to determine whether a patient is a "responder." If so, a full 30-day course (with 2–4-week taper) should be administered.
3. Lille score factors in age, albumin, creatinine, and change in total bilirubin (from initiation of steroids to day 7).
4. A Lille score of <0.45 is considered a poor prognostic sign, and in these cases, steroids should be discontinued and a goal of care discussion should be had, or in the right patient population, the role for early liver transplantation discussed.
5. Early liver transplantation for acute alcoholic hepatitis has far superior outcomes when compared to medical therapy.
6. For the boards, appropriate candidates for early LT for alcoholic hepatitis would have no prior liver decompensation (i.e. first offense), supportive family members, commitment to abstinence, and consensus among providers.

Notes

Once a contraindication, liver transplantation for acute severe alcoholic hepatitis has now become relatively commonplace. Alcohol is now the number one indication for LT in the US. Although transplantation in these patients raises many ethical questions, the superior outcomes when compared to medical therapy are undeniable.

Reference

Early liver transplantation for severe alcoholic hepatitis. PMID: 22070476.

Question 24

A 33-year-old female presents with a chief complaint of "coke colored urine." The patient says she has been feeling unwell for several days with nausea and nonbloody emesis, anorexia fevers, and diarrhea. She eventually is taken to the emergency room by her boyfriend when she was noted to be jaundiced.

Physical exam notes a temp of 100.4, HR 100, BP 110, 12, oxygen saturation 98%. She has marked scleral icterus; her skin is jaundiced. Mentation is normal without asterixis. Abdominal exam is notable for mild RUQ tenderness. There is no audible bruit or stigmata of chronic liver disease.

Laboratory studies:

WBC 11, Hb 15, Platelets of 330
TBili 11.7, AST 2300, ALT 3750, ALP 220; INR 1.3
Normal electrolytes and creatinine
Serologies: anti-HCV negative, HBsAg negative, anti-HBc total negative, anti-HBs negative, anti-HAV IgM positive, EBV IgM negative, CMV IgM negative; ANA, Immunoglobulins, smooth muscle antibody negative
Ceruloplasmin 23; Ferritin 670, Iron % saturation 44
Acetaminophen level negative
Ultrasound normal
The patient is discharged on hospital day 3 with a decline in her TBili to 8.6. The patient is seen in clinic 2 weeks postdischarge. She is feeling better, and her TBili is down to 3.3. The patient returns again for follow-up 10 weeks after her initial presentation. She is feeling relatively well but has noted dark urine again. On exam she has scleral icterus. Laboratory tests reveal: TBili of 5.8, AST 544, ALT 632, ALP 291.
Repeat serologies: anti-HCV negative, HBsAg negative, anti-HBc total negative, anti-HBs negative, anti-HAV IgM positive.
EBV IgM, CMV IgM negative.

▶ Question

Which of the following is FALSE?

A The relapsing variant of this infection can be seen in 3–20% of cases.
B Supportive care is the treatment of choice.
C The patient is no longer infectious.
D A liver biopsy is not necessary to make the diagnosis.
E Multiple relapses may occur.

C is the correct answer.

Commentary – Hepatitis A

Clinical Pearls: Hepatitis A

1. Acute hepatitis with fever and diarrhea? Think hepatitis A.
2. Classically fecal oral transmission, but can also be transmitted via sex and IVDU.
3. Jaundice in one third of cases; incubation periods is ~28 days.
4. Acute liver failure is rare (less than 1% of cases). When liver failure is seen, it is seen in the setting of undiagnosed underlying chronic disease (namely fatty liver and HCV; acute on chronic liver failure).
5. Hepatitis A never leads to chronic infection, but can have atypical manifestations.
6. Atypical manifestations of acute HAV.
   a. Relapsing
      i. Seen in 3–20% of cases, occurs after complete biochemical resolution of initial case; usually weeks 4–15, but can last up to a year.
      ii. Less severe.
      iii. HAV IgM reappears.
   b. Cholestatic variant
      i. Less than 5% of cases; elevated ALP.
      ii. Treat with UDCA and anti-pruritic agents; no role for steroids.
   c. Autoimmune
      i. Rarely HAV may serve as a trigger for AIH.

Notes

Every few years in the USA, there is an outbreak of hepatitis A. One of my first introductions to hepatology was the infamous HAV outbreak in Northwestern Pennsylvania. The culprit? Contaminated green onions from a (now bankrupt) Mexican restaurant. I will never forget one of my unfortunate patients with a total bilirubin of 93! I was a first-year medicine resident at the time, my co-author a first-year hepatology attending.

Reference

Relapsing hepatitis A. Review of 14 cases and literature survey. PMID: 1312659.

Question 25

In which of the following patients would you recommend the Hepatitis A vaccine?

A A 44-year-old male moving to Pakistan for a new job.
B A 34-year-old who works for the city sewage company.
C A 67-year-old elementary school cafeteria worker.
D A 26-year-old daycare worker.
E A 54-year-old with no known liver disease but morbid obesity (BMI 44) and diabetes.

A is the correct answer.

Commentary – HAV Vaccine

Clinical Pearls: HAV Vaccine

1. HAV vaccine is recommended for
   a. Children/adolescents aged 1–18 years.
   b. Infants aged 6–11 months who are traveling internationally.
   c. Those working in high-risk countries.
   d. Men who have sex with men (MSM).
   e. IVDU
   f. Those working with HAV-infected primates or in a HAV research lab.
   g. Homeless persons.
   h. Patients with chronic liver disease.
2. HAV is not routinely recommended for
   a. Those under 12 months of age.
   b. Childcare personnel.
   c. Health care worker.
   d. Food service worker.
   e. Sewage worker.
3. Passive immunization (immune globulin)
   a. Can decrease incidence of HAV infection by >90%. Preexposure protection is typically administered for anticipated risk of exposure from 1–2 months and is recommended for
   Adult travelers >40 years and infant travelers <6 months.
      Immunocompromised individuals who cannot mount immune response to vaccine.
   b. Immune globulin can be safely administered to mothers.
4. Postexposure prophylaxis (typically with vaccination) should be administered within 2 weeks of exposure to those who have not previously received HAV vaccine.

Reference

Hepatitis A. PMID: 34652109.

Question 26

A 27-year-old female presents to the emergency room with increasing abdominal distension and shortness of breath. The patient has no significant past medical or surgical history. She is single and sexually active. She does not drink or smoke. Despite the recent distension, she reports a 12-pound weight loss in the last three months.

Exam is notable for an ill appearing, female who appears older than her stated age. She is afebrile and her vitals are normal. Her body mass index (BMI) is 26 kg/m². Her abdomen is tense with a fluid thrill. Cardiovascular exam is normal.

Laboratory studies:

WBC 12, Hb 11, Platelets 320. Normal renal and hepatic function. INR 1
Albumin 3.3
A diagnostic tap is performed at beside yielding the following results:
Ascites albumin 2.9, total protein 2.8
WBC 333 with 78% monocytes and only 1 neutrophil
Cytology is pending.

▶ Question

What is the most likely diagnosis?

A Budd Chiari
B PVT
C Peritoneal Carcinomatosis
D Alcoholic cirrhosis
E Cardiac ascites

C is the correct answer.

Commentary – SAAG

Clinical Pearls: Serum Albumin to Ascites Gradient (SAAG)

1. SAAG is calculated by subtracting the ascites albumin from the serum albumin, for example in this case: 3.3–2.9 or 0.4; i.e. low SAAG ascites.
2. 1.1 is generally considered the cut-off.
3. ≥1.1, differential includes cirrhosis, alcoholic hepatitis, cardiac disease, fulminant hepatic failure, venous outflow obstruction (Budd Chiari, sinusoidal obstruction syndrome), portal vein thrombosis.
4. ≤1.1: peritoneal carcinomatosis, TB, pancreatic ascites, bile leak, nephrotic syndrome, serositis, myxedema.
5. 5% of ascites is "mixed," where SAAG may lose accuracy. This is especially true in patients with cirrhosis and severe malnutrition (very low serum albumin).
6. Cardiac ascites: high SAAG, high TP (usually >2.5), elevated BNP (usually >350).
7. Peritoneal carcinomatosis occurs when there is metastatic "caking" of the peritoneum; 150 cc examined for cytology has nearly 100% sensitivity.
8. Low SAAG, elevated total protein with a predominantly lymphocytic differential? Think tuberculosis (TB) peritonitis.
9. Gold standard for TB peritonitis is growth of mycobacterium on ascites or peritoneal biopsy; Adenosine deaminase (ADA) useful nonculture method with high sensitivity and specificity (using cutoff >39).
10. Chylous ascites is ascites rich in triglycerides; generally, use >200 as cutoff. Identification of chylomicrons using lipoprotein electrophoresis is gold standard. In USA, the most common cause is malignancy or cirrhosis; TB is the number one cause of chylous ascites in developing countries.
    a. If you are suspicious of a lymphatic leak as the cause of chylous ascites (postop, trauma etc.,) perform lymphoscintigraphy.
11. Pancreatic ascites: low SAAG, high TP, and ascites amylase >1000.
12. Hemorrhagic ascites is defined as RBC count >50,000 mm^3.
    a. Hemorrhagic tap is >10,000 RBC.
    b. 1 PMN should be subtracted for every 250 RBC when determining if patient has SBP.
    c. Example 5000 RBC; 1000 WBC; 50% neutrophils:
       i. 5000/250 = 20. Subtract 20 from 500. ANC = 480

High SAAG ascites: >1.1	Low SAAG ascites: <1.1
Cirrhosis	Peritoneal carcinomatosis
Alcoholic hepatitis	Tuberculosis
Cardiac	Pancreatic
Fulminant hepatic failure	Bile leak
Budd Chiari	Nephrotic syndrome
Sinusoidal obstruction syndrome	Serositis
PVT (although rarely presents with ascites)	Myxedema

Notes

Know the most common causes of low and high SAAG ascites; a table is provided. A young female with malignant ascites is a favorite board question. Cytology will confirm the diagnosis. On the other hand, cytology for routine ascites is almost never warranted.

Reference

Ascitic fluid analysis in the differential diagnosis of ascites: focus on cirrhotic ascites. PMID: 26357618.

Question 27

A 59-year-old African American male presents with fatigue and right upper quadrant pain for 1 week. He reports a 12-pound weight gain. The patient was recently diagnosed with multiple myeloma and 2 weeks ago was initiated on: cyclophosphamide, bortezomib, and dexamethasone.

Vital signs are normal with a BMI of 26 kg/m^2. Exam is notable for +scleral icterus, tender hepatomegaly with small ascites and mild asterixis.

Laboratory studies:

TBili 10.1, AST 98, ALT 78, ALP 544; INR of 2.2.
Ultrasound reveals mild hepatomegaly, small ascites, no intra or extrahepatic duct dilation, patent portal vein.
A transjugular liver biopsy is performed with the following results:

Wedge hepatic pressure of 22 mmHg, free hepatic pressure of 6 mmHg.
Histology: Pericentral congestion with dilation of sinusoids and necrosis of hepatocytes.

▶ Question

Which of the following is FALSE?

A This entity is seen most commonly in patients undergoing stem cell transplant.
B The most common presenting symptoms are jaundice, hepatomegaly, right upper quadrant pain, and ascites.
C Defibrotide is the only FDA-indicated medication for this disease.
D UDCA 2 weeks prior to therapy should be considered as prophylaxis in patients deemed to be high risk for this disorder.
E An US with Doppler can adequately rule out this disease.

E is the correct answer.

Commentary – Sinusoidal Obstruction Syndrome (SOS)

Clinical Pearls: Sinusoidal Obstruction Syndrome (SOS)/Hepatic Veno-Occlusive Disease (VOD)
1. SOS occurs most commonly as a complication of myeloablative regimens and most commonly in patient's undergoing stem cell transplant.
2. Medications to link with SOS for the boards: cyclophosphamide combined either with total body irradiation or busulfan; oxaliplatin.
3. Classic presentation is jaundice, tender hepatomegaly, weight gain (with or without ascites). Presentation is usually within 3 weeks of starting treatment.
4. Although not always required, the gold standard for the diagnosis is wedge hepatic vein pressures.
5. Other diagnostic findings: low antithrombin and protein c levels; high plasminogen motivator inhibitor levels.
6. Cirrhosis is generally considered a contraindication to high-dose myeloablative conditioning regimens.
7. Defibrotide is the only FDA-approved medication for SOS. It has antithrombotic and profibrinolytic activity.
8. UDCA beginning 2 weeks before stem cell transplant is commonly used as prophylaxis against SOS.

Reference

Sinusoidal obstruction syndrome (hepatic veno-occlusive disease). PMID: 25755580.

Question 28

A 21-year-old female with no significant past medical history is admitted with abdominal fullness. She does not drink, but occasionally smokes. No other habits. Her only medication is norgestimate and ethinyl estradiol. Twelve hours into her admission she has massive hematemesis. She undergoes EGD and banding of large bleeding esophageal varices.

▶ Question

The patient undergoes a CT scan (see images). The area circumscribed in red can be attributed to

A Mass like external compression on inferior vena cava.

B The liver venous drainage is preserved through the caudate lobe. The caudate vein receives blood not only from the caudate lobe but also from other parts of the liver through collateral vessels.

C Compensatory hypertrophy of this liver segment as a result of global atrophy of the remainder of the liver.

D Congestion related to outflow obstruction.

E Sequelae of rapidly progressive hepatic fibrosis.

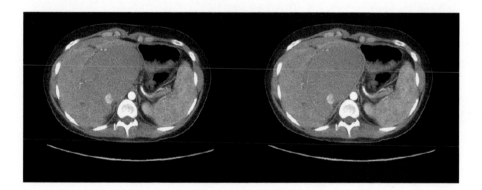

B is the correct answer.

Commentary – Budd Chiari

Clinical Pearls: Budd Chiari

1. Named after an internist (Budd) and a pathologist (Chiari) is an obstruction usually related to hepatic vein thrombosis.
2. Key histological findings: severe centrilobular congestion; sinusoidal dilation; thrombosis can sometime be visualized within the hepatic vein.
3. Caudate lobe hypertrophy is seen in ~50% of cases. It is due to the presence of patent caudate lobe veins that enter the IVC just below the ostia of the main hepatic veins. The liver venous drainage is preserved through the caudate lobe. The caudate vein receives blood not only from the caudate lobe but also from other parts of the liver through collateral vessels: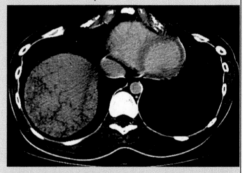
   a. Other radiographic findings include inhomogeneous liver enhancement (molted appearance, see image to the right), intrahepatic collaterals, and hypervascular nodules.
   Molted liver in corresponding segment to occluded hepatic vein.
4. It can present as acute liver failure in 5% of cases.
5. Up to 50% of cases will have an underlying chronic myeloproliferative disorder (polycythemia vera, essential thrombocythemia) and hypercoagulable state.
6. JAK2 tyrosine kinase (V617F) have been described in up to 50% of patients.
7. Other hypercoagulable states: factor V Leiden, Antiphospholipid syndrome, Anti-thrombin deficiency, Protein C deficiency, Protein S deficiency, paroxysmal nocturnal hemoglobinuria.
8. Oral contraceptives and pregnancy account for 20% of cases.
9. High risk of HCC especially those with IVC and HV thrombosis.
10. Rotterdam classification (I–III) can be used to help guide management. This scoring system takes into account: encephalopathy, ascites, PT, and bilirubin.
    a. Rotterdam I: Anticoagulation
    b. Rotterdam II: TIPS
    c. Rotterdam III: Transplant

Notes

A striking image of massive caudate lobe enlargement in a young female with Budd Chiari formed the basis for this question. This particular patient was actually diagnosed as having a "mass" at an outside hospital. Her course was complicated by a massive variceal bleed. The second image is from a young female who presented with an isolated right HV occlusion, causing corresponding vascular radiographic changes in her right lobe.

Reference

Update on the management of Budd-Chiari syndrome. PMID: 32691382.

Question 29

A 57-year-old male cirrhosis from alpha-1 antitrypsin deficiency is admitted to your hospital with confusion. He is afebrile and vitals are normal. Exam is notable for jaundice, asterixis, and shifting dullness. Home medications include furosemide, spironolactone, lactulose, and rifaximin. The patient is currently listed for liver transplant.

Laboratory studies:

WBC of 5.8 with 82% neutrophils. Platelets are 42K. Sodium 133 and Cr 1.3. TBili is 2.9 remainder of LFTs are normal. Albumin is 2.9, INR is 1.7.

▶ Question

What do you recommend?

A Triphasic CT scan of abdomen
B Empiric antibiotics
C Administer platelets and then perform diagnostic tap
D Administer platelets, FFP, and vit-K and then perform diagnostic tap
E Bedside diagnostic tap

Question 30

The patient in the question above undergoes a diagnostic bedside tap, yielding: 800 WBC with 70% neutrophils. Ascites culture is negative, and blood cultures are negative. Ascites albumin is 0.7 and total protein is 1.3. The patient is administered intravenous antibiotics and albumin. On hospital day 3, he is feeling much better with clear mentation. What do you recommend?

A Repeat diagnostic tap to confirm clearance of infection
B Ok to discharge home on diuretics; no antibiotics
C No need for repeat tap, complete IV antibiotics in house and discharge on prophylaxis
D Discontinue rifaximin and add a different antibiotic for prophylaxis
E Patient should be removed from transplant list indefinitely given diagnosis of infection

29 – E is the correct answer.
30 – C is the correct answer.

Commentary – SBP

Clinical Pearls: Spontaneous Bacterial Peritonitis (SBP)

1. The definition of SBP is an absolute neutrophil count (ANC) ≥250 **and** culture positive, but treatment is recommended regardless of culture results.
2. Up to 1/3rd of patients will have no obvious symptoms, and the general rule is if a patient is admitted to the hospital for any decline in clinical status with moderate/large ascites, they should have a diagnostic tap performed to rule out SBP.
3. Diagnostic tap should be performed at bedside. No need for products to reverse coagulopathy.
4. The only potential contraindications to performing a diagnostic tap? Overlying cellulitis or severe neutropenia.
5. Blood cultures should be sent on all patients with SBP.
6. A "day 3 tap" to ensure response to antibiotics is not required in patients who are otherwise clinically improving.
7. For the boards: weight-based albumin should be administered in addition to antibiotics on days 1 (1.5 g/kg) and 3 (1 g/kg) in "sick" cirrhotics. For the boards albumin will almost always be recommended when a diagnosis of SBP is made.
8. SBP prophylaxis is recommended for
   a. Prior history of SBP: indefinite prophylaxis or until time of transplant
   b. Ascites total protein less than 1.5: indefinite prophylaxis or until time of liver transplant
   c. All upper GI bleed (with or without ascites): in house prophylaxis
9. Most recommendations are for daily antibiotic prophylaxis (as opposed to weekly).
10. Infected hydrothorax: spontaneous bacterial empyema: ANC is ≥500 (versus 250 SBP).
11. Controversies unlikely to be tested on board at this time: SBP and PPI and SBP and b-blockers (some data to suggest stopping both when diagnosis of SBP is made).
12. Secondary peritonitis: more than one bug growing in culture by definition is not spontaneous bacterial peritonitis. Other characteristics of secondary peritonitis:
    a. Total Protein >1, LDH >upper limits of serum, Glucose <50, CEA >5, Alk Phos >240.
    b. Elevation of WBC in ascites fluid is not reliable to distinguish between SBP and secondary. However, if ascites WBC >10K think secondary.
    c. If you make diagnosis of secondary peritonitis, imaging is recommended to look for a potential source.
13. CA 125 should not be tested in patients with ascites. It will be elevated (in males and females) and many times leads to unnecessary testing.

Notes

All patients with moderate-to-large ascites who have a change in clinical status should undergo a diagnostic paracentesis to rule out SBP. Bedside taps are a safe and simple procedure but are becoming a lost art. Patients are routinely sent to radiology which may delay a diagnosis. Remember to inoculate ascites into culture bottles directly at bedside to increase the yield.

Reference

Spontaneous bacterial peritonitis in patients with cirrhosis: incidence, outcomes, and treatment strategies. PMID: 30666172.

Question 31

The only curative option for the autosomal recessive enzyme defect illustrated below is.

Hepatocyte

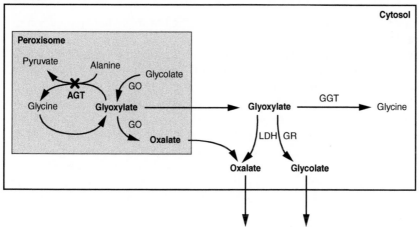

A High-dose pyridoxine
B Lumasiran
C Dialysis
D Liver transplantation
E Increase in dietary calcium

D is the correct answer.

Commentary – Primary Hyperoxaluria

Clinical Pearls: Primary Hyperoxaluria

1. There are three types of primary hyperoxaluria. The transplant hepatology boards will want you to know type I.
2. Primary hyperoxaluria 1 is due to defects in the gene that encodes the hepatic peroxisomal enzyme alanine glyoxylate aminotransferase (AGT), an enzyme which is involved in the transamination of glyoxylate to glycine.
3. This autosomal recessive inborn error of metabolism leads to overproduction of oxalate. The excess oxalate is excreted by the kidneys. This results in urinary calcium oxalate supersaturation leading to crystal aggregation, urolithiasis, and/or nephrocalcinosis with the potential of ultimately leading to end-stage kidney disease.
4. This disease usually manifests before the age of 21, with median age of onset of symptoms 5 years. It mostly affects patients of Northern African and Middle Eastern descent.
5. Other organ involvement: cardiac conduction defects, peripheral vascular disease, bone pain and spontaneous fracture, and oxalate deposition in joints and retina.
6. The diagnosis used to be confirmed by liver biopsy but now is done by genetic testing demonstrating an absent or significantly reduced AGT activity.
7. Medical management includes large fluid intake, inhibitors of calcium oxalate precipitation, avoiding foods high in oxalate (tea, chocolate, spinach, and rhubarb), high-dose pyridoxine (coenzyme of AGT), lumasiran, and oxalobacter formigens.
8. Liver transplantation is the only curative intervention for primary hyperoxaluria type I. There is some controversy regarding lone liver transplantation versus combined liver/kidney transplant.

Reference

Primary hyperoxaluria type 1: improved outcome with timely liver transplantation: a single-center report of 36 children. PMID: 11502971.

Question 32

A 26-year-old male from India presents with 1 week history of abdominal pain, itching, and dark urine. He is in town visiting his brother who is a medical resident. The patient says he has been feeling unwell for the last month with upper respiratory like symptoms, low-grade fevers, and an erythematous rash which eventually resolved. He has no past medical history and takes no herbals or medications. He does not drink, smoke, or use illicit drugs.

Exam: afebrile, HR 100, BP 128/64. He is jaundiced with chest excoriations. There is no asterixis. He is slightly tender in his RUQ. Labs revealed a TBili of 14, AST 1890, ALT 2652, ALP of 218; INR of 1.2. Seventy-two hours into the admission, the patient develops worsening mental status and somnolence, INR has increased to 1.7. An ultrasound is negative.

Serological studies are provided below.

Anti-HAV IgM negative, IgG positive; HBsAg negative, anti-HBc total positive, anti-HBs negative, anti-HCV negative, anti-HEV IgM positive, ANA negative, Immunoglobulins normal.

▶ Question

Which of the following is correct?

A   The patient should be started on ribavirin immediately.
B   The patient should be started on corticosteroids.
C   The patient should be transferred to a transplant center immediately.
D   The patient should be started on plasmapheresis.
E   An MRCP should be ordered.

C is the correct answer.

Commentary – HEV

Clinical Pearls: Hepatitis E Virus (HEV)

1. HEV outbreaks are usually related to contamination of drinking water with human fecal matter. Genotypes 1&2 (endemic).
2. Genotypes 3&4 in nonendemic areas. Usually seen in immunocompromised patients or those with chronic liver disease.
3. GT 3 can also cause a chronic infection in HIV patients, bone marrow transplant patients, and especially posttransplant patients. Treat by lowering immunosuppression and with Ribavirin × 12 weeks.
4. All immunocompromised patients with unexplained LFTs should be tested for hepatitis E.
5. Pigs are the predominant reservoir. Pig farmer on boards? Think hepatitis E
6. Acute hepatitis E is diagnosed with positive anti-HEV IgM. A total of 1–4% of patients develop ALF.
7. ALF seems to occur most frequently in third trimester pregnant females.
8. It is one of the most common causes of acute liver failure worldwide.
9. Treatment of acute HEV is supportive and self resolves in a large majority of patients.
10. HEV is associated with neurological disorders like Guillain–Barre syndrome.

Reference

Hepatitis E virus: epidemiology, diagnosis, clinical manifestations, and treatment. PMID: 33071523.

Question 33

Which of the following is FALSE regarding the systemic hemodynamics, renal dysfunction, and fluid retention in cirrhosis? There is:

A Sodium retention
B Reduced sodium excretion
C Splanchnic arterial vasoconstriction
D Increased cardiac output
E High ADH levels

C is the correct answer.

Commentary – Hemodynamics in Cirrhosis

Clinical Pearls: Systemic Hemodynamics, Renal Dysfunction, and Fluid Retention in Cirrhosis

1. Phase 1: Portal hypertension (PHTN) leads to splanchnic arterial vasodilation causing an increase in portal flow and maintains progression of PHTN.
2. Phase 2: Sodium retention causes water retention leading to ascites which causes an increase in cardiac output (hyperdynamic circulation) and reduced sodium excretion.
3. Phase 3: Cardiac output eventually starts to drop causing reduced renal, cerebral, and muscular blood flow.
4. Phase 4: Renal perfusion and glomerular filtration rate are lowered leading to dilutional hyponatremia and high ADH levels which can contribute to cerebral edema and encephalopathy.
5. Hepatorenal syndrome is in part related to intense renal vasoconstriction.

Notes

One of the reasons I was drawn to hepatology is because it just seems to make sense. Knowing some basic physiology behind the hemodynamics in cirrhosis and portal hypertension provides great insight into disease manifestation.

Reference

Relationship between systemic hemodynamics, renal dysfunction, and fluid retention in cirrhosis. PMID: 30992841.

Question 34

A 47-year-old alcoholic cirrhotic who continues to drink "a moderate amount," comes to your clinic upset that he is taking his water pills (200 mg of spironolactone and 80 mg of furosemide) as directed but continues to retain fluid. His mother confirms good compliance with his water pills. Exam reveals no scleral icterus, spider angiomata, palmar erythema, small ascites, no audible bruit, but 2–3+ bilateral edema with scrotal edema.

Laboratory studies:

Sodium 133, K 4.4; BUN 16, Cr 0.9
TBili 1, AST 47, ALT 24, ALP 119, gGTP 109
US reveals small perihepatic ascites, and patent vessels
Spot Urine Sodium 318, spot potassium 11
The major cause of the patient's persistent fluid retention is the following:

A Cardio-renal syndrome
B Diuretic responsive but unlikely following a 2 g sodium diet
C Diuretic resistant
D Diuretic responsive and adherent
E Noncompliance with diuretics

B is the correct answer.

Commentary – Ascites and Sodium Intake

Clinical Pearls: Assessment of Dietary Compliance: Spot Na/K Ratio

1. It is important to determine sodium compliance in order to avoid mislabeling patients with refractory ascites, when in fact their problem is inadequate dietary salt restriction.
2. Patients who are gaining weight despite excreting more than 78 meq of sodium in 24-hour period are not complaint with a low-sodium diet.
3. In the absence of diuretics, patient with ascites have very low sodium and high urine K (due to secondary hyperaldosteronism).
4. 90% of patients with a urine Na/K >1 in a random specimen are excreting more than 78 meq/day in a 24-hour urine collection.
5. On diuretics? Na/K >2.5 seems to have good sensitivity and specificity.
6. Na/K >1 and losing weight? Diuretic sensitive and adherent.
7. Na/K <1 and not losing weight? Diuretic-resistant.
8. Na/K >1 and not losing weight? diuretic-sensitive, but noncompliant.

Notes

The spot sodium to potassium ratio is a very simple but very underutilized test. Adhering strictly to a low sodium diet it is critical for maintenance of fluid balance in patients with cirrhosis. Checking a spot Na/K can be revealing, especially before pulling the trigger on TIPS.

Reference

Spot urinary sodium for assessing dietary sodium restriction in cirrhotic ascites. PMID: 19653340.

Question 35

A 32-year-old female patient, blood type A-positive, underwent liver transplantation for PSC. Her preliver transplant course was complicated by variceal bleeding requiring multiple blood transfusions and a TIPS procedure. The patient eventually underwent liver transplant receiving an ABO-compatible graft. Cold ischemic time (CIT) was 6.5 hours. On postoperative day 4, the patient was complaining of extreme fatigue and developed fever, hypotension, renal failure, and coagulopathy. A Doppler ultrasound revealed sluggish flow within the portal vein. The patient was listed for emergent re-transplantation. Gross examination of the liver revealed it to be enlarged, cyanotic, and mottled with areas of geographic necrosis. The patient did well and was discharged 2 weeks after her second transplant.

Explant analysis revealed: marked microvascular endothelial cell hypertrophy/ hobnailing and eosinophilic, neutrophils, monocytic microvasculitis; diffuse C4d staining in the microvasculature; portal/periportal edema, necrosis, and hemorrhage.

▶ Question

The most likely cause of the patient's primary nonfunction was

A Underlying hypercoagulable state and thrombosis of the portal vein
B Ischemic liver injury related to sepsis and hypotension
C T-cell mediated rejection
D Preformed anti-donor antibodies
E Ischemia-reperfusion injury

D is the correct answer.

Commentary – Antibody Mediated Rejection

Clinical Pearls: Antibody-Mediated Rejection

1. There are two types of rejection in organ transplant: T-cell mediated rejection (TCMR) and Antibody mediated rejection (AMR).
2. AMR is caused by preformed anti-donor antibodies, ABO incompatibilities (approximately 60% incidence), or de novo antibodies that develop after transplant.
3. ABO incompatible grafts and donor-specific antibodies (DSA) are responsible for AMR.
4. There are two main types of DSA: preformed DSA (pDSA) and de novo DSA (dnDSA). Preformed DSA approximately 5%; recipient factors associated with preformed DSA: previous transfusions, previous transplant, and female sex.
5. De novo donor-specific antibody has a reported incidence of 11% at 5 years: factors associated with dnDSA: female sex, recipient donor/sex mismatch, variation in immunosuppression, noncompliance, previous pregnancy, or younger age.
6. Hyperacute AMR presents with early graft failure within a few hours of transplant.
7. There are four criteria for establishing a diagnosis of acute AMR in liver allografts:
   a. positive serum DSA tests
   b. histopathologic findings consistent with AMR
   c. C4d staining
   d. clinical correlation to exclude other entities
8. If a patient has an episode of rejection that is unresponsive to steroids or if clear histopathological features of acute AMR are seen on biopsy before treatment, serum DSA testing, C4d staining, and exclusion of other causes should be performed.
9. Treatment should be focused on prevention by decreasing exposure to blood products and encouraging compliance with IS regimens.
10. Treatment of episodes of AMR require some combination of steroids, immune-modulating agents, IVIG, plasmapheresis, and proteasome inhibitors (example bortezomib).
11. There is evolving literature on AMR as a cause of chronic rejection following liver transplant, but histological features are not as specific, and it is unlikely to be tested on the boards at this time.

Reference

Antibody-mediated rejection of the liver allograft: an update and a clinico-pathological perspective. PMID: 34343613.

Question 36

Which of the following donor and recipient ABO blood type pairings would be expected to have the highest risk of AMR?

A Donor A to recipient AB
B Donor AB to recipient A
C Donor O to recipient B
D Donor A2 subtype to recipient O
E Donor AB to recipient AB

B is the correct answer.

Commentary – ABO Incompatible Transplant

> **Clinical Pearls: ABO-Incompatible Liver Transplant**
>
> 1. Blood-type AB is the universal recipient. AB blood type has both A and B antigens and so has no antibodies. O is the universal donor. O blood type has no A or B antigens, but has both A and B antibodies.
> 2. Using conventional immunosuppression (IS), ABO-incompatible (ABO-I) liver transplantation has generally been considered a contraindication due to high risk of antibody mediated, biliary, and vascular complications.
> 3. Organ shortage has led to the development of reducing immunosuppressive protocols in the hopes of utilizing ABO-I and expanding the donor pool.
> 4. Protocols vary per transplant center. If preliver transplant isoagglutinin titer is ≤1:8, then you may consider ABO-I transplant.
> 5. To reduce the risk of complications associated with ABO-I, perioperative: plasmapheresis, intensive induction IS and prostaglandin E1 administration have been used.
> 6. Rituximab and plasma exchange (both started several weeks before transplant) are being increasingly utilized with favorable outcomes in elective ABO-I liver transplants.
> 7. Blood-type A subgroups: A1 and A2. A2 phenotype has a lower cell surface expression of the A antigen. A2 donors elicit weaker immunogenic responses in ABO-incompatible recipients.
> 8. A2 donor to O recipient liver transplantation has been demonstrated to be safe in retrospective studies and some centers will treat these subtypes as ABO compatible.

Reference

ABO-incompatible liver transplantation: state of art and future perspectives. PMID: 32370710.

Question 37

A 62-year-old female with NASH cirrhosis underwent a balloon retrograde transvenous obliteration (BRTO) 4 years ago for large bleeding gastric varices. She has had no recurrent bleeding and has done relatively well until a few months ago when she began to develop increasing dyspnea on exertion. She says her breathing difficulties are worse on exertion. She denies platypnea. Exam is notable for an oxygen saturation of 87% on room air. She has spider angiomata, palmar erythema, splenomegaly, and small ascites.

Labs revealed a WBC count of 3.4, Hb of 17 and platelet count of 34K. TBili 1.3 with otherwise normal LFTs. Sodium 134, Cr 1.1. Serum albumin was 2.7, INR was 1.4. An ultrasound reveals a dilated portal vein and a spleen measuring 16 cm with small ascites. High-resolution CT scan of chest shows bilateral patchy ground glass opacities in the bases bilateral. Spirometry was normal except for a DCLO of 72% of predicted. A contrast echocardiogram with agitated saline reveals bubble appearance in the left atrium and left ventricle after the third cardiac cycle. Left ventricular size and function are normal. Pulmonary artery systolic pressure is estimated at 33 mmHg.
A room air ABG reveals a PaO_2 of 54 mmHg.

▶ Question

What is this patient's most likely diagnosis and what is the best treatment plan?

A Moderate porto-pulmonary HTN and bosentan
B Moderate HPS and TIPS
C Very severe HPS and referral to interventional radiology for closure of shunts
D Moderate porto-pulmonary HTN oxygen and anticoagulation
E Severe HPS and referral for liver transplant with MELD exception points

E is the correct answer.

Commentary – HPS

> ### Clinical Pearls: Hepatopulmonary Syndrome (HPS)
>
> 1. HPS is probably underdiagnosed with an estimated incidence of 5–32% in patients with cirrhosis and portal hypertension (PHTN). It felt to be the result of pulmonary vascular dilation resulting from an imbalance of vasodilators and vasoconstrictors.
> 2. All patients with cirrhosis and PHTN should be evaluated for HPS if their room air oxygen saturation is <96%.
> 3. Diagnostic criteria:
>   a. Portal hypertension (with or without cirrhosis).
>   b. Pulmonary vascular dilation as shows by positive contrast enhance echo or by radioactive lung-perfusion scan (showing brain shunt fraction >5%).
>   c. Partial pressure of oxygen <80 on room air or alveolar-arterial oxygen gradient (A-aO$_2$) ≥15 (>20 in patients above 60).
> 4. Severity:
>   a. Mild PaO$_2$ >80, Moderate 60–80, Severe 50–60, Very Severe <50 (or PaO$_2$ <300, while breathing 100% oxygen).
> 5. Clinical clues include cyanosis, digital clubbing, spider nevi:
>   a. Platypnea: worsening of dyspnea when moving from supine to upright position.
>   b. Orthodeoxia: decrease in PaO$_2$ of more than 5% when moving from supine to upright position.
> 6. The "late" appearance of microbubbles in the left atria, i.e.: between fourth and sixth cardiac cycles is consistent with HPS.
> 7. Radioactive lung perfusion scanning can help in diagnosis of HPS in the setting of concomitant lung disease. Brain shunt fraction of >5% is considered significant; >40% shunting may be a contraindication to liver transplant.
> 8. Pulmonary function tests may show decreased diffusion capacity for carbon monoxide (DLCO).
> 9. Definitive treatment for HPS is liver transplant. Patients with PaO$_2$ less than 60 may be eligible for MELD exception points. PaO$_2$ of less than 50 is associated with poor outcomes following liver transplant.
> 10. Hypoxemia may take up to one-year posttransplant to resolve.

> ### Notes
>
> HPS is an under-recognized, life-threatening complication of PHTN. HPS should be evaluated for in all patients with cirrhosis and PHTN whose room air O$_2$ sat is <96%.

Reference

Update on current and emergent data on hepatopulmonary syndrome. PMID: 29599604.

Question 38

A 63-year-old female is admitted to the hospital with complaints of dyspnea. Exam reveals multiple telangiectasias on her lips and tongue. Cardiac exam was notable for a mid-systolic murmur. A bruit was appreciated over the epigastrium. She has had issues with recurrent epistaxis for years. She recalls her mother having similar issues with bleeding and receiving numerous blood transfusions over the years.

Labs reveal a Hb of 8.2 with an MCV of 73. LFTs are normal. Anti-HCV is positive, but HCV RNA is negative. INR is 1.1.
CT scan is noted below.

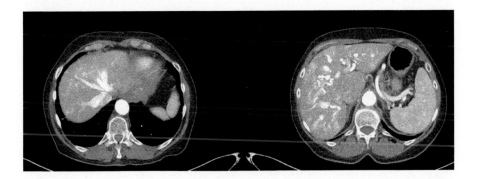

▶ Question

What is the most likely diagnosis?

A Multiple hepatic hemangiomas
B Hepatopulmonary syndrome
C Portopulmonary hypertension
D Hereditary hemorrhagic telangiectasia
E Hepatic sarcoidosis

D is the correct answer.

Commentary – HHT

Clinical Pearls: Hereditary Hemorrhagic Telangiectasia (HHT)

1. Also known as Osler–Weber–Rendu disease.
2. HHT is an autosomal dominant disorder characterized by multiple mucocutaneous telangiectasias.
3. The typical presentation includes recurrent epistaxis, GI bleeding, or iron deficiency anemia.
4. The classic triad is the following: recurrent epistaxis, mucocutaneous telangiectasia, and familial occurrence.
5. Mutations found in the ENG (endoglin; a membrane glycoprotein) gene that disrupts TGF-beta-mediated pathway in vascular endothelial cells. Treatment with bevacizumab (anti-vascular endothelial growth factor) has been reported to be effective in patients with heart failure with HHT.
6. There is a high prevalence of FNH in patients with HHT compared to the normal population.
7. Liver arterial-vascular-malformations (AVMs) can lead to high output heart failure, hypertension, and rarely, ischemic biliary disease. Liver AVMs are commonly seen in HHT patient but are symptomatic in less than 10% of cases.
8. The physiological mechanism in high output heart failure is related to systemic vascular resistance leading to activation of the renin–angiotensin–aldosterone system, causing salt and water retention. The shunting of blood through the AVMs leads to maldistribution of cardiac output. In order to maintain blood supply, cardiac output is increased.
9. Embolization of liver AVMs is not recommended given the high risk of postembolization necrosis and death.
10. In refractory cases, liver transplantation is the standard of treatment.

Notes

Early enhancement of a dilated IVC and hepatic veins as a result of contrast reflux from the right atrium into the IVC can be a radiographic clue suggestive of passive hepatic congestion or right sided heart failure. In this particular CT scan, it is a result of multiple hepatic AVMs in a patient with HHT.

Reference

Liver involvement in hereditary hemorrhagic telangiectasia. PMID: 29987403.

Question 39

A 47-year-old female with primary biliary cholangitis (PBC) complicated by large ascites and portosystemic encephalopathy is status postliver transplantation. The patient received a deceased donor graft from a 55-year-old male. Donor steatosis was 33%. Cold ischemic time (CIT) 10 hours, warm ischemic time (WIT) 122 minutes. On postoperative day 3, the patient remains intubated and on pressors. An ultrasound with Doppler and angiogram reveals patent vessels.

Laboratory studies:

TBili 2.7, AST 4400, ALT 1900, ALP 233; INR 3.3 with a lactate of 5.8. Sodium 132, Cr 1.6. WBC 11, Hb 9, Platelets 66.

What is the diagnosis?

A Hepatic artery thrombosis
B Obliterative portal venopathy
C Primary nonfunction
D ABO incompatible
E Biliary leak

C is the correct answer.

Commentary – PNF

Clinical Pearls: Primary Nonfunction (PNF)

1. PNF is a form of reperfusion injury resulting in irreversible graft failure leading to death or need for re-transplantation within 7 days without any detectable technical or immunological problems.
2. It is the most common cause for early retransplantation with an incidence of 4–8%.
3. For purposes of status 1 (liver transplant listing) designation, PNF should meet the following criteria:
   a. AST >3000
   b. INR >2.5
   c. Arterial pH <7.3 or lactate >4
   d. Hepatic artery, portal vein, hepatic vein, and caval outflow must be ruled out
4. Risk factors for PNF include donation after cardiac death (DCD), ABO mismatch, advanced donor age (>50), graft steatosis (typically >30%), small for size, CIT >12 hour, and WIT >90 minutes.

Reference

Primary non-function of the liver allograft. PMID: 33982912.

Question 40

A 37-year-old male patient presented with marked jaundice and acute tubular necrosis (ATN) renal failure. He was diagnosed with acute severe alcoholic hepatitis with a discriminant function of 98 on admission. He failed a course of steroids. He required dialysis for metabolic abnormalities and eventually underwent a deceased donor liver transplant with a pre-LT MELD of 40.

The patient's donor was a 28-year-old male who died of electrocution. The surgery was uneventful. Explant was consistent with alcoholic hepatitis with advanced underlying cirrhosis.

The patient was discharged on postoperative day 8. His kidney function had recovered. The patient's immunosuppression at discharge consisted of tacrolimus, mycophenolate, and corticosteroids.

Ten days after discharge the patient is brought to the emergency room by his girlfriend with 1 day of drowsiness and then onset of seizures.

WBC 12, Hb 12, Platelets 157. Normal BMP. Magnesium 0.9. LFTs normal. FK 14.6
T2 sequence of MRI is shown below shows hyperintensity involving the bilateral occipital lobes and parietal lobes.

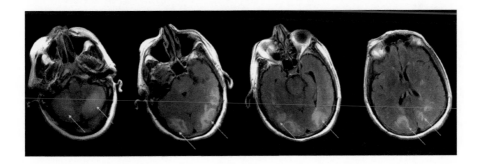

What is the diagnosis?

A Glioblastoma
B Posterior reversible encephalopathy syndrome
C Metastatic hepatocellular carcinoma
D JC virus
E *Cryptococcus neoformans*

B is the correct answer.

Commentary – PRES

Clinical Pearls: Posterior Reversible Encephalopathy Syndrome (PRES)

1. Posterior reversible encephalopathy syndrome (PRES) is a rare cliniconeuroradiologic syndrome attributed to calcineurin inhibitor (CNI) use.
2. The incidence is only about 1%.
3. The most common presenting symptoms is seizure, but PRES can also present with focal deficits, mental status changes, delirium, coma, headache, and visual changes.
4. The diagnosis is made on imaging revealing a distinct pattern involving the cortical and subcortical areas of the parietal or occipital lobes.
5. Concomitant hemorrhage can be seen in 15% of cases.
6. Pathophysiology of PRES remains controversial but likely centers around a vascular process. CNIs are powerful vasoconstrictors, increasing production of endothelin with overproduction of reactive oxygen species; it is associated with reversible vasogenic subcortical edema.
7. Risk factors may include pre-LT alcoholic liver disease, hypomagnesemia, and infection.
8. Mainstay treatment is lowering CNI levels, although not all patients with PRES will have supratherapeutic levels of CNI.

Notes

The T2 weighted MRI in this question stem shows T2 hyperintense lesions (arrows) involving the posterior fossa, cerebellar hemispheres, occipital, and parietal lobes.

Reference

Posterior reversible encephalopathy syndrome in liver transplant patients: clinical presentation, risk factors and initial management. PMID: 22494636.

Question 41

Which of the following statements is TRUE?

A Fluconazole inhibits CYP3a and increases calcineurin inhibitor (CNI) concentrations
B Rifampin induces CYP3a and increases mammalian target of rapamycin (mTOR) concentration
C Phenytoin inhibits CYP3a and increases CNI concentration
D Grapefruit juice induces CYP3a and increases mTOR concentration
E St. John Wort induces CYP3a and increases CNI

A is the correct answer.

Commentary – Drug Interactions with Immunosuppression Drugs

Clinical Pearls: Major Drug Interactions Post Liver Transplant

Drugs that **inhibit** CYP3a4/5 increase CNI and mTOR concentration include the following:

1. Macrolides: clarithromycin, erythromycin.
2. Antifungals: fluconazole, ketoconazole, voriconazole, clotrimazole.
3. Calcium channel blockers: verapamil, diltiazem, nifedipine.
4. Others: metoclopramide, amiodarone, danazole, protease inhibitors, grapefruit juice

Drugs that **induce** CYP3a4/5 decrease CNI and mTOR concentration:

1. Antibiotics: rifampin, rifampicin, rifabutin, nafcillin.
2. Anticonvulsants: phenytoin, phenobarbital, carbamazepine.
3. Other: St. John Wort.

Reference

Long-term immunosuppression and drug interactions. PMID: 11689777.

Question 42

A 26-year-old female presents to the emergency room with nausea and vomiting after an intentional ingestion of over 10 g of acetaminophen. The patient broke up with her boyfriend and admits to being depressed with minimal PO intake over the last several days.

Exam: A thin female with a flat affect. Abdominal exam is benign. She is lethargic but without asterixis.

HR 110, BP 100 systolic, 37.3, RR 14, O_2 sat 97% on room air; BMI 18.4

Laboratory studies:

Cr 1.3, Normal CBC; TBili 1.1, AST 18,888, ALT 20,780, ALP 156; INR 4.2
NH3 222

▶ **Question**

Regarding the figure – the patient's relative starvation affects which labeled portion below of acetaminophen metabolism, potentially exacerbating her liver injury?

Conjugation
A
Glucuronide ◀——— Acetaminophen

Moiety
(nontoxic)

B
P-450
2E1

Conjugation
E
———▶ Sulfate

Moiety
(nontoxic)

C
NAPQI (toxic)

NAC

D
Glutathione

Cysteine and mercapturic acid
conjugates (nontoxic)

Question 43

The patient in the question above is administered *N*-acetylcysteine (NAC) but develops worsening encephalopathy over the next 24 hours. pH is 7.36. Which of the following would fulfill King's College criteria for acetaminophen and warrant transplant evaluation?

A Grade IV portosystemic encephalopathy (PSE), INR 4.4, Cr 4.4
B Grade IV PSE, INR 11, TBili 12
C Grade III PSE, INR 9, Cr 3.9
D Grade III PSE, INR 5.5, Cr 5.5
E pH 7.41, INR 4.5, TBili 14

42 – A is the correct answer.
43 – C is the correct answer.

Commentary – ALF

Clinical Pearls: Acetaminophen Acute Liver Failure

1. Acetaminophen (*N*-acetyl-para-aminophenol, paracetamol, APAP) overdose is the number one cause of acute liver failure in the United States, accounting for nearly 40% of cases.
2. Nearly half of cases are suicide attempts and half are unintentional (therapeutic misadventure).
3. Overdose levels peak at 4 hours.
4. A majority (90%) of metabolism of acetaminophen primarily occurs though glucuronidation and sulfation; 2% is unchanged and excreted in urine. See diagram below:
5. The remainder (5–9%) is converted to the toxic metabolite *N*-acetyl-*p*-benzoquinone imine (NAPQI) via CYP2E1.
6. Agents that induce CYP2E1 lead to an increase in metabolism of acetaminophen and consequently increase production of NAPQI include isoniazid, rifampin, phenytoin, phenobarbital and smoking.
7. Hepatic glutathione removes a majority of NAPQI. But in cases of acetaminophen overdose the amount of NAPQI produced can exceed hepatic glutathione stores.
8. Situations that can lead to depletion of hepatic glutathione stores include chronic alcoholism, chronic liver disease, and malnutrition or starvation.
9. In addition, glucuronidation of acetaminophen is dependent on carbohydrate stores and more acetaminophen is converted to NAPQI in malnourished patients.
10. Histological features: causes zone 3 (centrilobular) injury/necrosis.
11. *N*-acetylcysteine (NAC) is nearly fully protective if given within 8 hours after ingestion. NAC reduces NAPQI back to acetaminophen and acts as a substitute for hepatic glutathione. NAC can be given oral: 18 doses q4 × 72 hours or IV: 20 hours of treatment.
12. For the boards, there is a role for activated charcoal if the patient presents within one hour of ingestion.
13. King's college criteria for acetaminophen: pH less than 7.3 or all three: (i) grade III/IV PSE, (ii) INR >6.5 and Cr >3.4.

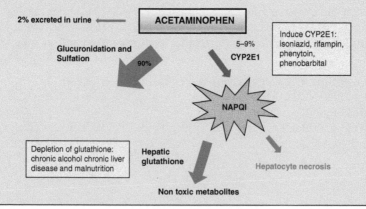

Notes
The association between fasting, ethanol use, and acetaminophen toxicity (the basis for this question) was first published by one of my mentors, Dr. David Whitcomb in a JAMA paper from 1994. David started his career with the liver and is now a world-renowned pancreatologist (who could predict moving to a lesser organ would pay such huge dividends!).

Reference

Acetaminophen-induced hepatotoxicity: a comprehensive update. PMID: 27350943.

Question 44

A 62-year-old female with cryptogenic cirrhosis is referred to your center for liver transplant evaluation. Her disease has been complicated by diuretic-controlled ascites, non-bleeding varices, and mild PSE. She is a Child Pugh C with a MELD score of 16.

INR 1.5, Cr 1.3, TBili 0.9, Na 135; LFTs are normal
On her review of systems, she does complain of leg cramps and dyspnea on exertion.
Exam is notable for mild ascites, spider angiomata, palmar erythema, and 1+ lower extremity edema.
O_2 Sat is 97%.

As part of her preop evaluation, the patient undergoes a transthoracic echo (TTE) revealing the following results:

Normal LV size and function with EF 62%, mildly dilated RV and right atrium with normal function, flattened IVC; PASP 72 mmHg
Normal saline contrast injection

A right heart catheterization (RHC) is performed revealing:

mean PASP 54
PCWP 9
PVR of 5.1 Woods

▶ Question

What is the best management strategy?

A Anticoagulation
B Endothelin-receptor antagonist
C TIPS
D B-blockade
E Liver transplantation

B is the correct answer.

Commentary – PPHTN

Clinical Pearls: Porto-Pulmonary Hypertension (PPHTN)

1. The prevalence of PPHTN is reported to be up to 15% of patients undergoing transplant evaluation.
2. The diagnosis of PPTN is confirmed on RHC:
   a. elevated mean PASP >20.
   b. normal or low pulmonary capillary wedge pressure <15.
   c. an elevated PVR >3 wood units (240 dynes).
3. The most commonly utilized medical therapy includes single agent or combination therapy of: phosphodiesterase type-5 inhibitor (sildenafil, tadalafil), endothelin receptor antagonist (bosentan, ambrisentan), and IV prostacyclin.
4. Liver transplantation should be considered in patients with mild-to-moderate PPHTN. Severe PPHTN (mPAP >50) is considered a contraindication to LT given the historical high perioperative mortality.
5. Up to 20% of patients with PPHTN may have persistently elevated pressures post LT and may require continued therapy.

Reference

Hepatopulmonary syndrome and portopulmonary hypertension: current status and implications for liver transplantation. PMID: 32905452.

Question 45

A 63-year-old male with NASH cirrhosis complicated by refractory ascites is status post liver transplant. His preoperative MELD score was 24. The patient underwent a right lobe live donor liver transplant from his 48-year-old cousin. Surgical procedure was without complications. The patient was administered basiliximab induction and is currently on combination prednisone, mycophenolate, and tacrolimus. WIT: 37 minutes, CIT 5 hours, and 12 minutes.

The patient has persistent ascites requiring drainage several times in his first week postop. At day 15, TBili is 11.4, AST 228, ALT 191, ALP 422; INR 2.4. The patient is confused with asterixis. An ultrasound with Doppler is normal. There is no evidence of infection. Viral serologies are negative.

A trans-jugular liver biopsy reveals a gradient of 17 mmHg. Histology shows hepatocyte ballooning, steatosis, centrilobular necrosis, and parenchymal cholestasis.

▶ Question

Which of the following is associated with this syndrome?

A Basiliximab induction
B Intraoperative portal pressure >19 mmHg
C Graft recipient weight ratio >1%
D Recipient MELD >30
E Answer choices B&C

B is the correct answer.

Commentary – SFSS

Clinical Pearls: Small for Size Syndrome

1. Small for size syndrome is a clinical syndrome that occurs when a partial graft (live donor or split) is inadequate to sustain the metabolic demands of the recipient.
2. The typical presentation is ascites, persistent jaundice, coagulopathy, and encephalopathy.
3. Other causes should be excluded (technical, anatomical, immunological, or hepatitis-related).
4. Biopsy findings include hepatocyte ballooning, steatosis, centrilobular necrosis, and parenchymal cholestasis.
5. Risk factors include MELD >20, donor age >38, and end portal venous pressure of >19 mmHg.
6. Graft Recipient Weight Ratio (GWRA) <0.8%.
7. Management may include modulation of portal inflow such as splenectomy, splenic artery ligation, portocaval shunts, and hepatic outflow modification.

Reference

Small-for-size syndrome in liver transplantation: definition, pathophysiology and management. PMID: 32646775.

Question 46

A 9-year-old boy is referred to your clinic by his pediatrician with jaundice and abnormal liver tests. The patient is originally from Kuwait. His parents moved to the United States four months ago. His medical care has not been consistent. Via the Arabic interpreter you learn that the patient has had chronic itching and clay-colored stools for years. He has a chronic cough. He has had multiple fractures over the years. In addition, he has difficulty seeing at night. The patient has no family history of liver disease. He has two healthy siblings. On exam, the patient is very thin with a BMI of only 14 kg/m². He has a broad forehand, deep set eyes, and a pointed chin. He has icterus and multiple excoriations. His liver is enlarged and firm. His spleen is palpable. Cardiac exam reveals amid systolic murmur.

Laboratory studies:

Viral serologies negative Ceruloplasmin 15; 24-hour urine copper is 19. Alpha1-antitrypsin 92, MZ phenotype WBC 3.4, Hb 11, Platelets 78K Normal renal function TBili 13, AST 72, ALT 59, ALP 422; Albumin 2.5 INR 1.4

▶ Question

The most likely diagnosis is the following:

A BRIC
B Cardiac cirrhosis secondary to congenital pulmonary stenosis
C Alagille syndrome
D Schistosomiasis
E Cystic fibrosis

C is the correct answer.

Commentary – Alagille Syndrome

Clinical Pearls: Alagille Syndrome

1. Alagille syndrome is a rare multisystem autosomal dominant disorder.
2. The disease is associated with mutations in the *JAG1* gene.
3. In addition to liver involvement other organs/manifestations include the following:
   a. cardiac: pulmonary stenosis, tetralogy of Fallot
   b. renal: renal dysplasia
   c. skeletal: butterfly vertebrae, pathological fractures of long bones
   d. ophthalmology: posterior embryotoxon
   e. facial findings: prominent broad forehead, deep-set eyes, prominent ears, triangular face with pointed chin, and broad nasal bridge
4. Hepatic manifestations: cholestasis (which can lead to fat soluble vitamin deficiency; for example, vitamin A deficiency leading to night blindness as was alluded to in the case question above) caused by paucity of biliary ducts (classic finding on liver biopsy), conjugated hyperbilirubinemia, pruritus.
   Cirrhosis/end stage disease is seen in up to 15% of cases.
5. Overall mortality is 10%.
6. Treatment is generally supportive. In cases of liver failure, liver transplant offer ~85% survival at 5 years follow-up.

Reference

Outcomes of liver transplantation for patients with Alagille syndrome: the studies of pediatric liver transplantation experience. PMID: 22454296.

Question 47

A 67-year-old female with NASH cirrhosis is referred to you for refractory encephalopathy despite good compliance with lactulose and rifaximin. The patient has diuretic-controlled ascites. She has large "isolated" gastric varices (IGV1) on EGD but has not bled.

Other past medical history includes morbid obesity with a BMI of 53 kg/m², diabetes, and sleep apnea.

The patient lives with her husband (who also has NASH cirrhosis but is well compensated). She has become dependent on him for activities of daily living. The patient has had four admissions in the last 8 months for encephalopathy including two severe bouts that required intubation. She was diagnosed with a UTI on one occasion, otherwise, no obvious precipitating event has been noted.

Laboratory studies:

Na 136, Cr 1; TBili 1.4, AST 22, ALT 24, ALP 128, Albumin 3.4
WBC 3.7, Hb 11, Platelets 63K
INR 1.2
A1C 7.7

▶ Question

Which of the following do you recommend?

A Referral for liver transplantation
B Addition of zinc
C Increase lactulose
D Prophylactic nitrofurantoin
E Cross-sectional imaging

Question 48

Cross-sectional imaging is obtained for the patient in the question above. Axial and coronal cuts are displayed below.

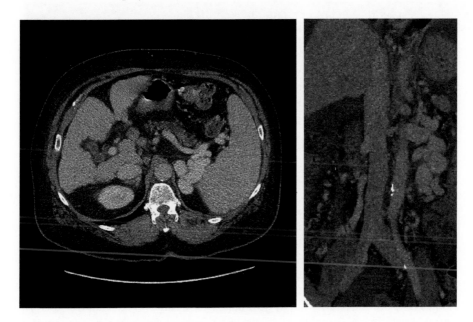

▶ Question

Based on the imaging findings, what would you recommend for this patient?

A IR consult for embolization
B Surgical meso-caval shunt
C Splenic artery embolization
D Transjugular intrahepatic portosystemic shunt
E L-Ornithine L-Aspartate (LOLA) and branch-chained amino acids (BCAA)

47 – E is the correct answer.
48 – A is the correct answer.

Commentary – Spontaneous Spleno-Renal Shunt

Clinical Pearls: Spontaneous Spleno-Renal Shunt (SRSS)

1. Portosystemic shunts are collateral blood vessels that form as a compensatory response to portal hypertension and divert blood flow to the systemic circulation.
2. Spontaneous splenorenal shunts (SSRSs) are a common type of portosystemic shunt occurring in up to 50% of patients with cirrhosis.
3. These collaterals decompress the portal circulation through the left renal vein and IVC.
4. SSRS can act as a point of access to the portal circulation in the angiographic obliteration of bleeding varices.
5. They can also be embolized or ligated to treat hepatic encephalopathy which is refractory to medical therapy.
6. Studies have suggested that up to 70% of patients with refractory HE show large SSRS upon radiological screening.
7. The diagnosis of SSRS as a cause of refractory PSE can be delayed on average by up to 1 year in patients.
8. In well-selected patients (MELD scores of 11 or less), embolization of dominant large SSRS is safe and effective.
9. A small proportion of patients may go on to develop clinically relevant worsening portal hypertension, namely ascites and less so varices. Surveillance EGD should be performed after closure of shunts.

Notes

I tell my fellows all the time, "if a patient is admitted multiple times for encephalopathy, there's a good chance there is a shunt present." Sometimes these shunts are so large, they will be mistaken for bowel by inexperienced observers. What separates a great gastroenterologist/hepatologist from an average one is the ability to read your own imaging. I can't emphasize how important it is to look at the imaging studies yourself. Start the habit early in your career. Look at the images yourself and *then* look at the official read.

Reference

Portosystemic shunts, and refractory hepatic encephalopathy: patient selection and current options. PMID: 30774483.

Question 49

A 51-year-old female is referred to your clinic for abnormal liver tests. The patient has had a mild elevation in alkaline phosphatase for over a year, but over the last 6–8 months it has steadily increased. The patient has no specific complaints, although on review of systems she does complain of dry eyes and dry mouth.

Laboratory studies:

Normal renal function and CBC
TBili 1.0, AST 43, ALT 39, ALP 288, GTP 303
Exam: 83 kg
Mild palmar erythema – Her primary care physician dew labs drawn one month prior: anti-HCV, HBsAg, anti-HBc, anti-HBs, anti-HAV total all negative CMV IgG negative, CMV IgM negative; EBV IgG positive, EBV IgM negative ANA negative IgG 1400, IgM 590, IgA 287.
An ultrasound is normal with a kPa of 5.32 on transient elastography. A liver biopsy is performed with a representative image shown below:

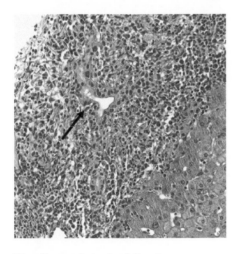

The diagnosis is the following:

A Hepatic sarcoidosis
B Primary biliary cholangitis
C CMV hepatitis
D Bartonella infection
E Small duct PSC

B is the correct answer.

Reference

Florid biliary duct lesions in an AMA – positive patient in absence of cholestatic liver biochemistry. PMID: 30975574.

Question 50

The patient in the question above is started on ursodeoxycholic acid (UDCA) at a dose of 1200 mg daily. The patient weighs 220 pounds. After 1 year the patient's ALP is 249.

▶ Question

What do you recommend now?

A Trial of steroids
B Obeticholic acid
C Increase UDCA to 1800 mg
D Repeat liver biopsy
E Addition of azathioprine

B is the correct answer.

Commentary – PBC

Clinical Pearls: Primary Biliary Cholangitis

1. Primary biliary cholangitis (the name was appropriately changed from primary biliary *cirrhosis* in 2014–2015) is an autoimmune disorder that leads to the gradual destruction of intrahepatic bile ducts.
2. The incidence is 9:1 female to male; generally middle-aged; there is a higher prevalence in first-degree relatives.
3. The diagnosis is made with two of three:
   a. Predominant elevation in cholestatic enzymes.
   b. Positive anti-mitochondrial antibody (positive in ~90% of cases). The anti-mitochondrial AB binds to lipoic acid containing the E2 component of the pyruvate dehydrogenase complex located on the mitochondria inner membrane.
   c. Liver histology consistent: destruction of bile ducts with predominant lymphocytic infiltration. Nonsuppurative destructive cholangitis or "florid duct lesion" is pathognomonic but only seen in ~15% of cases. Noncaseating portal granulomas (see image below).

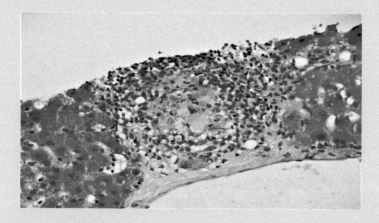

4. Many patients are asymptomatic; most common presenting symptoms are the following: fatigue, RUQ discomfort, and pruritus. Jaundice is typically only seen in late-stage disease.
5. Concomitant autoimmune diseases include the following: Sjogren (~25%), thyroid dysfunction 15% (Hashimoto's 10%), celiac (8%), CREST (5%), and rheumatoid arthritis (5%).
6. Other lab abnormalities include deficiency of fat-soluble vitamins (vitamins D, A, K, E), elevated cholesterol 50% cases which can manifest as xanthomas and xanthelasmas. Elevation in cholesterol does seem to predispose to increase in cardiovascular events.

Question 51

Which of the following is true regarding early stage (precirrhotic) portal hypertension in patients with PBC?

A Prehepatic with normal gradient
B Posthepatic with normal gradient
C Intrahepatic sinusoidal with elevated gradient
D Intrahepatic presinusoidal with normal gradient
E Intrahepatic postsinusoidal with elevated gradient

D is the correct answer.

Clinical Pearls: Primary Biliary Cholangitis

1. There are currently two FDA-approved medications:
   a. UDCA; standard dose being 13–15 mg/kg. Patients who "normalize" their ALP have excellent long-term prognosis; ~75% of patients with PBC will respond to UDCA. UDCA has recently been shown to be beneficial even in patients with PBC *cirrhosis* and preventing decompensated disease.
   b. patients who do not respond to lone UDCA should be given second-line agent. Obeticholic acid was approved as a second-line agent in 2016. It is a farnesoid X receptor (FXR) agonist (usually used in addition to UDCA). Side effect of worsening pruritus seen in up to 30% of patients. Can also cause dyslipidemia (increase in total cholesterol, LDL, triglycerides, and lowering of HDL)
   c. There is some emerging data on the role of fibrates.
2. Bone disease is common in patients with PBC. DEXA should be obtained at diagnosis.
3. Younger patients (less than 35-year-old) with PBC may have an accelerated course.
4. Surveillance for HCC is reserved for PBC patients with cirrhosis; incidence is ~2.5%. Some data to suggest male patients with PBC cirrhosis are at higher risk of HCC.
5. Recurrent PBC seen in 10–40% of patients post-LT; evidence suggests a benefit to "prophylactic" UDCA to prevent recurrence.
6. Strongest predictors of inadequate response to therapy: early age at diagnosis (less than 35) and advanced stage at presentation.
7. Patients with PBC can develop precirrhotic PHTN; initially as presinusoidal type. As the disease progresses, it is joined by a sinusoidal component.

   Intrahepatic presinusoidal: Normal Wedge – Normal Free – Normal Gradient.

Notes

PBC is a favorite disease of many hepatologists. It was one of the more common indications for liver transplantation when Dr. Starzl started his career. Now, largely in part due to medical therapy, it can be managed in a vast majority of patients. A special thanks to Dr. Marta Minervini (transplant pathologist) for many of the histology images provided in this book.

References

A placebo-controlled trial of obeticholic acid in primary biliary cholangitis. PMID: 27532829.
Primary biliary cholangitis. PMID: 33308474.

Question 52

Which letter corresponds to segment VI?

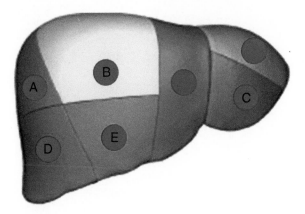

Question 53

In the Couinaud classification, this segment drains directly into the inferior vena cava (IVC) by one or more small hepatic veins.

A 1
B 8
C 4a
D 4b
E 7

Question 54

Resection of segments II and III would be categorized as:

A Right anterior segmentectomy
B Right posterior segmentectomy
C Left lateral segmentectomy
D Left hepatectomy
E Extended left hepatectomy

52 – D is the correct answer.
53 – A is the correct answer.
54 – C is the correct answer.

Question 55

The liver segment-colored green above represents:

A 2
B 4a
C 4b
D 5
E 8

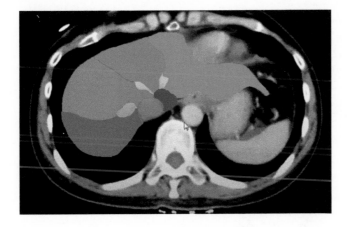

B is the correct answer.

Commentary – Hepatic Segments

Clinical Pearls: Couinaud Classification of Hepatic Segments

1. Named after French Surgeon Claude Couinaud (pronounced Keww-No) is the most widely used system to describe functional liver anatomy.
2. It divides the liver into eight independent functional units (termed segments).
3. The figure above (adopted from Pauli and colleagues) provides a "hand-y" tool to learn segmental liver anatomy.
4. The middle hepatic vein (MHV) demarcates the true right and left lobes.
5. The right lobe is further divided into anterior and posterior segments by the right hepatic vein (RHV). The left lobe is divided into the medial and lateral segments by the left hepatic vein (LHV).
6. Resection of segments 2 and 3: left lateral segmentectomy.
7. Resection of segments 2, 3, and 4: left hepatectomy.
8. Resection of segments 5, 6, 7, and 8: right hepatectomy.

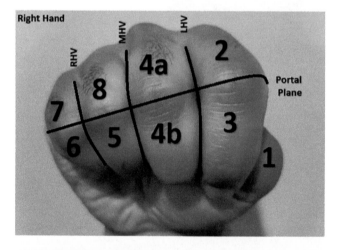

Notes

Human hands were not meant to mimic the lobes of the liver. I had a difficult time manipulating my 4th and 5th fingers to represent the larger right lobe. But hopefully the learning point comes across.

Reference

Clinical and surgical anatomy of the liver: a review for clinicians. PMID: 24453062.

Question 56

A 49-year-old female with decompensated alcoholic cirrhosis is undergoing liver transplant evaluation. She is a Child Pugh C with a MELD score of 28. During the evaluation she undergoes a transthoracic echo revealing a pulmonary artery systolic pressure of 53 mmHg. Per your center guidelines she is scheduled for a right heart catheterization (RHC).

Laboratory studies:

Platelets 41K, PT 24 (11–15), INR 2.6; PT 48 (23–34).
Cardiology is asking if any products should be administered prior to the RHC. You order a thromboelastrography (TEG); the tracing and results are provided below.

▶ Question

What do you recommend?

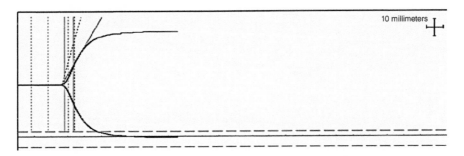

R: 13.8 min (4–9); K: 2.5 min (1–3); Angle deg: 63 (59–74); MA: 65 mm (50–75); LY30: 1.2% (0–8)

A Administer FFP
B Administer platelets
C Administer cryoprecipitate
D Administer tranexamic acid
E Administer Vit-K

A is the correct answer.

Commentary – TEG

Clinical Pearls: Thromboelastrography (TEG)

1. Thromboelastrography is a method of assessing efficiency of blood clot formation. It measures rate of clot formation, firmness, and stability of clot and eventually lysis and breakdown.
2. Interpretation of TEG can provide insight into potential deficiencies in the formation of and dissolution of blood clot.
3. As opposed to static measurements (PT, PTT, etc.) TEG allows for a real-time, in vivo assessment of clot capacity.

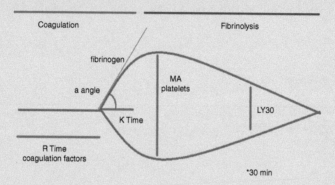

Phase	What it signifies	What influences it	Normal	Treatment
Reaction time	Time it takes for initiation of clot	Coagulation factors	5–10 min	R time >10 min: FFP
Kinetic time	Time it takes clot to reach a certain strength (20 mm)	Fibrinogen	1–3 min	K time >3 min: cryoprecipitate
Alpha angle	Speed of fibrin accumulation	Fibrinogen	53–72 mm	Alpha angle <53: Cryoprecipitate
Maximum amplitude	Highest vertical amplitude measured by TEG	Platelets	50–70 mm	MA <50: platelets
LY30	"% of clot dissolved at 30 min"	Plasmin	0–3%	LY30 >3% tranexamic acid

Notes

A labeled diagram of a TEG tracing is provided and a table on interpretation and how to treat the most commonly encountered abnormalities.

Reference

Thromboelastrography (TEG). PMID: 28804853.

Question 57

A 59-year-old female with PBC cirrhosis complicated by hepatocellular carcinoma undergoes an uneventful deceased liver transplant. The patient received an allograft from a 48-year-old donor who died in motor vehicle accident. Viral serologies from the donor are negative. The patient was discharged on combination tacrolimus, mycophenolate, and low-dose steroids. The patient returns to clinic on postoperative day 26 with 2 days of fever, diarrhea, and rash. Temperature is 38.4. There is an erythematous, macular papular rash with tenderness and blanching on the patient's neck and upper chest. Abdominal exam is benign. FK level is 11 ng/mL. WBC is 2.74, Hb 9.8, Platelets 78K; LFTs and Cr are normal. Chest X-ray is negative. Blood, stool, and urine culture are negative. CMV and EBV PCR are negative.

The patient is treated for cellulitis but returns 1 week later with progressively worsening rash and persistent fevers and diarrhea. The patient is admitted to the hospital. A skin biopsy reveals: vacuolar interface alteration of the dermal–epidermal junction with overlying lymphocytic infiltration and apoptotic keratinocytes.

Which of the following statements about this disease is FALSE?

A It is seen more commonly in stem cell transplant patients.
B It typically occurs within the first 100 days of transplant.
C First-line treatment is steroids.
D The presence of a large number of donor-derived T-lymphocytes in the patient's blood is strongly supportive of the diagnosis.
E Allograft rejection is the most common cause of death.

E is the correct answer.

Commentary – GVHD

Clinical Pearls: Graft Versus Host Disease (GVHD) Following Liver Transplantation

1. GVHD is frequently seen after hematopoietic stem cell transplantation but is very rare after liver transplantation, seen in only 1–2% of cases.
2. It has a very high mortality approaching 85% in patients with severe leukopenia. Sepsis is the number one cause of death.
3. GVHD occurs when lymphocytes from the donor liver are able to mount an immune response against the tissues of the host.
4. The presentation is usually within the first four months of transplant. The most common presenting symptoms are fever, rash, diarrhea, and leukopenia. Rash, diarrhea, and BM failure with a normal liver? think GVH.
5. Risk factors for GVHD include: HLA A/B mismatch, recipient age >65, delta of 40 years between recipient and donor, donor, and recipient gender disparity.
6. There are currently no widely accepted clinical or lab diagnostic tests for GVHD. Skin biopsy can help with diagnosis. Short tandem repeat (STR) loci is a method that can be used to quantitate the donor's contribution to any of the nucleated cell populations in the blood; STR level >20% is highly supportive of diagnosis of GVHD.
7. Corticosteroids are the mainstay of therapy. In patients with severe pancytopenia related to GVHD, broad spectrum antibiotics, antiviral, and antifungal prophylaxis should be administered.

Reference

Graft-versus-host disease after liver transplantation. PMID: 32226622.

Question 58

Patient A is 72-year-old male undergoing evaluation for liver transplant. He has a history of end-stage liver disease secondary to autoimmune hepatitis. Despite normal LFTs, he has developed decompensation in the last 8 months with the development of ascites requiring large volume paracentesis monthly, encephalopathy, and nonbleeding varices. Imaging shows no evidence of HCC. He is a Child Pugh Class C with a MELD-Na of 31. His BMI is 21 kg/m^2. As part of his evaluation, he undergoes a stress test which is negative. His estimated pulmonary artery systolic pressure (PASP) is 34 mmHg. His liver frailty index (LFI) is 5.02; his skeletal muscle index (SMI) is 37 cm^2/m^2.

   Patient B is a 49-year-old male with HCC secondary to hemochromatosis who is also undergoing evaluation for liver transplant. He is a Child Pugh Class A with a native MELD score of 8. His HCC on MRI measures 2.8 cm. His AFP is 109. He has no vascular invasion or evidence of metastases. BMI is 33 kg/m^2. Stress testing is negative. His estimated PASP is 29 mmHg. His LFI is 3; his SMI is 55 cm^2/m^2.

▶ Question

Which of the following scores has been demonstrated to incur a higher liver transplant waitlist mortality for patient A compared to B?

A MELD score
B Liver frailty index
C Skeletal muscle index
D A and B
E A, B, and C

E is the correct answer.

Commentary – Sarcopenia

Clinical Pearls: Sarcopenia

1. Sarcopenia is defined as the disproportionate loss of muscle mass leading to negative effects on physical performance and clinical outcomes.
2. The prevalence of sarcopenia in cirrhosis ranges from 40% to 70%. Sarcopenia can affect even those that are obese (up to 20–40% of cirrhotic patients listed for LT are obese).
3. Sarcopenia is a powerful predictor of poor quality of life, hepatic decompensation, mortality on the waitlist, longer hospital and ICU stay, higher incidence of infection, higher health care cost, and post-LT mortality.
4. Several quantitative tools are used to evaluate sarcopenia in cirrhosis. The most widely accepted are DEXA scan and muscle area quantification (at the level of the third lumbar vertebra) using abdominal CT scan (skeletal muscle index cut off $<50\,cm^2/m^2$ in men and $<39\,cm^2/m^2$ in women).
5. Sarcopenia should not be a sole criterion on which to determine candidacy for liver transplant.

Reference

A North American expert opinion statement on sarcopenia in liver transplantation. PMID: 31220351.

Question 59

A 39-year-old African American male is referred to your clinic for chronic elevation in liver function tests.

The patient works as a delivery driver. He does smoke but denies alcohol or illicit drugs. He has been experiencing increasing fatigue, an intermittent cough, and occasional itching.

TBili 0.8, AST 29, ALT 39, ALP 319, GTP 444.

Anti-HAV total negative, HBsAg negative, anti-HBc total positive, anti-HBs negative, anti-HCV negative.

EBV IgG and CMV IgG positive; IgM negative.

ANA 1 : 80, IgG 1200; ANCA negative; AMA negative.

A1-AT 216; Ceruloplasmin 39.

An ultrasound shows a slight increase in hepatic echotexture; gallbladder appears normal, and the common bile duct is measured at 4 mm without intrahepatic duct dilation. Hepatic and portal veins are patent with normal flow.

A random ultrasound guided; percutaneous liver biopsy is performed the results are shown below

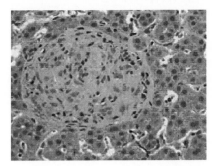

▶ Question

The most likely diagnosis is following:

A Sarcoidosis
B Tuberculosis
C Primary biliary cholangitis
D Primary sclerosing cholangitis
E Amyloidosis

A is the correct answer.

Commentary – Hepatic Granulomas

Clinical Pearls: Hepatic Granulomas

1. Granulomas are localized collections of inflammatory cells and are characterized by a central accumulation of macrophages with a surrounding rim of lymphocytes and fibroblasts.
2. They are found in 2–10% of patients who undergo liver biopsy.
3. The most common cause of hepatic granuloma in the United States is PBC.
4. In many cases, a cause will not be found.
5. Other causes include the following:
   a. Sarcoid
   b. Drug-induced (nitrofurantoin, allopurinol, phenytoin)
   c. Infection
      i. **Bacterial:** TB, brucellosis, listeriosis, mycobacterium avium, bacillus, rickettsia, Coxiella, Yersinia.
      ii. **Viral:** CMV, EBV, HAV, HBV, HCV
      iii. **Fungal:** histoplasmosis, coccidiomycosis, and cryptococcus
      iv. **Parasitic:** schistosomiasis, toxoplasmosis
   d. Crohn's disease
   e. Neoplastic disease and infections
6. Noncaseating epithelioid granuloma: sarcoid
7. Noncaseating granuloma near portal triad: PBC

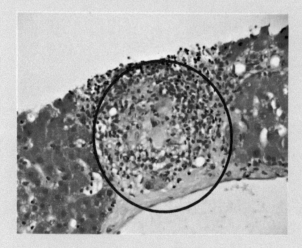

8. Caseating granuloma: TB

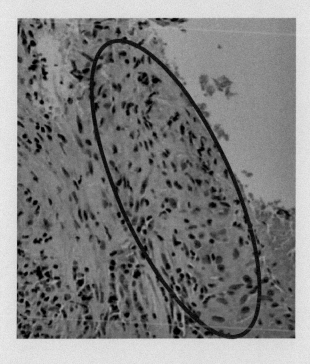

Notes

Hepatic granulomas are a favorite board question. Usually, the answer can be gleaned from the stem, but you should know that noncaseating granuloma are seen in both sarcoid and PBC. The granuloma in sarcoid are usually tighter and well formed. Granulomas in tuberculosis are caseating; areas of necrosis which cause the tissue to have a cheese-like appearance. *Need a way to remember? Tom Brady (**TB**) plays quarterback for Tampa Bay (**TB**) and his smile is **cheesy** (I'm a Steelers fan...what can I say?).*

Reference

Granulomas of the liver. PMID: 31041038.

Question 60

A 28-year-old female presents to the emergency room with nausea, vomiting, and abdominal discomfort. She noted dark urine 3 days prior to admission. She took some antibiotics in her mother's medicine cabinet, suspecting a urinary infection. Initially, the patient denied alcohol and illicit drugs, but eventually admits using intravenous drugs for the first time 5 weeks ago. The patient reports being clean now for 2 weeks. She has professional tattoos and has never received blood transfusions. She has two young children and was sharing drugs with the father of one of her children.

On exam appears well other than + icterus and jaundice. Temp 98.6, Pulse 88, Systolic BP 120; Abdomen is mildly tender in RUQ, negative Murphy's sign; there are no stigmata of chronic liver disease.

Normal WBC and BMP; Albumin 3.8
TBili 8.8, AST 785, ALT 814, ALP 203; INR 1.
Anti-HAV IgM negative, HBsAg negative, anti-HCV negative, HCV RNA pending; anti-HEV IgG positive, IgM negative.
ANA negative, IgG 1400, smooth muscle antibody negative.
An US shows gallbladder wall thickening but no ductal dilation.

The most likely diagnosis is the following:

A Acute severe alcoholic hepatitis
B HIV
C Cholangitis
D Acute HCV
E Acute HEV

D is the correct answer.

Commentary – Acute HCV

Clinical Pearls: Acute HCV

1. Acute HCV is defined as the first six months of infection.
2. The acute illness of HCV is typically mild and goes unrecognized.
3. Acute HCV will almost never present with liver failure and will not present as acute liver failure (ALF) on the boards.
4. For the boards acute HCV will present with a straightforward discrete, known, or suspected exposure: IVDU, needlestick exposure to HCV Infected blood, non-sterile tattoo, sexual contact – namely MSM.
5. Up to 25% of patients with HCV will spontaneously clear the infection within the first six months of acquisition of the virus; only 10% of patient's will spontaneously clear after six months.
6. Factors associated with spontaneous clearance include development of jaundice, elevated ALT, female sex, younger age and IL28B CC genotype.
7. HCV Ab can be negative for up to 6 weeks (as in the case presented here) and so if the clinical suspicion for acute HCV is high a PCR should be checked.
8. The HCV guidance panel recommends initiating direct acting anti-viral (DAA) therapy upon initial diagnosis of acute HCV (as opposed to awaiting possible spontaneous clearance), the rational mainly being to decrease the risk of transmission in high-risk populations. There is some emerging data on abbreviated DAA courses in patients with acute HCV.

Notes

For the boards, acute HCV will present with an identifiable risk factor in the stem. It will present as acute severe hepatitis with transaminases just under 1000 and a high TBili (but usually not above 10). It will not present with acute liver failure (ALF). Remember anti-HCV can take a few weeks to turn positive.

Reference

Acute hepatitis C: a systematic review. PMID: 18477352.

Question 61

Which of the following assessments is not factored into the liver frailty index (LFI)?

A Grip strength
B Skeletal muscle index
C Timed chair stands
D Balance
E Skin fold caliper measurements

E is the correct answer.

Commentary – Frailty

Clinical Pearls: Frailty and Liver Transplantation

1. Frailty is most often defined as a biological syndrome of physiological decline. Frailty is common in patients with cirrhosis (independent of age) and is a powerful predictor of mortality.
2. In patients with chronic liver failure, frailty represents the end manifestation of chronic undernutrition, muscle wasting (sarcopenia), and functional impairment. While sarcopenia is a central and dominant component of frailty in patients with cirrhosis, frailty is more multifaceted.
3. The prevalence of frailty in cirrhosis ranges from 18% to 43%.
4. The Liver Frailty Index (LFI) consists of three performance-based tests: (i) grip strength, (ii) timed chair stands, and (iii) balance. The LFI stratifies patients into robust, prefail, and frail.
5. An LFI ≥ 4.4 is considered as frail.
6. Frailty in decompensated liver disease has been associated with increased risk of falls, hospitalizations, removal from transplant waitlist, post-LT complications, and waitlist mortality.

Notes

Not surprisingly, measurements of frailty and sarcopenia have huge implications on outcomes in patients with chronic liver disease. Most transplant centers are incorporating some combination of these scores into their transplant evaluations.

Reference

Frailty in liver transplantation: an expert opinion statement from the American Society of Transplantation Liver and Intestinal Community of Practice. PMID: 30980701.

Question 62

A 73-year-old female with diabetes and NASH cirrhosis has been hospitalized four times in the last 6 months for recurrent encephalopathy. She lives alone. She reports good compliance to lactulose and rifaximin. No obvious precipitants for the bouts of encephalopathy have been identified. Cross sectional imaging shows no portal vein thrombosis or HCC. Her Na-MELD is 19. She is not interested in liver transplant. She is accompanied by her 37-year-old son who works full time. He tries to visit her daily but admits to having a difficult time caring for her. Reviewing her discharge papers, recommendations are to "limit protein intake." On exam the patient has muscle wasting. Her BMI is 31 kg/m^2; it was 34 kg/m^2 1 year ago. She is oriented × 2. She has no asterixis. She has small ascites, splenomegaly, and mild lower extremity edema. You notice a 2 × 2 cm open wound on her left leg. She admits to falling 2 days ago. The patient is reluctant to have any discussion about moving out of her house.

All of the following should be recommended EXCEPT:

A Palliative consult
B Continue protein restriction to 0.8 g/kg
C 10–15 g evening protein snack
D Physical therapy
E Screening for micronutrient deficiencies

B is the correct answer.

Commentary – Malnutrition and Liver Disease

Clinical Pearls: Malnutrition and Liver Disease

1. Malnutrition is defined as an altered body composition affecting quality of life. Its prevalence in cirrhosis has been reported as high as 75%:
   a. Malnutrition is associated with more frequent hospitalizations, longer hospital stays, delayed wound healing, higher prevalence of portal hypertension, and increased postoperative morbidity and mortality.
   b. Liver disease increases basal metabolic demands, causes inadequate caloric intake and systemic malabsorption. Consequently, muscle and adipose tissue are preferentially broken down. Ultimately, this results in muscle and fat wasting, sarcopenia, and frailty.
   c. The Royal Free Hospital-Nutritional Prioritizing Tool is liver-specific and includes variables of alcoholic hepatitis, fluid overload, and impact on dietary intake, BMI, unplanned weight loss, and reduced dietary intake.
   d. For nonobese individuals (BMI <30) optimal energy intake is 35 kcal/kg.
   e. Protein restriction is not necessary in patients with PSE; guidelines recommend 1.2–1.5 g/kg of protein daily.
   f. Emerging data on the benefits of an added evening/bedtime snack consisting of 10–15 g of protein.
   g. Patients with advanced liver disease are also at risk of micronutrient deficiencies: Zn, Mg; fat-soluble vitamins (especially in patients with cholestatic liver disease): Vitamins D, A, K, and E.

Reference

A practical approach to nutritional screening and assessment in cirrhosis. PMID: 28027577.

Question 63

Which of the following regarding liver transplant operative techniques is true?

A Mean intraoperative time would be expected to be higher in "traditional" caval resection versus piggyback technique.
B In conventional or classic liver transplant the donor IVC is completely resected.
C In piggyback liver transplant, the recipient IVC is left intact.
D Piggyback technique has been associated with reduced blood loss and improved kidney function.
E All of the above.

E is the correct answer.

Commentary – Operative Techniques

Clinical Pearls: Piggyback Versus Cava Resection

1. In "conventional" or "classic" liver transplant: the donor retrohepatic inferior cava is completely resected and reinserted into the recipient (i.e. recipients retrohepatic IVC is removed in addition to hepatectomy). See image.
2. Preservation of the recipients IVC with a side-to-side anastomosis is referred to as the piggyback technique. See image.
3. Piggyback technique allows maintenance of blood flow of the IVC. Piggyback technique (especially with elimination of venovenous bypass) may lead to:
   a. cardiovascular stability
   b. improved kidney function
   c. reduced blood loss
   d. reduced OR time (shorter warm ischemic time)
   e. shorter ICU stays

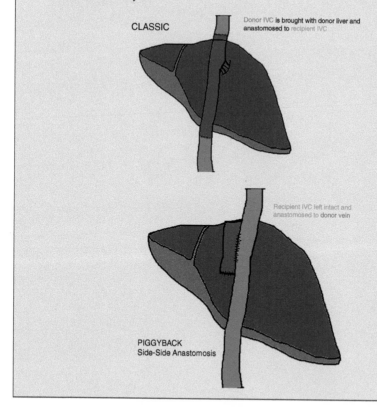

CLASSIC

Donor IVC is brought with donor liver and anastomosed to recipient IVC

Recipient IVC left intact and anastomosed to donor vein

PIGGYBACK
Side-Side Anastomosis

Reference

Comparison of surgical methods in liver transplantation: retrohepatic caval resection with venovenous bypass (VVB) versus piggyback (PB) with VVB versus PB without VVB. PMID: 20723178.

Question 64

Warm Ischemic Time is defined as follows:

A The time the organ is placed in preservation fluid to the time it is removed.
B The time from withdrawal of life support to initiation of cold organ preservation.
C Time from blood pressure of 80 or oxygen sat of less than 80 in the donor until after withdrawal of support.
D The time from removal from cold storage to establishment of reperfusion of liver graft.
E The time the donor organ is not at "body" temperature (98.6; 38 °C).

D is the correct answer.

Commentary – Ischemic Times

Clinical Pearls: Ischemic Times

1. Graft Cold ischemic time (CIT) is defined as the time from initiation of donor in vivo cold organ preservation to removal of the graft from 4 °C cold storage.
2. Donor Warm Ischemic Time (DWIT) is the time from withdrawal of life support (donor extubation) to initiation of cold organ preservation.
3. Donor Agonal time (DAT) also known as functional Donor Warm Ischemic Time is defined as the time starting at a specific donor blood pressure (usually 80 mmHg) or oxygen saturation (usually SaO_2 less than 80%) after withdrawal of support and ending in the in situ aortic cold perfusion.
4. Graft warm ischemic time (WIT): It is the time from removal from cold storage to establishment of reperfusion of the liver graft:
   a. In the event of brain-dead organ recovery (DBD), WIT is generally quite minimal because the time that the heart stops is essentially the same time the organs are cooled.
   b. For a donation after circulatory death (DCD; previously referred to as donation after cardiac death or non-heart beating organ donation), WIT includes the amount of time that the organ is not being properly perfused prior to death, the five-minute waiting period following death, and the time it takes for cannulation to occur and to get the flushes and icing started.
5. There are multiple factors that need to be taken into consideration, but optimum CIT is <6 hours (especially in extended criteria donors) and WIT <30 minutes.
6. Prolonged CIT is an independent risk factor for delayed graft function and primary nonfunction, likely by contributing to ischemia-reperfusion injury.
7. Limiting CIT, especially for extended criteria donors (elderly or steatotic) is essential as these organs are more susceptible to injury.

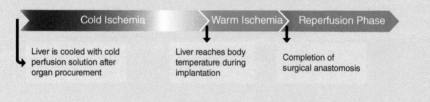

Cold Ischemia	Warm Ischemia	Reperfusion Phase
Liver is cooled with cold perfusion solution after organ procurement	Liver reaches body temperature during implantation	Completion of surgical anastomosis

Reference

Clinical implications of donor warm and cold ischemia time in donor after circulatory death liver transplantation. PMID: 30912253.

Question 65

A 29-year-old male with primary sclerosing cholangitis complicated by multiple bouts of recurrent cholangitis and worsening jaundice is called in for a potential transplant. The donor is a 63-year-old African American female with a long history of diabetes who was admitted 24 hours ago with a massive stroke. The patient is deemed to have irreversible brain damage. She is currently on mechanical ventilation in the Neuro ICU. The patient had previously declared herself an organ donor. The ICU team and family have agreed to withdraw care and remove her from ventilatory support and donate when her heart stops beating.

The most consistent complication leading to graft loss from such a donor would be

A Small for size syndrome
B Portal vein thrombosis
C Fibrosing cholestatic hepatitis
D Ischemic cholangiopathy
E De novo nonalcoholic steatohepatitis

D is the correct answer.

Commentary – Deceased Donors

> ### Clinical Pearls: Donation after Cardiac Death Versus Donation after Brain Death
>
> 1. Donation after brain/brainstem death (DBD) is from a patient whose death has been confirmed using neurological criteria. Brain injury in these cases has caused irreversible loss of the capacity of consciousness and irreversible loss of the capacity for respiration before terminal apnea has resulted in hypoxic cardiac arrest. This diagnosis is only possible in patients who are on mechanical ventilation.
> 2. Donation after circulatory death or donation after cardiac death (DCD, sometimes referred to as nonheart-beating) is a donor who has suffered an irreversible neurological injury and or irreversible brain damage but still has minimal brain function. They are unable to breathe without the aid of a ventilator. In controlled DCD, once the patient is removed from ventilatory support, the heart must cease beating within 60 minutes. If the patient's heart does not stop beating within 60 minutes, the donation is no longer an option, and the organs are not recovered.
> 3. Potential DCD patients can be classified according to the modified Maastricht classification:
>   I: dead on arrival: uncontrolled
>   II: unsuccessful resuscitation: uncontrolled
>   III: awaiting cardiac arrest: controlled
>   IV: cardiac arrest in brain stem donor: controlled
>   V: unexpected cardiac arrest in critically ill patient: uncontrolled
> 4. The main difference between DCD and DBD is the duration of WIT. DCD will by definition incur some degree of warm ischemia as there will be an interval after asystole, where organs are not being perfused and have not yet been cooled.
> 5. Numerous studies show worse outcomes with DCD donors compared to donors after brain death (DBD).
> 6. The most consistent complication leading to graft loss in DCD transplantation is ischemic cholangiopathy.
> 7. Expanded criteria donors (ECDs) is typically referring to a donor with:
>   a. Advanced age (>65)
>   b. Macrovesicular steatosis (>30–40%)
>   c. DCD
>   d. Organ dysfunction at time of procurement (ICU stay >7 days, serum Na >165, TBili >3, elevated LFTs, Vasopressor use)
>   e. Anoxic brain injury or CVA
>   f. Anti-HBc positive, HBsAg positive, HCV, HIV
>   g. Extrahepatic malignancy
>   h. CIT >12 hours

Reference

Extended criteria donors in liver transplantation. PMID: 28364814.

Question 66

A 49-year-old male with end-stage liver disease secondary to alcohol and hepatitis C, (genotype 4; treatment naïve) undergoes liver transplantation. His disease was complicated by PSE and bleeding varices. His pre–LT MELD-Na was 29. He receives a 33-year-old DCD graft. CIT is 8 hours, WIT 27 minutes.

The patient does well postoperatively. He is discharged on tacrolimus, mycophenolate, and low-dose prednisone.

The patient contacts his transplant coordinator 12 weeks posttransplant complaining of dark urine and increasing abdominal distension.

The patient is seen in the emergency room. He is ill appearing, but afebrile and vital signs are stable. He has marked scleral icterus and moderate ascites, his mentation is slow, but he has no asterixis. Liver is enlarged, but there is no audible hepatic bruit. There is no elevation in jugular venous pressure (JVP). Cardiac exam is normal. He has 1+ bilateral edema.

WBC 12.2, Hb 10.9, Platelets 108
Na 135, K 4.4; BUN 22, CR 1.6
TBili 11.7, AST 118, ALT 215, ALP 719, and gGTP 981
INR 1.4
HCV PCR: 63,000,000 IU/mL; HBsAg negative, anti-HBc negative, anti-HBs negative; anti-HAV IgM negative; anti-HEV IgM negative.
FK level 14.2; Urine metabolites for alcohol: negative.
An ultrasound reveals moderate ascites, but patent vessels and, otherwise, normal appearing allograft. Noncontrast MRCP shows no intra- or extrahepatic duct dilation.
Cultures are negative.
A transjugular liver biopsy is performed. Wedge pressure is 16 mmHg, free hepatic pressure is 4 mmHg.

▶ Question

The biopsy findings are most likely to reveal?

A Reticulin stain highlighting nodules but no significant fibrosis.
B Lymphoid inflammation of the portal tracts with ground glass cells on H&E.
C Sinusoidal dilation, congestion, edema, and hemorrhage.
D Ballooning of hepatocytes, minimal to no inflammation, cholangiocellular proliferation without bile duct loss.
E Severe macrovesicular steatosis (involving >80% of hepatic parenchyma) with ballooned hepatocytes surround by neutrophil rich inflammatory infiltrate with megmitochondria, Mallory's hyaline, and canalicular bile plugs.

D is the correct answer.

Commentary – FCH

Clinical Pearls: Fibrosing Cholestatic Hepatitis (FCH)

1. Fibrosing cholestatic hepatitis can be a fatal form of HBV or HCV in patients receiving immunosuppressive treatment.
2. The term was coined in 1991 to describe a subset of HBV patients post-LT. For the boards, it will almost certainly pertain to HCV postsolid organ transplant.
3. About ~10% of patients transplanted with active HCV will develop FCH posttransplant. Risk factors for the development of FCH (other than it occurs in the setting of an immunocompromised state) are not well established.
4. Clinically, it presents more than one month post-LT with marked jaundice (TBili >6 mg/dL), predominantly cholestatic liver injury pattern (ALP and GGT >5× ULN) and very high titers of viremia (sometimes in the 100 of millions) in the absence of surgical biliary complications or HAT.
5. Pathologically, FCH manifests as marked hepatocyte swelling, cholestasis, and periportal fibrosis with only mild inflammation.
6. If left untreated, the disease can progress to rapid liver failure and graft loss.
7. There are several case series and reports on the efficacy and safety of DAA therapy in patients with FCH post liver transplant.

Notes

FCH is a disease entity seen much more frequently in the interferon era. With the safety and efficacy of DAA regimens, we can now offer even patients with advanced disease therapy pre-LT. As most transplant centers are offering HCV organs (even to non-HCV recipients), being aware of this diagnosis remains important. Some of the highest HCV viral loads you will see are in FCH patients.

Reference

Fibrosing cholestatic hepatitis C in post-transplant adult recipients of liver transplantation. PMID: 277085109.

Question 67

Review the following five patients. Which one would carry the highest "donor risk index"?

Patient	Donor age	Donor Cause of death	DCD	Donor height (cm)
A	62	CVA	Yes	134
B	28	Trauma	No	170
C	49	CVA	Yes	155
D	53	Trauma	No	172
E	36	CVA	N0	166

A is the correct answer.

Commentary – DRI

Clinical Pearls: Donor Risk Index (DRI)

1. The donor risk index identifies seven donor and graft characteristics (all of which are known at the time of organ offer) that are significantly and independently associated with increased failure of deceased liver transplant.
2. The seven characteristics (listed in order of significance with corresponding relative risk):
   a. Age (especially >60): RR: 1.53-1.65
   b. Partial/Split graft: RR: 1.52
   c. DCD:RR: 1.51
   d. Cause of death (namely CVA or anoxia): RR: 1.16
   e. COD (*other than trauma, CVA or anoxia*): RR: 1.20
   f. African American Race: RR: 1.19
   g. Donor height (per 10 cm decrease): RR: 1.07

Reference

Characteristics associated with liver graft failure: the concept of a donor risk index.
PMID: 16539636.

Question 68

Please read the following hypothetical scenario:

Postliver transplant patients are at an increased risk of skin cancer. Patients educated on skin cancer prevention (sunscreen, protective clothing, yearly dermatology evaluations) are less likely to develop skin cancer.

A total of 1000 posttransplant patients receive a series of classes on skin cancer prevention.

A total of 1000 posttransplant patients receive no classes on skin cancer prevention.

Among those attending skin cancer education classes, 50 get skin cancer.

Among those who are not exposed to education, 200 get skin cancer.

What is the relative risk reduction of patients who receive skin cancer education?

A 25% relative risk reduction
B 50% relative risk reduction
C 75% relative risk reduction
D 100% relative risk reduction
E 175% relative risk reduction

C is the correct answer.

Commentary – Relative Risk

Clinical Pearls: Relative Risk

1. Explanation: of the 1000 patients taking the class on skin cancer prevention, 50 get skin cancer. The risk of a patient getting skin cancer who takes the class is 50/1000 or 0.05.
2. The risk of a patient getting skin cancer who does not take the class is 200/1000 or 0.2.
3. The risk ratio (or relative risk) is calculated by dividing the risk of the event (skin cancer) among those exposed to the intervention (class) by the risk of the event (skin cancer) among those not exposed (class):

   $$0.05/0.2 = 0.25$$

4. A relative risk of 1 would mean the risk is no different between the two groups.
5. A relative risk of less than 1 means patient's receiving the intervention have a lower risk.
6. A relative risk above 1 means patient's receiving the intervention have a higher risk.
7. The relative risk reduction is calculated is 1-risk ratio or in this case 1–0.25 which $= 0.75$.
8. Ie: patient's taking the class have a 75% risk reduction in skin cancer.
   Using 2×2 table:

	Disease (skin Ca)	No disease (no skin Ca)
Exposed (class)	**a** 50	**b** 950
Unexposed (no class)	**c** 200	**d** 800

   Relative risk = incidence in exposed/incidence in unexposed
   $$= a/(a+b) \, / \, c/(c+d) = (50/1000) \, / (200/1000) = 0.05/0.2 = \mathbf{0.25}$$

9. Relative risk below 1 indicates that the exposure is protective against the outcome.
10. Relative risk reduction is 1-RR or 1–0.25 which equals 0.75.

Question 69

Please review this hypothetical scenario.

Patients with Hepatitis B are at risk of developing HCC. Patients with HBV exposed to a newly discovered mushroom are at a higher risk of developing HCC.

There are 20 patients with HBV. Of the seven that have been exposed to the mushroom, four develop HCC. Of the 13 that have not been exposed to the mushroom, 4 develop HCC. See filled in 2 × 2 table:

	Disease (HCC)	No disease (no HCC)
Exposed (mushroom)	a 4	b 3
Unexposed (no mushroom)	c 4	d 9

What is the increased risk of HCC in HBV patients exposed to the mushroom?

A 16%
B 84%
C 26%
D RR = 1, no increased risk
E 116%

B is the correct answer.

$$\text{Relative risk} = 4/(4+7)/4\,(4+9) = 0.57/0.31 = 1.84$$

Exposure to mushroom increases risk of HCC by 84%.

Reference

Clinicians' guide to statistics for medical practice and research: part I. PMC3121570.

Question 70

A randomized placebo-controlled trial is performed to determine the effect of a new drug on prevention of variceal bleeding in cirrhotic patients with "large" varices.

From the 400 patients in the placebo arm, 100 suffer a variceal bleed.
From 400 patients receiving the study drug, only 50 end up developing the variceal bleed.

What is the number needed to treat?

A 8
B 18
C 28
D 4
E 20

A is the correct answer.

Commentary – NNT

Clinical Pearls: Number Needed to Treat (NNT)

1. The number needed to treat is the number of patients you need to give therapy to for the duration of the study in order to prevent one bad outcome:
   a. Conversely, the Number Needed to Harm is the number of patients who, if they received the intervention in question, would lead to one person being harmed.
2. NNT = 1/Absolute Risk Reduction (ARR).
3. Absolute Risk Reduction = the absolute value of control event rate – experimental even rate:
   a. **In this particular example** the *control event rate* is the number of patients suffering a variceal bleed in the control arm: 100/400 = 25%.
   b. The *experimental event rate* is the number of patients suffering a variceal bleed in the "drug" arm: 50/400 = 12.5%
   c. ARR = 25%–12.5% = 12.5%
   d. 1/12.5% = 1/0.125 = 8

Notes

I've never been great with statistics, but they are of critical importance when critiquing and interpreting medical literature. We included some of the more commonly tested points. Know some of the basics and you can pick up some easy points on your exam.

Reference

Clinicians' guide to statistics for medical practice and research: part I. PMID: 21765796.

Question 71

A 44-year-old male with cryptogenic cirrhosis complicated by ascites and variceal hemorrhage is referred to your center for liver transplant evaluation. The patient's medical history is notable for long-standing pancytopenia and osteoporosis with fractures. A bone marrow biopsy performed one-year prior reveals tri-lineage hematopoiesis with no evidence of myelofibrosis.

Viral serologies are negative.
Ceruloplasmin 22 with 24-hour urine copper less than 50.
ANA, smooth muscle, and IgG are all within normal limits. Alpha-1 AT level is 216. He does not drink alcohol. His father died of "liver" disease at the age of 41 years that was attributed to alcohol.
On exam, he has mild scleral icterus, spider angiomata, small ascites, lower extremity edema, and gray hair. The patient has a lacy reticular hyperpigmentation involving his upper chest and neck. MELD score is 22.
During evaluation the patient undergoes pulmonary function tests revealing a reduced diffusing capacity and imaging revealing ground glass opacities with fibrotic interstitial lung disease.

The patient is referred to the lung transplant team for "clearance". Which of the following tests would clinch the diagnosis?

A Phenotyping for alpha one
B Lung biopsy
C Transjugular liver biopsy
D Telomere length analysis
E MRCP

D is the correct answer.

Commentary – TERT

Clinical Pearls: Telomerase Reverse Transcriptase (TERT) and Liver Disease

1. Telomeres are specialized structures that form at the ends of human chromosomes. The main function of telomeres is to maintain chromosomal stability and integrity.
2. Telomeres shorten as a consequence of cell division. This limits the proliferative life span of cells (including hepatocytes). Studies have demonstrated that telomere shortening is a general marker of liver fibrosis and cirrhosis.
3. Mutations in telomerase can cause accelerated telomere shortening and are responsible for some rare genetic diseases including forms of dyskeratosis congenita which is considered the prototypic short telomere syndrome. It is a bone marrow failure syndrome with a classic triad of skin pigmentation, nail dystrophy and oral leukoplakia.
4. Other clinical clues include premature graying and hair loss, osteopenia, developmental delay, short stature, and esophageal stricture.
5. Cancers, especially head and neck, stomach/esophageal, skin; less often, HCC.
6. Liver disease has been reported in ~7% of cases. Cirrhosis usually presenting in 4th or 5th decade.
7. 10% of cases of familial idiopathic lung disease are associated with telomerase mutations, in most cases, mutations are found in the telomerase reverse transcriptase (TERT).
8. Pulmonary fibrosis, bone marrow hypoplasia and premature aging? think telomere disorder.
9. The diagnostic testing consists of telomere length analysis and genetic testing for specific mutations. Average telomere length below the 1st percentile for age is considered indicative.

Notes

My pulmonary transplant colleagues send me a handful of these cases a year. Another under-recognized disease entity. We provide some helpful clinical clues that should raise the suspicion for TERT mutation.

Reference

Telomerase gene mutations are associated with cirrhosis formation. PMID: 21520174.

Question 72

A 24-year-old graduate student is referred to you by his inflammatory bowel disease specialist for abnormal liver function tests. The patient was diagnosed with Crohn's disease 4 years previously and has done well on weight-based azathioprine.

On review of systems the patient does complain of mild fatigue. He denies pruritus. There is no history of ascites or encephalopathy. The patient takes levothyroxine for hypothyroidism.

Laboratory studies:

TBili 1.6, AST 67, ALT 48, ALP 439
IgG 2100, IgM 211, IgA 304
ANCA positive
ANA, smooth muscle antibody negative
Viral studies negative
Ceruloplasmin 47, Alpha-1 AT 128
An MRI/MRCP shows a normal liver and biliary tree without any duct abnormalities. You recommend a liver biopsy which reveals: periductal fibrosis, periductal inflammation, portal edema, ductular proliferation, and cholestasis.
The most likely diagnosis is the following:

A IgG-sclerosing cholangitis
B Lymphoma
C Fibrosing cholestatic hepatitis
D Autoimmune cholangitis
E Small duct PSC

E is the correct answer.

Commentary – Small Duct PSC

Clinical Pearls: Small Duct Primary Sclerosing Cholangitis

1. Small duct PSC is defined as individuals with biochemical and histological features of PSC but with normal cholangiography. This variant is seen in less than 10% of patients with PSC.
2. Small duct PSC may represent an earlier stage of disease. Studies suggest that up to 25% of patients with small duct disease will progress to "classic" PSC over a 10-year time frame.
3. The incidence of IBD in small duct disease is similar.
4. Patients with small duct disease seem to have a less aggressive course and very good long-term survival.
5. Cholangiocarcinoma does not seem to occur in patients with small duct disease.

Reference

Small-duct primary sclerosing cholangitis: A long-term follow-up study. PMID: 12029635.

Question 73

With regards to quality of life (QOL) in patients with cirrhosis, which of the following statements is TRUE

A Patients with cirrhosis do better in generic (SF-36) questionnaire, but worse in disease-specific questionnaires (CLD-Q) compared to controls.

B The Chronic Liver Disease Questionnaire (CLD-Q) is a 29-question survey that asks for responses based on the last 2 weeks in domains including emotional function, fatigue, and abdominal symptoms.

C Treatment of complications of cirrhosis but not liver transplant can improve patient's HRQL.

D Portosystemic encephalopathy does not seem to affect QOL scores in patients with cirrhosis.

E The severity of liver disease (Childs and MELD) is associated with significant HRQL, but symptoms of cirrhosis, specifically muscle cramps, fatigue, and pruritus are not.

B is the correct answer.

Commentary – Quality of Life

Clinical Pearls: Quality of Life and Liver Disease

1. Health-related quality of life (HRQL) assesses the impact of a disease or a condition on an individual's well-being and is an important patient-reported outcome in those with liver disease. HRQL worsens with the severity of liver disease.
2. HRQL can be assessed using both:
   a. Disease specific instruments focus on a specific illness. The two most used in hepatology are: Chronic Liver Disease Questionnaire (CLD-Q) and the Liver Disease Quality of Life Questionnaire.
      i. The CLD-Q is a 29-question survey that evaluates seven different domains over the last 2 weeks including fatigue, activity, emotional function, abdominal symptoms, systemic symptoms, and worry.
   b. Generic instruments provide an assessment that can be compared across a variety of chronic diseases. These include Medical Outcomes Survey Short Form 36 which consists of 36 questions (SF-36), the sickness impact profile (SIP), and the Nottingham Health Profile.
3. Depression, especially in patients with HCV and alcohol liver disease, is higher than in the general population.
4. Numerous studies have shown that patients with hepatic encephalopathy have diminished HRQL.
5. Symptoms of cirrhosis, especially muscle cramps and pruritus are associated with HRQL impairment (some studies suggest even more so than ascites and PSE).
6. Interventions to improve the aforementioned complications (PSE, ascites, fatigue, depression, itching, and muscle cramps) also improve patient's HRQL.
7. Liver transplantation leads to substantial improvement in HRQL.

Reference

Health-related quality of life in liver cirrhosis patients using SF-36 and CLDQ questionnaires. PMID: 30603670.

Question 74

A 61-year-old Hispanic male with diabetes and biopsy proven NASH cirrhosis is admitted to the hospital with abdominal and lower extremity swelling. On review, he complains of dyspnea on exertion and a 15-pound weight gain. He has a history of non-bleeding esophageal varices and refractory ascites. Seven days prior to admission he underwent a large volume paracentesis for 6L. Physical exam is notable for mild scleral icterus, moderate-to-large ascites with caput and 2+ bilateral lower extremity edema. Cardiac and pulmonary exam are normal. The patient has grade I PSE but is oriented x 3. Outpatient medications include metformin, lactulose, rifaximin, and nadolol. He is not on diuretics.

Labs reveal: WBC 4, Hb 10, Platelets of 68K. Na 132, Cr 1.4. TBili 2.2, AST 29, ALT 33, ALP 121; INR 1.7. A large volume paracentesis for 4L is performed; there is no evidence of spontaneous bacterial peritonitis. His beta-blocker is discontinued. He undergoes an EGD and prophylactic banding of medium, high-risk varices. His creatinine is worsening in house, and he is started on treatment for hepatorenal syndrome with combination albumin, octreotide, and midodrine.

As part of an expedited inpatient transplant evaluation a dobutamine stress echocardiogram is ordered.

Results Are as Below

Dobutamine was infused in increasing doses up to a maximum of 50 mcg/kg/min. Atropine 0.5 mg total was given during the dobutamine infusion. Handgrip exercise was performed during the dobutamine infusion to augment the cardiac rate response.

Peak HR achieved was 160 beats/minute which was 92% of predicted heart rate. Baseline BP was 108/54. Blood pressure response to stress was hypertensive. Baseline EKG was NSR without ischemic changes during stress. There were rare PVCs during stress.

Baseline 2-D Echocardiography

LV size and function is normal with an estimated EF of 55%. The global LV longitudinal strain is −12%. RV size and function is normal. Left atrial volume index is 24 mL/m^2. Right atrial area is 14 cm^2.

Normal saline contrast injection without evidence of right to left intracardiac or intra-pulmonary shunt.

Spectral Doppler

There is mild MR and TR. The mitral inflow E velocity is 100 cm/sec. The mitral inflow A velocity is 63 cm/sec. The mitral annular E velocity is 11 cm/sec. The mitral inflow E/A ratio is 1.1. The mitral inflow E to annular E ratio is 9. The peak tricuspid regurgitant velocity is 2.5 m/sec with an assumed RALP of 3 mmHg, the estimate PASP is 34 mmHg.

Color Flow Doppler: mild MR, TR, and PR

Stress: LV global systolic function response to stress was normal.

Which of the following echo findings in this patient are consistent with a diagnosis of cirrhotic cardiomyopathy?

A EF 55%

B Left atrial ventricular index 24 mL/m^2

C PASP 34 mmHg

D Peak TVR 2.5 m/sec

E Global longitudinal strain −12%

E is the correct answer.

Commentary – Cirrhotic cardiomyopathy

Clinical Pearls: Cirrhotic Cardiomyopathy

1. The characteristic cardiovascular finding in end-stage liver disease is hyperdynamic function with low systemic vascular resistance and high cardiac output.
2. Although left ventricular ejection fraction remains an important measure of global systolic function additional surrogates are needed in patients with cirrhosis to assess cardiac contractility.
3. "Strain" categorized into circumferential, longitudinal, radial, and transverse can provide a more comprehensive assessment of contractive function.
4. Global longitudinal strain (GLS) expresses myocardial longitudinal shortening percentage (change in length during systole as a proportion to baseline length at diastole) and is typically described as a negative number.
5. Diminished LVEF (<50%) or diminished GLS (absolute number <18) in the absence of known cardiac disease should be considered diagnostic of CCM.
6. Assessment of LV diastolic function is part of the routine echocardiographic evaluation of LV function. Diastolic dysfunction (sometimes referred to as heart failure with preserved EF; HFPEF) occurs when the LV myocardium is noncompliant and not able to accept blood return in a normal fashion from the right atrium.
7. Diastolic dysfunction is grade I–IV. Grade II and higher is pathological.
8. The E-wave on Doppler echo represents the early, passive filling of the LV. The A-wave represents the active filling during atrial contraction. On Doppler analysis, the first peak in diastole is the E wave the second peak is the A wave.
   a. Normal diastolic function E/A >0.8
   b. Diastolic dysfunction E/A <1
      i. Mild <0.8
      ii. Moderate 0.8–2
      iii. Severe >2

Normal E to A ratio is illustrated here:

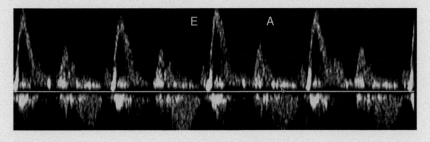

(Continued)

(Continued)	
Updated proposed criteria for cirrhotic cardiomyopathy:	
Systolic dysfunction (Any of the following)	**Advanced diastolic dysfunction** ≥3 of the following
LV EF ≤50%	Septal e′ velocity <7 cm/sec
Absolute GLS <18% or >22%	E/a′ ratio ≥15
	LAVI >34 mL/m²
	TR velocity >2.8 m/sec

Notes

I ran this question by my two older brothers who are both cardiologists. They approved of both the question-and-answer choice. Any complaints can be directed towards them.

Reference

Cirrhotic cardiomyopathy consortium. redefining cirrhotic cardiomyopathy for the modern era. PMID: 31342529.

Question 75

A 24-year-old white female is referred to your outpatient liver clinic for abnormal liver function tests. The patient says she has had abnormal LFTs since she was a child. Reviewing her medical records, she has had AST/ALT 1–1.5 times upper limit of normal for years. Her most recent tests: TBili 0.5 AST 53, ALT 58, ALP 108.

Viral serologies, testing for AIH, Ceruloplasmin, and A1AT are normal.
Her Hb is 9.8, and she is iron deficient. She has regular menses. An EGD 1 year previously done elsewhere was reportedly normal.
An US is normal with a kPa of less than 3.
A capsule endoscopy is performed to evaluate chronic abdominal bloating and anemia.

Images are shown below.

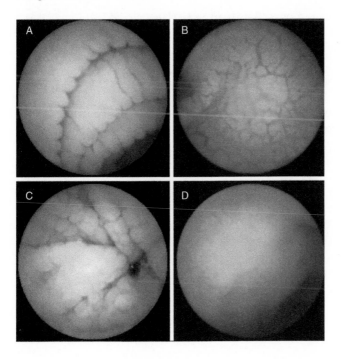

Which of the following would help establish the diagnosis of this disease?

A Liver biopsy
B Antineutrophil Cytoplasmic Antibody (ANCA)
C MRI/MRCP
D Abnormal D-xylose absorption test
E Tissue transglutaminase antibody IgA (tTG-IgA)

E is the correct answer.

Commentary – Celiac Disease

Clinical Pearls: Celiac Disease

1. Celiac is a chronic immune-mediated disease of the small bowel induced by an allergy to wheat, barley, and rye. This results in villous atrophy and crypt hyperplasia of the small intestine affecting absorption.
2. Classic endoscopic features include fold with visible fissures/scalloping with a granular and nodular appearance as well as absence of villi.
3. Abnormal LFTs have been reported in up to 50% of patients with celiac disease; conversely celiac is present in up to 9% of cases of chronic unexplained elevation in LFTs.
4. Enzyme elevation is usually modest (less than 5× ULN) usually AST/ALT.
5. Some studies suggest that celiac disease may be associated with increased risk from liver disease and should be excluded before a patient is labeled "cryptogenic."
6. LFTs will normalize when subjects adhere to a gluten free diet in up to 95% of patients after 1 year.
7. Liver biopsy findings are frequent, but are nonspecific and mild and not diagnostic.
8. The reported prevalence of celiac disease in patients with PBC is 0–11%, it has also been associated with AIH.
9. Tissue transglutaminase IgA Antibodies (TTG IgA) has near 95% sensitivity and specificity.

Notes

This question stem includes beautiful images of the classic "scalloping" that can be seen in celiac disease. Celiac, thyroid, and muscle injury are three "non-liver" diseases that can cause an elevation in liver enzymes.

Reference

The liver and celiac disease. PMID: 30947869.

Question 76

A 53-year-old male is admitted to the hospital with shaking fevers and chills. He is diagnosed with cholangitis. This is his fourth episode, despite prophylactic antibiotics. The patient has undergone two previous liver transplants, the last one was 7 years ago. He has a Roux-en-Y choledochojejunostomy. He has a medical history significant for diabetes, osteopenia, and CRI (1.4). His medications include 2.5 mg of prednisone and tacrolimus.

The patient's blood cultures are negative. He is treated with IV antibiotics and is feeling better.

The patient has no history of ascites or PSE. EGD reveals "small" esophageal varices.

Labs reveal. Sodium 138, Cr 1.6; TBili 2.3, AST 47, ALT 88, ALP 143, GGT 214. WBC 9, Hb 9.8, Platelets 135. INR 1.2. Albumin 3.3. FK 2.1

Blood cultures are negative. MRCP reveals recurrent PSC without evidence of dominant stricture.

The patient is now listed for a third liver transplant. He receives a liver from a 63-year-old deceased donor. CIT is 340 minutes.

▶ Question

According to the survival outcomes following liver transplantation (SOFT) score, which factor in this patient would incur the highest risk of mortality following liver transplant.

A MELD score
B PSC
C 63-year-old donor
D Third liver transplant
E Cold ischemic time

D is the correct answer.

Commentary – SOFT Score

Clinical Pearls: Survival Outcomes following Liver Transplantation (SOFT) score

1. The survival outcomes following liver transplantation (SOFT) score combines donor, recipient, and operative factors to accurately predict recipient posttransplant survival at 3 months.
2. Recipient and donor factors are allocated points. A total score of >36 predicts a high risk of posttransplant mortality. A score greater than 40 suggests "futility" with a 3-year survival of ~25%.
3. Recipient risk factors incurring the highest risk include (from highest to lowest):
   a. More than one previous transplant
   b. Life support pretransplant
   c. ICU pretransplant
   d. Portal bleed 48 hours pretransplant
   e. PVT
   f. Age >60
4. Factors lowering the SOFT score and providing a good prognosis postliver transplant include the following:
   a. CIT 0–60 minutes
   b. Donor aged 10–20 years

Reference

Survival outcomes following liver transplantation (SOFT) score: a novel method to predict patient survival following liver transplantation. PMID: 18945283.

Question 77

A 69-year-old male with HCC is called in for a liver transplant. The patient's current upgraded MELD score is 30. The potential donor graft is from a 49-year-old male who died in a motor vehicle accident.

The transplant surgeon calls you and is concerned that the donor liver appears fatty on gross examination. A liver biopsy is performed revealing a liver with 70% macrovesicular steatosis and 10% microvesicular steatosis.

▶ Question

Which of the following statements should you tell the surgeon?

A >60% macrovesicular steatosis is an absolute contraindication to transplant.

B Microvesicular steatosis should be differentiated from macrovesicular steatosis when determining graft outcomes.

C >70% macrovesicular steatosis is considered mild to moderate.

D The increased risk of short-term mortality in patient's receiving grafts with severe steatosis can be mitigated by limiting them to patients with BMI less than 25 kg/m².

E The sampling error with biopsy for fatty liver is too high to be reliable and should not be factored into the decision-making process.

B is the correct answer.

Commentary – Donor Steatosis

Clinical Pearls: Donor Steatosis

1. Hepatic steatosis is one of the more common findings in "extended-criteria donors" (ECD).
2. Steatosis is divided into micro and macrovesicular.
3. Microvesicular steatosis does not seem to affect graft or patient outcomes.
4. Macro is further subdivided into the following:
   a. Mild <30%
   b. Moderate 30–60%
   c. Severe >60%
5. Donor biopsy can be performed to aid in the decision to use the allograft.
6. The available literature is conflicting regarding outcomes using moderately steatotic livers and remains somewhat controversial. The use of severely steatotic livers, however, has been shown to increase the risk of delayed graft function and primary nonfunction.

Reference

Moderately macrosteatotic livers have acceptable long-term outcomes but higher risk of immediate mortality. PMID: 33931249.

Question 78

A 54-year-old alcoholic cirrhotic is admitted to your hospital with melena. In the emergency room, he has witnessed hematemesis. He is intubated and started on an IV proton pump inhibitor.

Vitals: Temperature 38, HR 110, BP 110, RR 14; 99% on 40% Fi02. On your arrival, the patient is sedated. He has mild scleral icterus, spider angiomata, palmar erythema, and an enlarged firm liver but no ascites.

The patient has a history of encephalopathy and is on lactulose and rifaximin. He is on low-dose diuretics.

WBC 12, Hb 7.8, Platelets 63. Na 134, Cr 1.2. Albumin 3.2. TBili 3.3, AST 78, ALT 38, ALP 89. INR 1.7

You should do all of the following EXCEPT?

A Prepare for an urgent EGD within 12–24 hours of arrival.
B Transfuse Hb to ~9–10.
C Administer octreotide.
D Obtain a stat RUQ ultrasound with Doppler to assess vessel patency.
E Continue PPI and broad-spectrum antibiotics.

Question 79

You perform an urgent EGD on the above patient within 12 hours of his arrival (see image) Endoscopy reveals a nipple sign on a medium sized varix.

You perform esophageal band ligation and send the patient for a transjugular intra-hepatic shunt.

▶ Question

Which of the following is FALSE regarding early or preemptive TIPS?

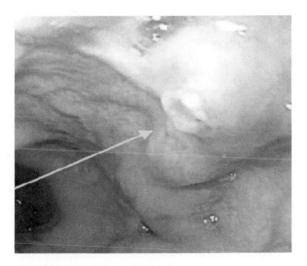

A Early TIPS should be considered within 72 hours of endoscopic therapy

B Early TIPS should be considered in patients with Childs B and active bleeding at the time of endoscopy or patients with Childs C (up to score of 13).

C Encephalopathy is a contraindication to early TIPS.

D Early TIPS decreases the risk of early rebleeding, ICU/hospital stay, and one-year mortality compared to standard endoscopic therapy.

E PTFE covered stent is preferred over uncovered stent.

78 – B is the correct answer.
79 – C is the correct answer.

Commentary – Early TIPS for Variceal Bleeding

Clinical Pearls: Early Tips/Pre-emptive TIPS

1. TIPS for "salvage" is very effective in control of bleeding (>90%), but mortality in this group remains upwards of 25–50%.
2. This was the basis for the early TIPS study, published in NEJM in 2010.
3. This was a randomized study looking at standard endoscopic/medical care versus "early" or preemptive (p) TIPS in high-risk cohort defined as: Child C (but less than 13) or Child B with active bleeding at time of endoscopy.
4. Early TIPS performed within 72 hours using covered stents; initially dilated to 8 mm (up to 10 if pressure did not decrease to less than 12 mmHg).
5. A total of 17.5% of patients admitted with acute variceal hemorrhage met inclusion criteria and were randomized.
6. Risk of re-bleeding, mortality (up to 24 months), hospital, and ICU LOS and ascites were significantly less in the early TIPS cohort.
7. There was no difference in PSE between the two groups.

Notes

In my opinion the "early TIPS" paper is one of the most important hepatology publications in the last 10 years; June 24, 2010, to be exact. I remember when the data was presented at AASLD, there was an audible buzz in the audience. The US has not yet widely adopted the practice of early TIPS, despite what appears to be consistent overwhelming evidence of its benefits.

Reference

Early TIPS (Transjugular Intrahepatic Portosystemic Shunt) Cooperative Study Group. Early use of TIPS in patients with cirrhosis and variceal bleeding. PMID: 20573925.

Question 80

The mechanism of action of octreotide is?

A Selectively causes splanchnic and extrarenal vasoconstriction by stimulation of V1 receptors.
B Dopamine receptor blockade.
C Nonselective adrenergic blocker with peripheral vasodilating effects.
D Releases nitric oxide, an endothelium-derived relaxing factor which dilate blood vessels.
E A somatostatin analogue which causes splanchnic arterial vasoconstriction and subsequent portal venous dilation.

E is the correct answer.

Commentary – Therapy of Active Variceal Hemorrhage

Clinical Pearls: Active Variceal Hemorrhage

1. EGD should ideally be performed within 12 hours of arrival.
2. Generally, five factors predict risk of variceal bleeding in patients with cirrhosis:
   a. Location (GE junction more risk than mid/proximal esophagus).
   b. Size (large>small).
   c. Appearance (nipple/fibrin plug, red wale, hematocystic spots).
   d. Clinical features of patient (Child C.A; high MELD> low MELD); prior history of variceal bleed.
   e. HVPG (risk of bleeding is greater than 50% when pressure is greater than 16 mmHg).
3. Current guidelines recommend antibiotics (ceftriaxone 1 g/day for 5–7 days), vasoactive drugs (octreotide 50 mcg bolus then 50 mcg/hr gtt for 5 days), and endoscopic therapy (band ligation preferable to sclerotherapy).
   a. Antibiotics have been shown to decrease mortality and risk of re-bleeding.
   b. Antibiotics are administered to all cirrhotic patients with UGIB (variceal or non) with or without ascites.
   c. Octreotide is a somatostatin analogue. It causes splanchnic arterial vasoconstriction and consequently portal venous dilation, i.e. lowers portal vein pressure:
      i. Terlipressin (not YET FDA approved in USA) has shown to provide mortality benefit in variceal bleeding.
4. Treatment failure remains 10–20%.
5. The most important variable consistently associated with treatment failure:
   a. HVPG >20.
   b. Active bleeding at time of EGD.
   c. Severity of liver disease.
6. Consider TIPS in high-risk patients:
   a. If your center does not have TIPS capability, there is role for balloon tamponade as a temporary bridge until definitive treatment can be offered:
      i. Minnesota (has four ports, one extra for esophageal aspiration) versus Blakemore (has three ports). See illustration below.
      ii. Typically, only the gastric balloon is inflated (up to 500 cc of air).
         1. It is recommended that the balloon not be kept up for more than 12–24 hours, given the risk of mucosal ischemia.

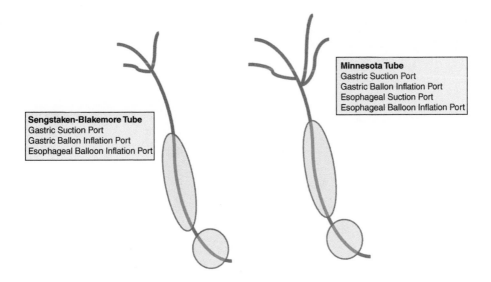

Sengstaken-Blakemore Tube
Gastric Suction Port
Gastric Ballon Inflation Port
Esophageal Balloon Inflation Port

Minnesota Tube
Gastric Suction Port
Gastric Ballon Inflation Port
Esophageal Suction Port
Esophageal Balloon Inflation Port

Reference

Management of acute variceal hemorrhage. PMID: 31281637.

Question 81

A 61-year-old female with NASH cirrhosis complicated by ascites is admitted to the hospital when routine labs revealed a creatinine of 2.5 (GFR 28). Her other notable past medical history includes diabetes (glycosylated hemoglobin of 8.2). On admission her home diuretics (50 mg of spironolactone and 20 mg of furosemide) were discontinued. A diagnostic tap was negative for SBP. She was administered IV albumin and within 48 hours her Cr dropped to her baseline of 1.6 (GFR 48).

The patient is followed regularly in clinic. She is requiring an LVP monthly. Six months after her admission for AKI she is admitted again this time for a bout of PSE. You recommend a simultaneous liver-kidney transplant.

Laboratory studies:

WBC 4, Hb 10, Platelets 67. Sodium 132, K 4.4; BUN 29, Cr 1.7 (GFR 44). TBili 3.8, AST 41, ALT 28, ALP 111.
INR 1.6.
MELD-Na is 25.
Cystatin C: 1.67.
24-hour urine protein is 0.8 g.

▶ Question

The patient would meet criteria for SLK based on:

A Baseline GFR less than 60 for 6 months
B GFR at time of listing less than 45
C Cystatin C level greater than 1.5
D Type II HRS
E The patient does not meet criteria for SLK at this time

E is the correct answer.

Commentary – Indications for SLK

Clinical Pearls: Indication for Simultaneous Liver Kidney (SLK) Transplant	
If the candidate's transplant nephrologist confirms a diagnosis of:	**Then the transplant program must document in the candidate's medical record:**
CKD with a measured GFR less than or equal to 60 mL/min for greater than 90 consecutive days	At least one of the following 1. That the candidate has begun regularly administered dialysis as an ESRD patient in a hospital based, independent non-hospital based, or home setting 2. That the candidate's most recent measured or calculated CrCl or GFR is less than or equal to 35 mL/min at the time of registration on the kidney waiting list
Sustained AKI	At least one of the following 1. That the candidate has been on dialysis for at least 6 consecutive weeks 2. That the candidate has a measured or calculated CrCl or GFR less than or equal to 25 mL/min for at least 6 consecutive weeks and this is documented in the candidate's medical record every 7 days beginning with the date of the first test with this value That the candidate has any combination of 1 and 2 above for 6 consecutive weeks
Metabolic disease	An additional diagnosis of at least one of the following 1. Hyperoxaluria 2. Atypical HUS from mutations in factor H and possibly factor I 3. Familial non-neuropathic systemic amyloid 4. Methymalonic aciduria

1. If a patient meets SLK medical eligibility criteria, the patient will be prioritized ahead of kidney alone candidates at the time of their liver offer.
2. The role of pretransplant kidney biopsy in liver transplant recipients has not been established:
   a. Some studies suggest performing dual transplant when glomerulosclerosis exceeds 40% and interstitial fibrosis exceeds 30%.
3. Cystatin C is a protein produced by all nucleated cells and catabolized by the renal tubular cells after passing the glomerular filter. Some studies suggest that it may be more sensitive for detecting a reduced GFR in cirrhotic patients compared to creatinine. Values >1.25 mg/L suggest reduced GFR.

Reference

Simultaneous liver kidney transplantation. PMID: 30548094.

Question 82

What is the "safety net" with regards to liver transplant?

A Patients with HCC beyond Milan criteria can undergo imaging following down-staging of cancer prior to being removed from the liver transplant list.

B Liver transplant recipients who are either on dialysis or who have an eGFR ≤ 20 mL/min between 60–365 days after liver transplant will receive priority on the kidney waiting list for donors.

C A patient has a right to refuse a donor offer if they deem the donor is "not safe" or high risk.

D Patients with metastatic neuroendocrine tumor (NET) to the liver are, given status 1a listing if the original tumor is removed, and the metastatic lesions are confined to the liver

E If a patient is removed from the liver transplant list, they have six months to officially appeal the decision of the transplant center.

B is the correct answer.

Commentary – Safety Net

Clinical Pearls: Safety Net

1. The simultaneous liver kidney (SLK) criteria were implemented in August 2017 and were expected to reduce the number of SLK transplants by 19%.
2. One of the key features of the new SLK policy is the so-called "safety net" provision.
3. Under this policy liver transplant recipients who are either on dialysis or who have a GFR $\leq$20 mL/min between 60–365 days after liver transplant will receive priority on the kidney waiting list for donors with a kidney donor profile index (KDPI) between 20 and 85%.
4. The Kidney Donor Risk Index (KDRI) combines a variety of donor factors to summarize the risk of graft failure after kidney transplant into a single number. The KDRI expresses the relative risk of kidney graft failure for a given donor compared to the median kidney donor from last year; values exceeding 1 have higher expected risk than the median donor and vice versa.
5. The KDPI is a remapping of the KDRI onto a cumulative percentage scale, such that a donor with a KDPI of 80% has higher expected risk of graft failure than 80% of all kidney donors recovered last year.

Reference

Simultaneous liver kidney allocation policy and the Safety Net: an early examination of utilization and outcomes in the United States. PMID: 33884677.

Question 83

The Model for End Stage Liver Disease (MELD) Score is a "weighted" calculation. Which laboratory parameter is given the most "weight"?

A INR
B Total bilirubin
C Creatinine
D Albumin
E Sodium

A is the correct answer.

Commentary – MELD Score

Notes
One of my favorite rounding questions. Residents not well acquainted with the MELD score will end up choosing bilirubin.

Reference

The model for end-stage liver disease (MELD). PMID: 17326206.

Question 84

Which of the following patient scenarios would produce the biggest "delta" MELD (assuming the other parameters are equivalent)?

A A patient with an INR of 1.2 versus a patient with an INR of 2.8.
B A patient with a MELD of 20 and serum sodium of 124 versus a patient with a MELD of 20 and a sodium of 118.
C A patient with a total bilirubin of 18 (conjugated 7) versus a patient with a total bilirubin of 25 (conjugated 21).
D A patient with a Cr of 4 versus a patient on hemodialysis.
E A patient with a 1.5 versus a patient with a Cr of 2.5.

A is the correct answer.

Commentary – MELD Score

Clinical Pearls: The MELD Score

1. The MELD score was originally developed in 2001 to predict three-month mortality following TIPS placement.
2. The equation is: MELD $= 3.78 \times \ln[\text{serum bilirubin (mg/dL)}] + 11.2 \times \ln[\text{INR}] + 9.57 \times \ln[\text{serum creatinine (mg/dL)}] + 6.43$.
3. INR is weighted more than creatinine which is weighted more than bilirubin.
4. In 2002, it was adopted by UNOS for prioritization of patients awaiting liver transplantation.
5. The incorporation of sodium into the MELD became official in January 2016.
6. The other three parameters include INR, TBili, and Cr. The MELD-Na score ranges from 6 to 40.
7. A creatinine of 4 should be inputted for patients on dialysis.
8. INR has the largest weight in the MELD score. Patients on systemic anticoagulation may have artificially elevated MELD. To adjust for this discrepancy, a MELD without INR (MELD-XI) has been proposed.
9. Hyponatremia is associated with mortality independent of MELD; a score between 125 and 137 increases the MELD score:
   a. Hyponatremia (<130) has also been associated with high rates of neurological disorders, infectious complications, and renal failure during the first month post-LT and a reduced 3-month survival.
10. MELD score does have good accuracy in predicting short-term survival in patients with cirrhosis: A MELD of 40 ~70% predicts a 3-month mortality (minus liver transplant).
11. Pre LT-MELD is a poor predictor of posttransplant outcomes.
12. The MELD score has been used to predict survival in patients undergoing surgical procedures, patients with ALF, alcoholic hepatitis, and acute on chronic liver failure.

Notes

The MELD score was first devised as a model to predict survival post-TIPS. The original 2001 paper has been cited >5000 times!

Reference

The MELD-Plus: a generalizable prediction risk score in cirrhosis. PMID: 29069090.

Question 85

You are evaluating a 19-year-old female for a live donor liver transplant. She is hoping to donate to her 26-year-old brother with Wilson disease. The recipient's current MELD score is 22. The recipient's weight is 100 kg.

The donor is healthy appearing. She is 5′4 and weighs 128 pounds (58 kg).

As part of routine preoperative evaluation, a CT scan is performed on the potential donor.

You are asked to calculate the graft to recipient weight ratio for a right donor liver transplant.

The morphology of the liver is normal. No focal hepatic lesions are identified. The total hepatic volume is 874 cc. The volume of the right lobe is 553 cc. The volume of the left medical segment is 153 cc; volume of the left lateral segment is 149 cc; the volume of the caudate lobe is 19 cc.

▶ Question

The calculated GRWR is and based on the results what do you recommend regarding the donor?

A GRWR .55; decline donor
B GRWR .87; ok to proceed
C GRWR .30; decline donor
D GRWR .55; ok to proceed
E GRWR .87; decline donor

A is the correct answer.

Commentary – GRWR

Clinical Pearls: Graft to Recipient Weight Ratio (GRWR)

1. Graft to Recipient Weight Ratio (GRWR): graft volume in kg/recipient weight in kg × 100.
2. Ideally GRWR should be >0.8. Most transplant centers utilize this threshold.
3. Because of this, the use of left lobe grafts has been limited.
4. Consequently, the right lobe is the graft of choice in adult LDLT.
5. Low GRWR has been associated with poor prognosis for patients following living donor liver transplantation especially in terms of 1- and 3-year survival rates and the development of small for size syndrome (SFSS).
6. Some centers will use small grafts (<0.8) only in patients with low MELD (<20), donor age less than 45 with no signs of hepatic steatosis and portal inflow modulation (via splenic artery ligation or splenectomy).

Notes

We have two GRWR questions in the book. More practice for a subject that will almost certainly be on your exam in some manner.

Reference

Association of graft-to-recipient weight ratio with the prognosis following liver transplantation: a meta-analysis. PMID: 32306226.

Question 86

A 72-year-old female with PSC cirrhosis is admitted with worsening abdominal pain, nausea, and nonbloody emesis × 48 hours. Her PSC was diagnosed over 10 years ago. Her liver disease is complicated by bleeding esophageal varices, treated with combination beta-blocker and variceal band ligation, diuretic controlled ascites, and mild portosystemic encephalopathy. She has a history of ulcerative colitis, which is quiescent. Her outpatient medications include nadolol, furosemide, and spironolactone. She has a remote history of breast cancer.

On exam she is uncomfortable. Her temperature is 99.2 F, hr 100, bp 112/62 she is breathing 16/min and her O_2 saturation on 98% on 2 L oxygen. She has mild scleral icterus, muscle wasting. Abdominal exam is notable for a large umbilical hernia which is erythematous and tender to palpation. It cannot be reduced. She has a fluid thrill.

Laboratory studies:

WBC 12, Hb 10, Platelets 58K. 87% Neutrophils and 2% bands. Sodium 133, K 4.9; BUN 21, Cr 1.4.
TBili 3.3, AST 18, ALT 22, ALP 254. INR 1.6
A CT scan shows a partial small bowel obstruction and an incarcerated umbilical hernia without strangulation or radiographic evidence of ischemia. There is a moderate amount of ascites, and large varices and collaterals throughout the entire abdomen.
The surgery service is reluctant to take her to the operating and asks you to document her "surgical risk". You use the MAYO surgical risk which predicts a 30-day mortality of 15%.

▶ Question

Which of the following clinical/laboratory parameters is NOT taken into account when predicting this mortality score?

A Age
B Etiology of liver disease
C Degree of ascites
D ASA score
E Creatinine

C is the correct answer.

Commentary – Surgical Risk Assessment in Cirrhotic Patients

Clinical Pearls: Surgical Risk Assessment in Cirrhotic Patients

1. Underlying liver disease has effects on the risk of morbidity and mortality after surgery. The magnitude of the risk depends on etiology of liver disease, severity, surgical procedure, and type of anesthesia.
2. High-risk patients with liver disease for any type of surgery include the following:
   a. Childs C
   b. MELD >15
   c. Acute liver failure
   d. Acute alcoholic hepatitis
   e. High serum bilirubin (>10 mg/dL)
3. High-risk surgery includes abdominal surgery, cholecystectomy (open), colectomy, gastric surgery, liver resection, cardiothoracic surgery, emergent surgery of any type, and surgery with high anticipated blood loss.
4. The most used risk assessment is the MAYO MELD surgical risk calculator. This online calculator factors in the MELD score (INR, Cr, TBili) in addition to age, ASA class, and etiology of liver disease to predict mortality in patients undergoing moderate-/high-risk surgical procedures (of note laparoscopic cholecystectomy was not included in the original paper formulating this risk score):
   a. https://www.mayoclinic.org/medical-professionals/transplant-medicine/calculators/post-operative-mortality-risk-in-patients-with-cirrhosis/itt-20434721
5. A more recent "Vocal-Penn" Cirrhosis Surgical Risk Score was specifically designed to improve on limitations of the Mayo Risk Score. This score also predicts postoperative mortality but uses a larger set of parameters including age, albumin, total bilirubin, platelet count, BMI, NAFLD, ASA score, emergency, and type of surgery.
   a. http://www.vocalpennscore.com/

Notes

The MAYO surgical risk score is more widely utilized in clinical practice but is limited by lacking parameters of portal hypertension. The VOCAL–Penn score factors in a surrogate of PTHN by incorporating platelet count.

Reference

Preoperative risk assessment for patients with liver disease. PMID: 1957712.

Question 87

A 67-year-old female with NASH cirrhosis is referred to you for increasing shortness of breath. The patient has a history of ascites but has not required paracentesis in six months. She has grade II esophageal varices but could not tolerate a beta-blocker with complaints of dyspnea. She has a history of encephalopathy requiring one admission (necessitating intubation).

A chest-ray reveals a large right effusion. A diagnostic and therapeutic thoracocentesis is arranged. Her pleural fluid albumin and total protein are less than 1 g/dL. You start her on diuretics but are forced to discontinue, given worsening hyponatremia. The patient and family are not interested in pursuing liver transplant. After a lengthy discussion, you mutually decide to proceed with a TIPS.

Laboratory studies:

WBC 4, Hb 11, platelets 67K
Na 131, K 4.8; BUN 14, Cr 1.2
TBili 2.3, AST 88, ALT 47, ALP 119; INR 1.6
CT: cirrhotic liver with patent vessels; splenomegaly and scant ascites
EGD: grade II esophageal varices
TTE: PASP 67 mmHg (mean 49)

▶ Question

Which of the following in this patient is considered an absolute contraindication to TIPS in this patient?

A Age of 67 years
B Prior bout of PSE necessitating intubation
C MELD-Na of 22
D PASP
E Hyponatremia

D is the correct answer.

Commentary – Contraindications to TIPS

Clinical Pearls: Contraindications to TIPS Procedure

1. The risk associated with TIPS must always be balanced with the severity of the complication from which the patient is suffering and the likelihood of the patient surviving (ideally to receive a liver transplant). Although transplantation candidacy is not necessarily required for a TIPS procedure.
2. Contraindications are divided into: Absolute and Relative.
3. Absolute contraindications:
   a. Primary prevention for variceal bleeding
   b. Multiple hepatic cysts
   c. Sepsis
   d. Unrelieved biliary obstruction
   e. CHF, severe TR, severe PHTN (defined as mean PASP >45 mmHg)
4. Relative contraindications
   a. Central HCC
   b. Obstruction of all hepatic veins
   c. Complete PVT
   d. Severe coagulopathy (INR >5)
   e. Severe thrombocytopenia (<20)
   f. Moderate pulmonary HTN
5. Caution should be taken in proceeding with TIPS in the following patients:
   a. MELD score >15–18; TBili >5
   b. Refractory PSE
   c. Severe hyponatremia
   d. Age >65
   e. Sarcopenia

Notes

Until live donor liver transplant becomes more widely utilized, I anticipate the boundaries of TIPS will be pushed more and more. Be cautious, however, of the pre-TIPS variables that may portend a poor outcome.

Reference

TIPS Special Conference. Consensus conference on TIPS management: techniques, indications, contraindications. PMID: 27884494.

Question 88

A 27-year-old male is referred to you from the pediatric cardiology clinic for evaluation of abnormal liver tests. The patient has a history of complex congenital heart disease with a hypoplastic left ventricle. He underwent a Fontan procedure at the age of 10.

Laboratory studies:

WBC 4.5, Hb 14, Platelets of 151. Na 132, Cr 0.7. Albumin 4.4. TBili 1.7, AST 20, ALT 13, and ALP of 87. Ultrasound findings show a coarsened liver. Elastography reveals a kPa of 10.4.

▶ Question

Which of the following statements regarding Fontan and liver disease are TRUE?

A >95% of patients with Fontan procedure will develop biochemical abnormalities in the liver enzyme but will never develop histological injury.

B Histological changes typically reveal sinusoidal dilation and perisinusoidal edema in centrilobular hepatocytes as a result of chronic passive congestion.

C The risk of HCC in patients with Fontan associated liver disease and advanced fibrosis is exceedingly rare, and so surveillance for HCC is not warranted

D The Fontan procedure creates a conduit by which blood from the IVC is routed directly into the pulmonary vein.

E HVPG measurement in these patients should be considered the gold standard for the presence of portal hypertension even in the presence of collaterals and shunting.

B is the correct answer.

Commentary – Fontan-Associated Liver Disease

Clinical Pearls: Fontan-associated Liver Disease

1. The Fontan procedure is a "palliative" procedure for patients born with single functional ventricle due to complex congenital heart disease.
2. The surgery includes techniques that divert systemic venous return to the pulmonary arterial system (inferior vena cava is connected through an artificial conduit to pulmonary artery), avoiding the right ventricle.
3. Although survival rates are 80% at 20 years post-Fontan, multiple consequences arise including arrhythmia, heart failure, thromboembolic events, protein-losing enteropathy, and liver disease.
4. Elevated systemic venous pressure leads to inefficient blood drainage of the liver resulting in chronic passive congestion. This state leads to sinusoidal dilation and blood hyperinflation causing perisinusoidal edema and hypoxia in centrilobular hepatocytes.
5. Hepatic damage following Fontan surgery is universal and patients operated on more than 10 years ago should be evaluated for liver-related complications.
6. Liver biopsy remains the gold standard for the assessment of fibrosis in patients with Fontan-associated liver disease. HVPG measurements can be difficult to interpret because of the high incidence of collateralization. There is emerging data on the role of elastography in these patients.
7. Studies suggest that up to 40% of patients will develop advanced fibrosis 30 years after Fontan operation.
8. The development of portal hypertension is associated with ascites and varices. The development of encephalopathy has been infrequently reported.
9. HCC is now a well-established complication of advanced fibrosis in patients with Fontan associated liver disease.
10. The role of transplantation (heart, liver, or combined) is now well established and requires institutions with experience and a multidisciplinary approach.

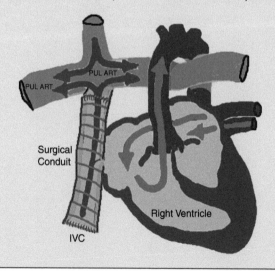

Notes

Fontan liver disease will become more frequently encountered in the next decade as many children with complex congenital heart disease survive into adulthood. They are an incredibly challenging subset of patients, especially when it comes to the role of transplantation. The illustration above shows a "surgical conduit" connecting the IVC directly to the pulmonary artery. One of the consequences of "Fontan circulation" includes the almost universal development of liver disease.

Reference

Fontan-associated liver disease: a review. PMID: 30928109.

Question 89

An 18-year-old healthy college student is interested in being a live donor to her 78-year-old grandmother with NASH cirrhosis complicated by recurrent encephalopathy. The potential recipient has a MELD score of 14.

▶ Question

What ethical principles should be weighed as part of the decision to proceed or not?

A Autonomy
B Nonmaleficence
C Beneficence
D All of the above
E None of the above

Question 90

A 37-year-old male is admitted with severe acute alcoholic hepatitis. This is his first episode. His course has been complicated by ascites and encephalopathy. He is currently in the ICU with renal failure. He has failed steroids. His MELD score is 40. You refer him for transplantation. You overhear a group of nurses discussing whether he should be transplanted.

▶ Question

Ethical considerations when it comes to Early Liver Transplantation for Alcoholic Hepatitis attempts best to balance what two ethical principles?

A Autonomy and utility
B Acuteness and severity
C Competence and understanding
D Beneficence and justice
E Nonmaleficence and fairness

89 – D is the correct answer.
90 – D is the correct answer.

Commentary – Ethics and Transplant

Clinical Pearls: Ethics and Liver Transplantation

1. Autonomy: Patient makes their own decision
2. Nonmaleficence: Avoiding the causation of harm
3. Beneficence: Balancing benefits against risk and costs
4. Justice: fair distribution of benefits, risk, and costs
5. Utility: greatest benefit for all
6. Five elements of informed consent
   a. Competence
   b. Disclosure
   c. Understanding
   d. Voluntariness
   e. Consent
7. National Organ Transplant Act: 1984 (NOTA)
   a. It shall be unlawful for any person to knowingly acquire, receive, or otherwise transfer any human organ for valuable consideration for use in human transplantation.
8. Ethnic and racial disparities in liver transplantation:
   a. Disparities are present regarding racial minorities to access, referral, pretransplant mortality, and transplantation rates.
   b. Disparities are also prevalent in posttransplant outcomes.

Notes

Ethics, racial disparities, quality of life, and the role of palliative services will be a handful of questions on your exam. We outlined some key points.

Reference

Liver transplantation in the USA: ethical issues. PMID: 31818469.

Question 91

Which of the following statements regarding azathioprine is TRUE?

A It is considered a class B pregnancy drug.
B It causes pancreatitis by increasing formation of gallstones.
C Patients with high TPMT levels can be started at standard dose of the medication.
D Xanthine oxidase inhibitors increase the production of the inactive metabolite 6-Thiouric acid.
E Standard starting doses in AIH are 5–10 mg/kg.

C is the correct answer.

Commentary – Azathioprine

Clinical Pearls: Azathioprine

1. Azathioprine is an inactive or prodrug. It is converted to its active form 6-MP (see illustration).
2. 6 MP is converted to TIMP by Hypoxanthine-guanine phosphoribosyltransferase (HBPRT). TIMP which eventually is converted to 6—Thioguanine (6-TG):
   a. 6-TG Interferes in "S" phase of cycle of B and T cell proliferation
   b. Also induces T cell apoptosis
3. Xanthine oxidase (XO) converts Azathioprine to 6-Thiouric Acid which is inactive.
4. Xanthine oxidase inhibitors prevent conversion of azathioprine to 6-Thiouric Acid (Inactive) and lead to greater production of 6-MP and so more active metabolite and so increased toxicity:
   a. Allopurinol is a XO inhibitor. Allopurinol and AZA increase levels of 6-MP and can lead to toxicity.
5. Thiopurine methyltransferase (TPMT) is the main enzyme responsible for inactivating 6-MP (remember 6-MP is "active") into 6-MMP (inactive):
   a. Patients who are deficient in TPMT will produce more TIMP and potential side effects.
6. Current recommendations are to check TPMT levels prior to the initiation of azathioprine in patients with AIH. Studies suggest using metabolite levels can optimize treatment regimens, maintaining biochemical response, and resulting in fewer adverse drug reactions.
   a. Activity test (phenotype)
      i. Normal: >12 (nmol/hr/mL RBC)
      ii. Intermediate; heterozygote or low metabolizer: 4–12
      iii. Low; homozygote deficient range <4
   b. Genetic test (genotype)
      i. Most people have two copies of "wild type" and produce sufficient TPMT
      ii. 10% are heterozygous and have intermediate activity
      iii. 1/300 (0.3%) of people are homozygous and have no enzyme activity
7. Side effects of azathioprine include myelosuppression, skin cancer, lymphoma, photosensitivity, and pancreatitis.
8. Pregnancy class: D, but increasing evidence to suggest its safety.

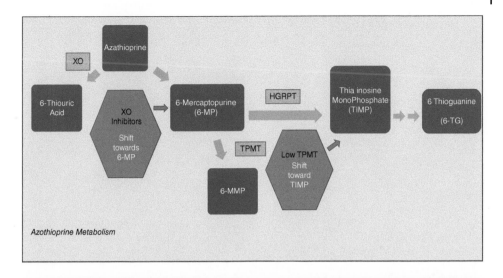

Azothioprine Metabolism

Notes

Azathioprine metabolism is a topic that will be covered in both the GI and transplant boards. Pay special attention to the "red-stop" signs in the illustration above on how different factors shift metabolism.

Reference

A physician's guide to azathioprine metabolite testing. PMID: 28210198.

Question 92

A 27-year-old male with no significant past medical history presents to his local emergency room with progressively worsening abdominal discomfort over the last month. He also complains of nausea and early satiety. He has lost 12 pounds.

The patient is married and lives with his wife and 2-year-old daughter. He works at a shipping yard. He chews tobacco but has no other habits.

On exam the patient is anxious. He is mildly tender in his right quadrant. His liver is palpable 4 cm below the right costal margin. The remainder of his exam is normal.

TBili 1.5, AST 22, ALT 28, ALP 66, gGTP 88; CBC and renal function are normal. CEA 1.2, CA 19-9 1.2, and AFP 2. Viral serologies are negative.

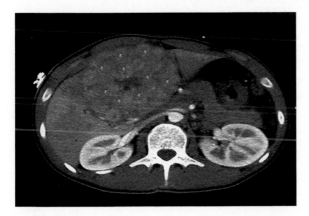

A CT scan above shows a large mass with a central scar with scattered calcification in an otherwise normal appearing liver. A biopsy is obtained confirming the suspicion of malignancy.

▶ Question

Which of the following is true regarding this tumor?

A   A majority of cases occur in patients less than the age of 40.
B   It occurs in the setting of a "noncirrhotic" liver and liver tests are typically normal.
C   AFP is normal in a majority of cases.
D   These are rare tumors and account for less than 1% of primary liver cancers.
E   All of the above.

E is the correct answer.

Commentary – Fibrolamellar Hepatocellular Carcinoma (FLHCC)

Clinical Pearls: Fibrolamellar Hepatocellular Carcinoma (FLHCC)

1. FLHCC is a rare and accounts for less than 1% of primary liver cancers.
2. Unlike "typical" HCC, these occur in the setting of otherwise "normal" livers; risk factors are not well identified.
3. An alteration in chimeric transcript DNAJB1-PRKACA has been suggested as a genetic cause contributing to tumor pathogenesis.
4. More than 85% of cases are reported in patients less than 35 years of age. Equal frequency amongst genders.
5. About 75% of cases will have a prominent central scar.
   a. Central scar and calcification? think FLHCC.
6. Microscopically: well, differentiated malignant cells with large central nuclei, eosinophilic cytoplasm, abundant fibrous stroma arranged in thin parallel lamellae around tumor cells. Background liver is normal.
7. Masses are large at time of presentation (usually >10 cm); 70% have lymphadenopathy and 50% have metastatic disease.
8. The cornerstone of treatment is surgical resection and lymph node dissection. About 50–75% cure rate has been reported.
9. Chemotherapy has shown varying degrees of response.
10. Liver transplant can be considered; nearly ½ of cases recur at 3.5 year follow-up.
11. Young patient, no liver disease, large tumor with central scar, with calcifications, biopsy shows cancer: think FLHCC.

Notes

The CT scan image shown here is classic for fibrolamellar HCC: a large tumor in a normal liver with a central scar and calcifications. Remember focal nodular hyperplasia (FNH) also has a central (stellate) scar.

Reference

Fibrolamellar hepatocellular carcinoma: current clinical perspectives. PMID: 27508204.

Question 93

A 57-year-old male with cirrhosis secondary to hemochromatosis is referred to your center for liver transplant evaluation. His cirrhosis has been complicated by HCC. He has three Li-Rads 5 lesions on imaging: 2.5 cm, 2.5 cm, and 3 cm. The patient has undergone TACE × 1 with partial treatment response on all three lesions. There is no evidence of vascular invasion on imaging or extrahepatic spread. The patient's pre-LT AFP is 1078 ng/dL.

The patient undergoes liver transplant. Explant analysis reveals three partially treated tumors, the largest being 2.4 cm and microvascular invasion.

▶ Question

Which of the following factors is associated with the highest risk of recurrent HCC post LT?

A Number of tumors
B AFP level
C Etiology of liver disease
D Microvascular invasion
E Total size of tumor burden

B is the correct answer.

Commentary – Recurrent Disease After Transplant

Clinical Pearls: Recurrent Disease Post LT

1. Autoimmune hepatitis (AIH): recurrence: 17–33% median ~5 years:
   a. The only modifiable risk factor is steroid withdrawal posttransplant. Guidelines do recommend low-dose corticosteroids post-LT in patients transplanted for AIH.
   b. A total of <5% of patients with recurrent AIH will require re-transplant
2. Primary Biliary Cholangitis (PBC): recurrence 20% at ~5 years:
   a. UDCA can be used for recurrent disease.
   b. Recent study suggests prophylactic UDCA can prevent recurrence.
3. Primary sclerosing cholangitis (PSC): 20% at ~5 years:
   a. Diagnosis: Cholangiographic findings >90 days posttransplant.
   b. Rule out: Ischemic cholangiopathy, anastomotic stricture, ABO incompatibility.
   c. Studies suggest a significantly decreased risk of recurrent PSC in patients who have had a pretransplant colectomy.
   d. Increase risk of recurrent PSC when ulcerative colitis is present post-LT.
   e. Up to 25% of those with recurrent PSC will receive a second transplant:
      i. Cholangiocarcinoma has also been reported post LT for PSC.
4. NASH
   a. Risk factors: BMI, PLNPLA 3, diabetes, post-LT hypertriglyceridemia, and Pan-hypopituitarism
   b. Diagnosis of NASH post-LT requires biopsy
   c. Studies suggest recurrent NASH 35–50% at 7-year follow; graft cirrhosis is less than 5% at 10 years follow-up.
   d. Treatment: weight loss and optimize hypertension (target goal of 130/80), HLD (LDL <100), DM (A1c goal <7%), OSA treatment.
5. Alcohol
   a. Relapse ~15%.
   b. Relapse into heavy drinking is associated with allograft loss (HR 2.5).
   c. Risk factors for relapse: short length of sobriety of LT, psych comorbidity, multiple failed treatment attempts, poor social support, illicit drug use, no rehab, or counseling.
6. HCC
   a. Recurrence of 5–15% at mean of 1 year.
   b. Sites: lung, liver, bone, adrenal gland, LN:
      i. Risk factors for recurrent HCC
         1. Pre-LT AFP
         2. Tumor beyond Milan
         3. Tumor differentiation
         4. Stage at explant
         5. Micro/macro invasion

     ii. RETREAT model for recurrent HCC:
       1. Alfa fetoprotein (AFP) >1000 Hazard Ratio (HR): 4.45
       2. Microvascular invasion HR 3.8
       3. Largest viable tumor diameter (cm) and number of visible tumors
   c. Surveillance chest and abdominal CT q6 months for 3 years and AFP (if elevated pre-LT).
   d. SILVER study showed that sirolimus-based immunosuppression likely does *not* decrease risk of recurrence.
7. Perihilar cholangiocarcinoma:
   a. Risk of recurrence: 20% median at 2 years.
   b. Risk factor: the need to perform Whipple because of distal bile duct involvement, residual tumor, LN invasion, vascular or perineural invasion on explant, elevated Ca 19-9, total PV encasement.
8. Neuroendocrine tumor:
   a. Recurrent NET in 30–80%:
     i. Criterion for LT for met NET:
       1. Well-differentiated NET with Ki-67 indexes <10%
       2. Primary tumor removed prior to LT
       3. <50% liver involvement
       4. Stable disease for >6 months
       5. Age <55
       6. Exclusion of extrahepatic disease with somatostatin receptor imaging
     ii. Post-LT surveillance:
       1. Imaging, chromogranin A, and tumor marker q3 months ×1 year than annually.
       2. Annual somatostatin receptor imaging (111-In pentetreotide or 68-Ga DOTATATE).
       3. Switch to everolimus-based IS.

Notes

In this section, we discuss recurrent disease post-transplant for the most common etiologies. HBV and HCV recurrence are covered in a separate section.

Reference

Recurrent nonviral liver disease following liver transplantation. PMID: 19485808.

Question 94

A 67-year-old is being seen in your liver clinic after a recent hospitalization for his third bout of cholangitis this year. He has a history of PSC and underwent his first liver transplant 24 years ago. He has a Roux limb. Liver biopsy shows proliferation of interlobular bile ducts with mononuclear cells with nodule formation; there is no strong histological evidence of rejection. The patient now has recurrent PSC with diffuse intrahepatic disease on imaging; there is scant ascites, collaterals, and splenomegaly. Vessels are all patent.

Laboratory studies:

TBili 4.6, AST 78, ALT 56, ALP 322, GGT 290. WBC 4, Hb 9, Platelets 57K. Albumin 3.1. INR 1.7. Na 133, Cr 1.3.

▶ Question

The patient and family are inquiring about the role for re-transplantation. Which of the following can you tell them?

A Based on the patient's current lab, he would not derive survival benefit from re-transplantation.
B The likely cause of this patient's need for re-transplantation is HAT.
C The cause for this patient's graft failure is rare, occurring in less than 5% of patient's transplanted for PSC.
D Graft survival with retransplant is worse compared to the first transplant.
E This patient should be considered for a combined liver/kidney transplant.

D is the correct answer.

Commentary – Re-transplant

Clinical Pearls: Re-Transplantation

1. Rate of retransplant (for all comers) has decreased from 8% (2006) to 4% (2016):
    a. Graft survival is worse compared to first transplant (69% versus 82% at 5 years).
    b. Early causes of re-transplant:
       i. Primary nonfunction and hepatic artery thrombus (up to 50% will require re-tx); portal vein thrombosis (rare):
          1. Can be listed as status 1 if within the first 7 days.
 2. Late causes of re-transplantation:
    a. Recurrent disease, chronic rejection, biliary complications (DCD), allograft cirrhosis with decompensation.
 3. Survival benefit in re-transplantation is MELD of 21 or above (as opposed to 15 for index transplant).

Reference

Liver retransplant for primary disease recurrence. PMID: 24907715.

Question 95

The highest incidence of PTLD is associated with which transplant?

A Multivisceral
B Heart–lung
C Pancreas
D Liver
E Bone marrow

A is the correct answer.

Commentary – Multivisceral Transplant

Clinical Pearls: Multivisceral Transplant

1. Full multivisceral transplant is defined as follows: stomach, duodenum, pancreas, intestine, and liver
   a. When feasible the native pancreaticoduodenal complex or spleen is preserved to reduce infection, posttransplant lymphoproliferative disorder (PTLD), and diabetes.
2. Simultaneous liver without advanced cirrhosis or overt hepatic failure should not be entertained solely because of the biological privilege of the simultaneously transplanted liver.
3. Standard of care for patients with irreversible gut failure who can no longer be maintained on parenteral nutrition.
4. Leading indications for multivisceral transplant:
   a. Short-gut syndrome due to mesenteric ischemia.
   b. End-stage Crohn's disease.
   c. Congenital disorders in pediatric population:
      i. Volvulus is the most common indication in children.
   d. Global gut dysmotility.
   e. Neoplastic disorders.
   f. Primary or secondary enterocyte dysfunction.
   g. Bariatric associated gut failure.
5. Despite periodic changes in UNOS regulations and organ allocation, the log relative risk of mortality for liver-intestine continues to be threefold that of liver-only candidates.
6. Three essential components of posttransplant care:
   a. Management of immunosuppression.
   b. Monitoring of allograft function:
      i. Protocol ileoscopy with random biopsies and serial measurement of donor specific antigen (DSA).
   c. Diagnosis with prompt treatment of infection.
7. Outcomes
   a. Patient survival 85% 1 year, 61% at 10 years. Graft survival 80% and 50%, respectively.
      i. Leading cause of death is infection. 94% of recipients develop bacterial infection posttransplant.
   b. Acute rejection ~40%:
      i. DSA has been reported in ~25% of patients has been associated with chronic rejection.
   c. PTLD is seen in up to 30% of patients.
   d. Reported risk of PTLD based on organ:

 i. Multivisceral up to 30%
 ii. Heart–lung 9%
 iii. Lung 2–8%
 iv. Heart 2–5%
 v. Liver 2–5%
 vi. Pancreas 2%
 vii. Kidney 1%
 viii. Bone marrow <1%
 ix. Graft Versus Host Disease (GVHD) 5–7% with mortality rate of 70%.
8. The two factors most strongly associated with patient and graft survival are: social support (hazard ratio: 6) and absence of liver as part of transplant (hazard ratio 3).

Reference

Composite and multivisceral transplantation: nomenclature, surgical techniques, current practice, and long-term outcome. PMID: 30471738.

Question 96

Which of the following is regarded as an absolute contraindication to liver transplantation?

A Complete PV thrombosis
B Delta infection
C Methadone use
D Graft failure from recurrent HCV
E None of the above

E is the correct answer.

Commentary

> ### Clinical Pearls: Contraindications to Liver Transplantation
>
> 1. Active bacteremia/fungemia/sepsis
> 2. Lack of social support
> 3. Lack of compliance; inability to cooperate with lifelong medical supervision
> 4. Extrahepatic malignancy not meeting oncologic criteria for cure:
>   a. Colorectal cancer can be an exception under center study protocol.
>   b. A period (2–5 years) of waiting is desirable in elective LT patients with a history of preexisting malignancy.
> 5. Intrahepatic cholangiocarcinoma:
>   a. Only under center protocol. Typically done in combination with adjuvant chemotherapy.
> 6. Hemangiosarcoma is a contraindication to transplant:
>   a. Epithelioid hemangioendothelioma, however, can be transplanted.
> 7. Severe cardiac disease:
>   a. Severe pulmonary HTN.
> 8. Severe respiratory disease.
> 9. Active IVDU.
> 10. AIDS.
> 11. Severe neurological impairment.
> 12. ALF with sustained ICP >50 mmHg or cerebral perfusion pressure <40 mmHg.
> 13. Anatomic abnormalities that preclude transplantation:
>   a. Extensive PVT with extension into SMV (appropriate patients may need to be considered for multivisceral transplantation).

Reference

Indications and contraindications for liver transplantation. PMID: 22007310.

Question 97

Which of the following is considered a risk factor for the most common malignancy post-LT in the United States?

A Red hair
B EBV status
C Barrett's esophagus
D Episodes of rejection
E Pre LT obesity

A is the correct answer.

Commentary – Malignancy After Transplant

Clinical Pearls: Extrahepatic Malignancy and LT

1. The risk of de novo malignancy is 2–3× higher after LT and contributes to lower long-term survival. The risk is due to prolonged IS.
2. Risk of all de novo cancer post-LT at 10 years has been reported 10–25%.
3. In western countries, the most common post LT cancers are the following:
   a. Nonmelanoma skin cancer, Kaposi's sarcoma, PTLD, head & neck, esophagus, colo-rectal cancer, lung.
4. Duration of exposure and intensity of immunosuppression is related to the risk of cancer post-LT. Specific risk factors include
   a. Skin cancer highest in PSC followed by alcohol (22 and 18% at 10 years compared to 10% for other etiologies); risk increases with age and smoking.
   b. Alcohol/smoking are associated with: lung, head & neck and esophageal cancer.
   c. Barrett's is associated with esophageal cancer: esophageal.
   d. PSC/IBD: CRC.
      i. Patients with IBD and PSC should undergo **yearly** colonoscopy with biopsy post-LT:
         1. PSC/UC LT population has 7× increased risk of CRC development compared to general population
            a. LT itself does not seem to be associated with an increased risk of CRC development in all other etiologies
   e. Higher age, male, red hair, alcohol and cyclosporin use are all associated with an increased risk of skin cancer post LT: Skin
   f. EBV, age of donor and recipient, rejection episodes are associated with increased risk of PTLD: PTLD
5. There is limited data available regarding the impact of pretransplant extrahepatic malignancies on outcomes of LT; most of the recommendations are derived from kidney transplant population.
6. A period (2–5 years) of waiting is desirable in elective LT patients with a history of preexisting malignancy.
7. However, in carefully selected sick patients, LT can be performed if the malignancy is proven to be or can be eradicated at the time of LT and type/stage of neoplasm is not associated with poor prognosis (this is most encountered with certain skin cancers, renal cell carcinoma, and prostate cancers).

Reference

Extrahepatic malignancies and liver transplantation: current status. PMID: 34276155.

Question 98

A 41-year-old male presents to the emergency room with 12 hours of nausea and vomiting. The patient is confused and unable to give a coherent history. The patient's partner reports he has been unwell for at least 2 weeks and has not worked in the last 7 days. He has been complaining of night sweats and anorexia. He has lost 12 pounds.

On exam, temperature is 38 F, pulse 110, blood pressure 126/64, O_2 saturation 96% on room air: BMI 27 kg/m^2.

He has scleral icterus, and his liver is palpable five fingerbreadths below the costal margin with a firm edge; no splenomegaly or ascites is appreciated. There is mild lower extremity edema. He is arousable but is drifting to sleep. He has asterixis.

Laboratory studies:

WBC 10, Hb 10, Platelet count 62K. Sodium 129, Cr 1.9. TBili 7.8, AST 258, ALT 314, ALP 740, GGT 986. INR 3.1. Acetaminophen level is negative. Serum ammonia level is 157.

A noncontrast CT was obtained in the emergency revealing hepatosplenomegaly and suggestion of diffuse lymphadenopathy. There is no obvious ascites.

The patient is administered NAC and IV antibiotics. He is intubated and transferred to your center. Anti-HAV IgM, HBsAg, and HCV RNA are negative. Testing for acute CMV/EBV and HSV are negative. IgG is 2300, ANA and smooth muscle are negative. Ceruloplasmin is 29.

The patient is seen by the transplant surgeon who recommends listing for liver transplant. What do you recommend?

A Status IA listing for liver transplant
B Transjugular liver biopsy
C Plasma exchange
D Exploratory laparotomy
E ERCP

B is the correct answer.

Commentary – ALF

Clinical Pearls: Acute Liver Failure

1. Defined by liver injury and coagulopathy (INR >1.5) and clinical encephalopathy (typically grade II or greater)
2. All patients with ALF should be transferred or discussed with a transplant center
3. Most common causes of ALF in the US
   a. Acetaminophen 43%
   b. Indeterminate 30%
   c. Other Drugs 8%
   d. Virus 7%
      i. Viral etiology is the most common cause worldwide
      ii. India: Hep E accounts for ~40%
         a. HEP E and pregnancy high incidence of ALF
   e. Other 13%
      i. Amanita phalloides (death cap mushroom)
         1. Early administration of activated charcoal is recommended
         2. Silibinin (milk thistle) and penicillin G are additional therapies
      ii. Methylenedioxymethamphetamine (MDMA; more commonly known as Ecstasy) synthetic derivative of amphetamine, used as a recreational drug. Clinical clues in the presentation may be hyperthermia and hypotension/collapse.
4. Chronic liver diseases that can present acutely
   a. Wilson
   b. AIH
   c. Budd Chiari
   d. HBV reactivation
   e. Alcoholic Hepatitis
5. Clinical clues/caveats
   a. ALF presenting with ascites think Budd Chiari
   b. Coombs negative hemolytic anemia, high bilirubin and low Alk Phos think Wilson
   c. Think AIH in a patient with other AI diseases, elevated gamma globulins and autoantibodies
6. Role of liver biopsy is limited. When performed, typically should be performed via transjugular to lower the risk of bleeding
   a. Main indication to perform biopsy is to rule out malignant infiltration, for example: lymphoma, as was the case in the 41-year-old male in this question stem.

Notes

Acute liver failure is one of the more dramatic presentations in all of medicine. Fortunately, it is not that common with only ~2,000 reported cases annually in the USA. Nearly half of these are acetaminophen-related. Prompt identification and referral to a transplant center is critical. It is interesting to note that liver tests are not in the definition of acute liver failure, an important point for medical students. Several prognostic scoring systems are available to identify which patients will ultimately require liver transplantation.

Reference

Acute liver failure etiology is an independent predictor of waitlist outcome but not post transplantation survival in a national cohort. PMID: 34081838.

Question 99

This product of ammonia metabolism plays a major role in the development of brain edema in patients with ALF:

A Glutamine
B *N*-acetyl-*p*-benzoquinone (NALPQI)
C Citrate
D Arginine
E Ornithine

A is the correct answer.

Commentary – ALF Management

Clinical Pearls: Management of Acute Liver Failure

1. Management
   a. Acetaminophen, ischemic injury, and HAV have the most favorable outcomes with spontaneous recovery rates ~60%
      i. Compared to drugs, autoimmune and indeterminate with only 20% recovery rates.
   b. The use of NAC in patients with acetaminophen live injury is a standard of care. Although somewhat controversial, if the boards provide a nonacetaminophen ALF case and NAC is offered as a therapeutic option – it should be chosen.
   c. Hypoglycemia increases mortality and should be corrected.
   d. Hyponatremia is detrimental and sodium levels should be maintained 140–150.
   e. Early institution of renal replacement therapy should be considered for hyper-ammonemia, control of hyponatremia, metabolic abnormalities, fluid balance, and potentially temperature control.
   f. Fresh frozen plasma (FFP) and other coagulant factors should be avoided and limited to insertion of lines and intracranial pressure (ICP) monitoring.
   g. Prophylactic antibiotics and anti-fungals have not been shown to improve survival.
   h. Regular periodic surveillance of cultures should be performed.
   i. Grade III–IV PSE should prompt intubation.
      i. Ammonia levels >200 have been associated with increased incidence of intracranial hemorrhage.
         1. Glutamine, a product of ammonia metabolism, plays a major role in the development of brain edema in ALF.
   j. Trans-cranial doppler is a useful noninvasive tool to monitor for ICP elevation and should be considered in patients with grade IV PSE and rapidly progressing grade III.
      i. Signs of ICP elevation: systemic hypertension, bradycardia, and irregular respirations (Cushing's triad).
   k. Mannitol or hypertonic saline should be administered for surges of ICP (>25 mmHg):
      i. Sustained ICP (>50) is a contraindication to transplant.
   l. Plasma exchange has been shown to improve transplant-free survival in patients with ALF and should strongly considered in nontransplant candidates.

Reference

Clinical Practical Guidelines on the management of acute (fulminant) liver failure.
   PMID: 28417882.

Question 100

All the following are poor prognostic markers in patients with acute liver failure EXCEPT?

A pH 7.14
B Phosphate 2.3
C AFP 2
D PT 71
E Interval of jaundice to onset of encephalopathy less than 7 days

B is the correct answer.

Clinical Pearls: Acute Liver Failure Prognostication

1. Nonacetaminophen Kings College (acetaminophen covered elsewhere):
   a. INR >6.5 or
   b. Three out of the following five:
      i. Etiology: indeterminate, drug-induced
      ii. Age <10 or >40
      iii. Interval jaundice-encephalopathy >7 days
      iv. TBili >17 mg/dL
      v. INR >3.5
2. Clichy
   a. PSE grade 3 or 4
   b. Factor V <20% of normal if age <30 years or
   c. Factor V <30% if age >30 years
3. An elevated or rise in AFP (marker of liver regeneration) may be associated with favorable outcome in patients with ALF.
4. Hypophosphatemia (less than 2.5) has been associated with good prognosis in ALF.
   a. Hypothesized that this is related to metabolic and synthetic demands of a liver with capacity to regenerate.

Reference

Acute liver failure: prognostic markers. PMID: 15025260.

Question 101

A 66-year-old male with NASH cirrhosis is found down. He is brought to the emergency room by ambulance. On arrival, he is barely arousable. Vitals reveal a temperature of 98.1F, HR 108, and systolic BP 88. His respirations are shallow. On examination, he has scleral icterus and spider angiomata. He has crackles in both lung bases. Abdomen is moderately distended with a shifting dullness. He has 1+ edema bilaterally.

The patient is intubated with an FiO_2 of 80% and is requiring two pressors to maintain a MAP of 60.
Sodium 121, Cr is 4.4. Lactate is 14.
WBC 22, Hb 9 with platelets of 24K. MCV is 108.
TBili is 14, AST 222, ALT 89 with an ALP of 181; Ammonia level is 357.
INR is 4.6 with a PTT of 88.
Serum alcohol level is negative.

▶ Question

How many organ failures would this patient be categorized as having?
What is the projected 28-day mortality?

A 2, 21%
B 3, 33%
C 4, 47%
D 5, 57%
E 6, 87%

E is the correct answer.

Commentary – ACLF

Clinical Pearls: Acute on Chronic Liver Failure (ACLF)

1. Syndrome characterized by acute decompensation of chronic liver disease associated with organ failures and high short-term mortality (28-day mortality).
2. Systemic inflammation is the hallmark of ACLF; elevated WBC, C-Reactive Protein, IL-6, IL-1B, IL8.
3. Identifiable triggers:
   a. Sepsis
   b. Active alcohol
   c. Viral hepatitis
   d. ½ of cases, no trigger is identified
4. Organ failure is defined based on organ-specific parameters (see table):
   a. Liver (bilirubin)
   b. Kidney (creatinine)
   c. Brain (encephalopathy)
   d. Coagulation (INR)
   e. Circulation (mean arterial pressure)
   f. Respiratory (PaO_2/FiO_2)
5. >3 organ failure translates in to 28-day mortality >80%.
6. Management is supportive and identification of the precipitating factor (bacteria/fungal infection, GI bleeding, alcohol, drug toxicity, viral infection).
7. If no contraindications, all patients admitted with ACLF should be evaluated for LT:
   a. Studies suggest only a minority of patients ~10–15% will get to transplant.

The chronic liver failure-consortium organ failure scale.

Organ system	Variable	Assigned points		
		1	2	3
Liver	Bilirubin	<6	6–12	>12
Kidney	Creatinine	<1.5	2–3.5	>3.5 or RRT
Brain	Encephalopathy grade	0	I–II	III–IV or Intubation for HE
Coagulation	INR	<2	2–2.5	>2.5
Circulation	Mean arterial pressure	>70	<70	Vasopressors
Respiration	PaO_2/FiO_2	>300	>200 to <300	<200
	SpO_2/FiO_2	>357	>214 to <357	<214 Or Mechanical ventilation

Source: Acute-on-chronic live Failure. PMID: 32459924.

Notes

There has been a large amount of literature on "acute-on-chronic liver failure" in the last decade. The most common precipitants are infection and alcohol. The prognosis minus liver transplant for patients with three or more organs failing is not good. Unfortunately, many times active infection will preclude transplantation. A table is provided based on the chronic liver failure-consortium organ failure scale.

Reference

Acute-on-chronic liver failure. PMID: 32459924.

Question 102

Review the liver biopsy slide below (hematoxylin and eosin stain 40×) in particular the structures outlined by yellow dashed lines.

▶ Question

Which of the following statements regarding this disease is FALSE?

A This disease is seen much more frequently in children than adults.
B It can recur after liver transplantation.
C The diagnosis is made based on the presence of four to five nuclei in Kupffer cells.
D The disease has been associated with various potential causes including infectious, autoimmune, drugs, and hematologic disorders.
E There is no approved treatment for this disease.

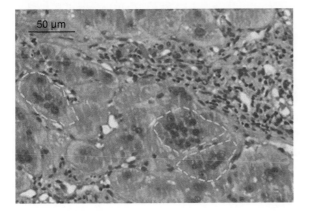

C is the correct answer.

Commentary – Giant Cell Hepatitis

Clinical Pearls: Giant Cell Hepatitis

1. The liver biopsy above reveals hepatocytes with multinucleated giant cells; more than 4–5 should be seen in a single lobule combined with other features of hepatitis.
2. The condition is rare in adults with <200 reported cases in the literature.
3. The histological findings of giant cells in adults seem to be a manifestation of hepatic stress as opposed to primary hepatic injury.
4. Giant cell hepatitis in adults has been linked with various etiologies including viral, autoimmune, drugs and hematologic disorders.
   a. Patients with an underlying AIH may respond to immunosuppressive therapy
5. Injury is variable with some patients only manifesting elevated liver tests while other develop acute liver failure and leading to death or necessitating liver transplant.
6. Recurrence of GCA after liver transplantation is not uncommon.

Notes

The liver biopsy above is from a 40-year-old female with Giant Cell Hepatitis. The dashed yellow lines outline three multinucleated giant cells. This particular patient was refractory to medical therapy and developed liver failure and is currently listed for liver transplant.

Reference

Post-infantile giant cell hepatitis: a single center's experience over 25 years. PMID: 31966907.

Question 103

All of the following are TRUE regarding liver transplantation for NASH EXCEPT?

A There is a higher incidence of diabetes and obesity at the time of liver transplant.
B The average age at listing is lower when compared to HCV and alcohol.
C The incidence of PVT is higher compared to other causes of cirrhosis.
D Despite a higher incidence of cardiovascular disease in NASH patients, the 1- and 5-year survival are comparable to the other most common indications for LT.
E NASH cirrhosis is the number one indication for LT in females.

B is the correct answer.

Commentary – NASH and LT

Clinical Pearls: NASH and LT

1. NASH is now the second leading indication for LT in the USA (behind alcohol, but in front of HCV).
2. It is the number one indication for LT in females.
3. NASH patients at the time of liver transplant are older, heavier, more diabetic, more hypertensive, with more CV disease, and renal insufficiency with a higher incidence of sarcopenia and PVT.
4. Despite these factors, the long-term outcomes are essentially equivalent (5-year survival near 80%).
5. There is data to suggest that NASH patients are more likely to be declined listing for LT due to comorbidities.
6. There are studies to suggest a "high-risk" cohort with worse outcomes: NASH patients with age >60, BMI >30 with pre-LT DM and HTN.
7. The number one cause of death in patients undergoing LT for NASH is infection; there is conflicting data on whether there is an increased risk of cardiovascular mortality post-LT.
8. NASH is the fastest growing cause of HCC in LT candidates.
9. NASH recurrence is ~35–50% at 7 years follow-up.
   a. Graft cirrhosis, however, is relatively low: less than 5% at 7 years of follow-up.
10. NAFLD in donor grafts many times precludes transplant; >30% macrovesicular steatosis is increased risk for short-term mortality following LT.

Notes

My coauthor and I were fortunate to be involved in the sentinel paper on NASH and LT. The high-risk cohort we identified (point 6 above) has come up in board questions. Although certainly not an absolute contraindication to liver transplant, caution should be taken with this subset of patients.

Reference

Outcome after liver transplantation for NASH cirrhosis. PMID: 19344467.

Question 104

The number one cause of death in noncirrhotic NASH patients is?

A HCC
B Nonliver cancer
C Variceal bleeding
D Cardiovascular disease
E Hepatorenal syndrome

D is the correct answer.

Notes
This is an incredibly important question and answer. We can't be so "liver-centric" and dismiss patients with early NAFLD because their short-term liver outlook is largely favorable. By far the number one cause of death in these patients is cardiovascular and guidance must be provided to primary care physicians in addressing risk factors. It also seems naïve to think that medications designed to treat the "liver alone" in patients with NASH, without addressing all the metabolic derangements will provide much benefit to the patient as a whole.

Reference

Non-alcoholic fatty liver disease and incident major adverse cardiovascular events: results from a nationwide histology cohort. PMID: 34489307.

Question 105

A 57-year-old female is referred to your clinic for abnormal LFTs and abnormal imaging. She has a history of type II diabetes (glycosylated Hb 8.3) and is on metformin. She also has dyslipidemia and is on a statin.

LFTS: TBili 0.4, AST 212, ALT 326, ALP 118.
A chronic workup reveals negative ANA, smooth muscle of 87, negative AMA, and IgG of 3100. US with elastography is suggestive of at least moderate fatty infiltration; kPa is 9.6 with an IQR of 11%.

Which of the following do you recommend?

A Discontinue statin
B Discontinue metformin and start pioglitazone
C MRI with PDFF and elastography
D Liver biopsy
E Vitamin E 800 IU/day

D is the correct answer.

Commentary – NAFLD

Clinical Pearls: NAFLD

1. Alcohol thresholds to exclude NAFLD: men >21 standard drinks per week. Women >14.
2. NASH defined as >5% steatosis with inflammation and hepatocyte injury (e.g. ballooning) with or without fibrosis.
3. When to biopsy remains controversial. Noninvasive testing can help to determine patients with more progressive disease.
   a. Enzymes with typical NASH 2–4× upper limits normal (ULN).
   b. Low-level autoimmune markers are not uncommon.
   c. More moderate enzyme elevations (2–300 range as in the question above) should prompt liver biopsy to rule out concomitant autoimmune hepatitis.
   d. For the boards, biopsy is required before any medical therapy is instituted.
4. Fibrosis-4 (FIB-4) and nonalcoholic fatty liver disease fibrosis (NFS) useful tools for identifying patients with NAFLD and bridging or cirrhosis.
   a. FIB4: Uses Age, AST, ALT, and platelet count.
   b. NFS: Uses Age, BMI, diabetes y/n, AST, ALT, platelet count, and albumin.
5. Weight loss of 3–5% can improve steatosis; 7–10% can improve fibrosis
6. Pharmacological therapy should generally be limited to those with biopsy proven NASH
   a. Pioglitazone improves liver histology (diabetes and non-diabetics) with biopsy proven NASH.
   b. Vitamin E 800 IU/day for nondiabetic patients with biopsy proven NASH.
   c. Obeticholic acid (OCA) in phase 3 trial showed significant improvement fibrosis after 18 months of therapy (25 mg).
   d. Subcutaneous semaglutide has been shown in a recent phase II trial to result in significantly higher NASH resolution compared to placebo (but no improvement in fibrosis).
   e. Regular coffee consumption has been shown to be beneficial in patients with chronic liver disease, in particular those with NAFLD.
7. Bariatric surgery can be considered, but it is premature for NASH to be the primary indication. Stable cirrhotic patients can be considered on a case-by-case basis.
8. Statins are safe in NASH, but should be avoided in decompensated disease.
9. *Primary* fatty liver is related to obesity and the metabolic syndrome.
10. Lysosomal acid lipase deficiency (LAL-D). A rare lysosomal storage disease. Consider this diagnosis in pediatric patients with elevated liver tests, fatty liver on imaging, and high LDL and low HDL. Defect in the LIPA gene. Should also be considered in lean young adults with fatty liver. Microvesicular steatosis is a classic feature on histology.

11. Patients with hypopituitarism and hypothalamic commonly develop metabolic syndrome. These patients can develop progressive fatty liver in a much shorter timeframe than typically NAFLD patients.
12. Rarer causes of fatty liver (other than alcohol) include
    a. HCV GT 3
    b. Wilson
    c. Lipodystrophy
    d. Starvation
    e. TPN
    f. Abetalipoproteinemia
    g. Medications (amiodarone, methotrexate, tamoxifen, steroids)

Reference

Non-alcoholic fatty liver disease. PMID: 33894145.

Question 106

The most important histological feature of NAFLD associated with long-term mortality is the following:

A Macrovesicular steatosis
B Ballooning degeneration
C Lobular inflammation
D Apoptotic bodies
E Fibrosis

E is the correct answer.

Commentary – NAFLD

Clinical Pearls: NAFLD

1. The worldwide prevalence of NALFD is estimated at 25%:
   a. Prevalence is highest in the Middle East and South America ~30%
   b. Lowest Africa 14%
2. Ethnic differences in NAFLD may be related to genetic variation related to patatin-like phospholipase domain-containing protein 3: *PNPLA-3* gene
3. Prevalence of NASH (the progressive form of NAFLD) in the general population is ~5%.
4. Patients with NAFLD have increased overall mortality.
5. The most common cause of death is cardiovascular.
   a. Followed by malignancy and the liver-related complications.
6. The most important histological feature of NAFLD associated with long-term mortality is fibrosis.
7. There is some data on the risk of HCC in noncirrhotic NAFLD:
   a. Guidelines, however, recommend limiting surveillance imaging to those with cirrhosis.
8. Up to ~70% of patients with cryptogenic cirrhosis are suspected to have "burned out" NAFLD.

Reference

Epidemiology, pathogenesis, diagnosis and emerging treatment of nonalcoholic fatty liver disease. PMID: 33334622.

Question 107

A 26-year-old mother is referred to your clinic when prenatal testing reveals a positive anti-HCV and anti-HBc. She is in her third trimester and is doing well other than some mild lower extremity edema.

Further testing reveals: TBili 0.6, AST 19, ALT 21, ALP 167, GGT 32.
HCV RNA 1.3 million IU/mL; HIV negative; HBsAg negative, anti-HBs 0.

The mother is concerned about the transmission of HCV to her child. Which of the following would you recommend?

A An elective C-section in order to decrease transmission rate.
B She should not breastfeed after delivery for fear of increasing transmission rate.
C Her elevated ALP is cause for concern and a discussion should be had regarding HCV therapy with combination Peg-IFN and Ribavirin during her pregnancy.
D Her ALP is likely related to ICP which has been associated with HCV and the baby should be delivered at 37 weeks to decrease fetal respiratory complications.
E Her child should be tested for HCV by testing anti-HCV after 18 months.

E is the correct answer.

Reference

Hepatitis C virus in neonates, and infants. PMID: 34030818.

Question 108

A 67-year-old African American female is seen in your clinic to discuss treatment options for her chronic HCV. The patient was diagnosed 7 years ago but never sought treatment. She is obese with a BMI of 36 kg/m^2 and poorly controlled diabetes. She has been clean from all illicit drugs for 4 years. She does admit to daily marijuana and averages about 4–6 beers daily.

Blood work reveals: HCV RNA 3.9 million, GT 3a disease.
HBsAg negative, anti-HBc total positive, anti-HBs 39.
HIV negative.

All of the following patient factors have been linked with progression to cirrhosis EXCEPT:

A Diabetes and obesity
B Alcohol consumption
C Female sex
D GT 3 disease
E Age

C is the correct answer.

Commentary – HCV

Clinical Pearls: Natural History of HCV

1. Hepatitis C was discovered in 1989.
2. HCV infection becomes 'chronic' in ~50–80% of those infected.
   a. 10–20% of patients will end up developing end-stage disease and complications over a period of 20–30 years.
3. Global prevalence of HCV in 2015 was 1%.
4. Six countries account for >50% of cases: China, Pakistan, Nigeria, Egypt, India, and Russia.
5. The World Health Organization (WHO) set a target of 90% reduction in incident cases and 65% reduction in mortality by 2030.
6. Risk factors for HCV include the following:
   a. IVDU
      i. Data show efficacy and cost-effectiveness of opioid substitution therapy and needle and syringe programs in reducing primary infection and re-infection.
   b. Vertical transmission ~6% (can be as high as 15% in mothers coinfected with HIV):
      i. Children born to HCV-positive mothers should undergo anti-HCV testing after the age of 18 months.
   c. Sexual
      i. Patients with high-risk sexual activity (heterosexual >50 partners) or men who have sex with men should be tested annually.
      ii. All patients with HIV or HBV.
      iii. Blood transfusion prior to 1992.
      iv. Long-term hemodialysis.
      v. Reusing glass syringes.
      vi. Needlestick injury.
      vii. Unregulated tattoo.
7. In 2012 CDC recommended screening all baby-boomers (born in the birth cohort: 1945–1965) and expanded it to all adults over age 18 (and all pregnant women during each pregnancy) in 2020.
8. Currently, there are eight known genotypes with 86 subtypes:
   a. GT 3 seems to run a more aggressive course including increased risk of HCC.
   b. GT 3 has emerged as the most difficult HCV genotype to treat.
9. Patients with HCV + cirrhosis have a 4–5% cumulative annual incidence of HCC.

---

10. Progression to cirrhosis is accelerated by the following factors:
    a. Older age
    b. Male sex
    c. Alcohol
    d. Coinfection (HBV, HIV) or other infectious agents (schistosomiasis)
    e. DM
    f. concomitant hepatic steatosis
    g. GT 3 disease

Reference

History of hepatitis C. Gastroenterol Clin North Am. PMID: 26600216.

Question 109

A 33-year-old male patient recently relocated to your area and establishes care with a PCP. The patient was diagnosed with HCV 18 months ago. He has not used drugs for nearly 4 years. The patient was found to have HCV GT 2 disease. His pretreatment viral load is 57K. A pretreatment ultrasound with elastography reveals a normal appearing liver with a kPa of 3.1 with an IQR of 10%. He completed an 8-week course of glecaprevir/pibrentasvir 6 months ago.

Laboratory studies:

WBC 8, Hb 14, Platelets 356. LFTs are normal. HIV is negative. HBsAg negative, anti-HBc negative, anti-HBs >1000.
His physical exam is normal.
Anti-HCV is 32. HCV RNA is undetectable.
The PCP refers the patient to you. You recommend?

A Annual HCV PCR for an additional 4 years (document a total of 5 years of UD virus).
B No further liver-related follow-up is necessary.
C Check HCV GT to confirm clearance.
D Six-month US and AFP for HCC surveillance.
E Repeat US with elastography to ensure stability or regression in kPa.

Question 110

Which of the following is FALSE regarding Sofosbuvir?

A It is a NS5B polymerase inhibitor.
B It is not FDA-approved for patients with CKD stage 4 or 5.
C It is contraindicated in patients postkidney transplant.
D It exhibits a high barrier to the development of resistance.
E The combination of Sofosbuvir/Voxilaprevir/Velpatasvir should not be administered in patients with Childs C cirrhosis.

Question 111

You are evaluating a 53-year-old male patient for HCV therapy. The patient is a veteran of the Gulf War. He was diagnosed with HCV 10 years ago. He is treatment naive. Exam reveals palmar erythema and a palpable spleen and mild edema.

Laboratory studies:

WBC 6, Hb 13.5, Platelets 78K. TBili 2.3 (unconj 1.6), AST 48, ALT 48, ALP 152. Na 140, Cr 1; Albumin 3.4, INR 1.3
HCV GT 3 with a HCV RNA of 57K. HBsAg negative, anti-HBc total negative, anti-HBs negative. HIV is negative.
NS5A resistance testing returns positive.
An ultrasound reveals coarsened hepatic echotexture with hepatofugal flow and enlarged spleen and small ascites. EGD shows no varices and mild portal hypertensive gastropathy.
What HCV regimen would give this patient that highest chance of achieving an SVR?

A Defer on treatment and refer for liver transplant
B Glecaprevir/Pibrentasvir × 16 weeks
C Glecaprevir/Pibrentasvir and low-dose Ribavirin (600 mg) × 12 weeks
D Sofosbuvir/Velpatasvir and weight-based Ribavirin × 12 weeks
E Pegylated interferon and weight-based Ribavirin × 24 weeks

109 – B is the correct answer.
110 – C is the correct answer.
111 – D is the correct answer.

Commentary – HCV Treatment

Clinical Pearls: HCV Treatment

1. HCV treatment should be offered to all infected individuals.
   a. The only exception is those with a life expectancy of 1 year or less.
2. The goal of therapy is to achieve a sustained virological response (SVR) defined as negative viral load 12 weeks after completion of therapy:
   a. SVR is associated with improved liver morbidity and mortality and all-cause morbidity and mortality including a significant reduction in risk of HCC:
      i. Those with METAVIR score of $\geq$3 require continued surveillance for HCC.
   b. Improvement in Quality-of-Life Scores.
   c. Improvement in cardiovascular, renal, and metabolic diseases.
3. Direct acting anti-virals (DAA) target three proteins involved in the HCV life cycle:
   a. NS3/4A protease
   b. NS5B polymerase
   c. NS5A protein
4. Protease inhibitors includes suffix – *previr*: Glecaprevir, Voxilaprevir, Grazoprevir.
5. NS5A inhibitors include the suffix – *asvir*: Ledipasvir, Velpatasvir, Elbasvir.
6. NS5B polymerase inhibitors include the suffix – *buvir*: Sofosbuvir.
7. Some form of pretreatment noninvasive fibrosis testing is recommended for all individuals.
8. Resistance testing: AASLD currently recommends baseline testing for the nonstructural protein-5A (NS5A) Tyr93His RAS (Y93H) in GT 3 cirrhotic patients:
   a. If Y93H is present, ribavirin should be added to the SOF-VEL (Epclusa) or SOF-VEL-VOX (Vosevi) regimen to maintain an SVR >95%.
   b. Those without evidence of resistance can be treated with 12-week regimen.
   c. Similar testing is recommended if using elbasvir–grazoprevir (Zepatier) for patients with GT 1a infection.

Regimens

1. Current simplified treatment regimen for noncirrhotic patients.
   a. Glecaprevir/Pibrentasvir (G/P) $\times$ 8 weeks.
   b. Sofosbuvir/Velpatasvir (SOF/VEL) $\times$ 12 weeks.
   c. No liver-related follow-up is recommended for noncirrhotic patients who achieve SVR.
2. Simplified treatment for compensated cirrhosis:
   a. G/P $\times$ 8 weeks GT 1-6
   b. SOF/VEL $\times$ 12 weeks, GT 1-6
3. Decompensated cirrhosis (Childs B/C):
   a. should be treated by experts in the field or transplant centers.
   b. protease inhibitors are contraindicated in decompensated cirrhosis.

    c. Ribavirin eligible:
        i. Sofosbuvir/Ledipasvir and Ribavirin (Riba) × 12 weeks.
        ii. SOF/VEL and Riba × 12 weeks.
    d. Ribavirin ineligible:
        i. SOF/LED × 24 weeks.
        ii. SOF/VEL × 24 weeks.
    e. Prior failure of SOF or NS5A-based treatment failure:
        i. SOF/LED and Riba × 24 weeks
        ii. SOF/VEL and Riba × 24 weeks
4. SOF-based treatment failures:
    a. SOF/VEL/Voxilaprevir (VOX) × 12 weeks
    b. G/P × 16 weeks
5. G/P treatment failures
    a. G/P and SOF and Riba × 16 weeks
    b. SOF/VEL/VOX × 12 weeks:
        i. For those with compensated cirrhosis recommendation to add Riba.
6. SOF/VEL/VOX failures:
    a. G/P and SOF and Riba × 16 weeks.
    b. SOF/VEL/VOX and Riba × 24 weeks
7. Drug-Drug-Interactions to be aware of for the boards:
    a. Phenytoin, Phenobarbital, Carbamazepine, Rifampin, and St. John Wort (all CYP3A inducers) should not be administered with SOF containing regimens or G/P as they can decrease DAA and potentially lower chances of SVR.
    b. Ethinyl estradiol should not be administered with G/P given risk in ALT elevation.
    c. Amiodarone should not be administered with any SOF containing regimen given risk of severe bradycardia.
    d. Caution with statins and G/P as the combination can increase the concentration of statins and lead to myopathy and rhabdomyolysis.

Notes

Direct-acting antivirals have completely changed the landscape of liver disease. HCV therapy nowadays is relatively simple in clinical practice. That being said, it is a difficult subject to condense given the multiple available regimens. We focused on the most commonly prescribed regimens and nuanced points that the boards may test you on; see "caveats" to the HCV therapy section.

Reference

Hepatitis C guidance: AASLD-IDSA recommendations for testing, managing, and treating adults infected with hepatitis C virus. PMID: 26111063.

Question 112

A 37-year former intravenous drug user is referred to your clinic for HCV therapy. The patient has been clean from drugs for 8 months. He is accompanied by his partner who you also manage for HBV.

The patient complains of fatigue and joint pains and is anxious to get started on treatment.

Physical exam is normal.

Laboratory studies:

HCV GT 1a, VL 6.2 million. HIV negative. HBsAg positive, anti-HBc total positive, anti-HBs negative, HbeAg negative, anti-HBe positive; HBV DNA negative
WBC 6, Hb 12, Platelets 222. TBili 1.1, AST 44, ALT 57, ALP 121. AFP 3. Cr 1.
An ultrasound normal with elastography: kPa of 7.7; IQR 13% no lesions. The liver appears normal.

What do you recommend?

A Initiate tenofovir concurrently with Glecaprevir/Pibrentasvir (G/P) × 8 weeks. Discontinue tenofovir 12 weeks after DAA therapy is completed.
B G/P × 8 weeks.
C SOF/LED × 12 weeks.
D Defer on treatment until patient is clean from drugs × 1 year.
E Tenofovir lead in (4 weeks) and then concurrently with G/P for an additional 8 weeks.

A is the correct answer.

Reference

Hepatitis B virus reactivation during direct-acting antiviral therapy for hepatitis C: a systematic review and meta-analysis. PMID: 29371017.

Question 113

A 56-year-old male with HIV/HCV is referred to your clinic for HCV therapy. The patient's HIV is under good control with an undetectable viral load and CD-4 count of 440. His other medical history includes anal condyloma, diet-controlled diabetes, HTN, depression, and recurrent UTIs. The patient lives with his partner. He does enjoy a few glasses of wine on weekends.

He is HCV GT 1a with a VL of 83,000 IU/mL. HBsAg negative, anti-HBc total positive, anti-HBs 3. Anti-HAV total positive. An ultrasound is normal and bedside FibroScan reveals a kPa of 7.7 with an IQR of 12%; CALP is 218 dB/m. CBC and renal function are normal. TBili 1.0, AST 63, ALT 71, ALP 108.

His exam is normal. BMI is 28 kg/m^2.

His current medications include combination HIV medication (bictegravir, emtricitabine, tenofovir alafenamide) and lisinopril.

What do you recommend for treatment?

A G/P and Entecavir × 12 weeks
B G/P × 12 weeks
C G/P and Entecavir × 8 weeks
D G/P × 8 weeks
E G/P 8 weeks; Entecavir × 24 weeks

D is the correct answer.

Commentary

Clinical Pearls: Caveats to HCV Treatment for the Boards

1. Coinfection with HIV:
   a. Up to 25% of patients with HIV have coinfection with HCV.
   b. For the most part treatment regimens are similar to non-HIV patients.
   c. Treatment of HIV/HCV coinfected patients does require attention to complex drug–drug interactions between DAA and antiretroviral medications, but it is unlikely that these will be tested on.
2. Renal failure:
   a. The major metabolite of sofosbuvir, GS-331007 accumulates during renal impairment.
   b. SOF is not recommended in patients with stage 4 or 5 CKD.
3. Coinfection with HBV:
   a. HBsAg, anti-HBc total, and anti-HBs should be checked on all patients before DAA therapy.
   b. Studies suggest reactivation of HBV can be as high as 24% in HBsAg-positive patients:
      i. 1.4% in patients with resolved HBV.
   c. If HBsAg is positive, concurrent HBV nucleoside analogue therapy is advised. Treatment should be continued 12 weeks after DAA therapy is stopped.
   d. Monitoring of LFTs is reasonable in patients who are HBV isolated anti-HBc total positive.
4. Pediatric populations:
   a. FDA has approved G/P for adolescents (aged 12–17).
   b. SOF and LED have been approved for children 3 years or older with GT 1, 4, 5, and 6.
5. Decompensated disease, when to treat?
   a. BE3A score: BMI, PSE, ascites, ALT, and albumin identifies patients who will benefit from DAA therapy.
   b. Patients with decompensated cirrhosis who have MELD scores of 18–20 or higher will benefit from transplant first than DAA therapy.
   c. Protease inhibitors should be avoided in decompensated cirrhosis.
6. If HCV is active at time of transplant, recurrence of HCV in allograft is universal:
   a. DAA therapy is safe and effective after solid organ transplantation with similar SVR rates without increased risk of rejection.
7. Use of HCV positive donors:
   a. Expands donor pool, increases access, and is cost-effective.
   b. Given high rate of SVR, HCV-positive organs can be considered for HCV positive and negative recipients.

---

c. The use of HCV donor grafts does require detailed informed consent about risk of FCH and membranous nephropathy and also requires histological assessment of liver graft quality and assured early access to DAA therapy posttransplant.

8. HCC
   a. SVR with DAA reduces the individual risk of HCC by 63%.
   b. Risk of de novo HCC is reduced after SVR.
   c. The risk of recurrent HCC is *not* increased after DAA therapy.
   d. AGA recommends deferring DAA therapy for 4–6 months to confirm response to therapy in patients who undergo treatment for HCC.
   e. Despite achievement of SVR, all patients with cirrhosis should continue standard surveillance.

Reference

AASLD-IDSA recommendations for testing, managing, and treating adults infected with hepatitis C virus. PMID: 26111063.

Question 114

All of the following extrahepatic disease have been linked with HCV infection EXCEPT:

A Type II cryoglobulinemia
B B-cell Non-Hodgkin's lymphoma
C Fatigue and decreased quality of life score
D Pulmonary sarcoidosis
E Necrolytic acral erythema

D is the correct answer.

Commentary – Extrahepatic HCV

1. Renal disease:
   a. Type I MPGN
   b. FSGS
2. Lymphoproliferative disease:
   a. Essential mixed cryoglobulinemia (also called type II cryo):
      i. Leads to deposition of circulating immune complexes into small and medium blood vessels. 90% of patients with essential mixed cryo have HCV:
         1. Leukocytoclastic vasculitis with palpable purpura and petechiae, arthralgia, renal disease (usually MPGN), neurological disease, and hypocomplementemia (see images below).

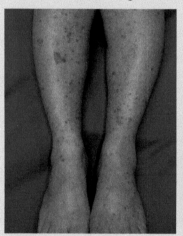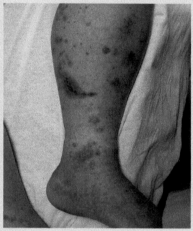

   b. B-cell non-Hodgkin lymphoma (including diffuse large B cell, marginal zone, splenic, MALT and hepatosplenic T-cell lymphoma).
      i. Prevalence of HCV in patients with NHL ~15%.
3. Skin disease:
   a. Porphyria cutanea tarda (see image of hands below):
      i. Disease caused by markedly reduced hepatic uroporphyrinogen decarboxylase resulting in accumulation of uroporphyrins in blood and urine:
         1. Blistering photosensitivity; photosensitivity to sun leads to erythema, vesicles, and bullae.
      ii. All patients with PCT should be investigated for HCV (prevalence up to 50%) in addition to HIV and genetic hemochromatosis.

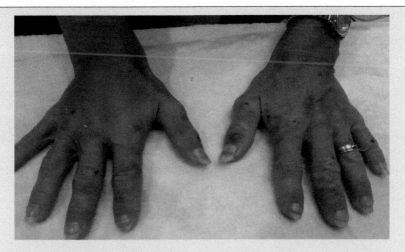

b. Lichen Planus (see images below): Flat-topped, violaceous, pruritic papules with generalized distribution. Can involve mucus membranes, hair, and nails.

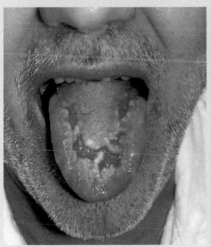 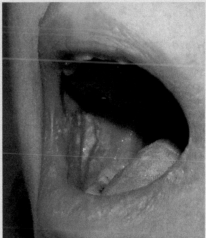

   c. Necrolytic acral erythema: Rare cutaneous disease associated with HCV: violaceous plaques extend from the distal interphalangeal joint to fingertips.

4. Eye disease:
   a. Sjogren's syndrome
   b. Mooren's ulcer
5. Thyroid disease:
   a. Antithyroid antibodies are present in 5–17% of patients with HCV.
6. ITP and Autoimmune hemolytic anemia.
7. Atherosclerotic coronary disease.
8. There is an association with HCV and insulin resistance and diabetes (OR 1.7).

(Continued)

(Continued)

9. Fatigue.
10. Lower health-related quality of life (QOL):
    a. QOL improves after SVR.

Notes

Extrahepatic manifestations of viral hepatitis are always a favorite board subject and a favorite "wards" question to ask on rounds. I want to thank dermatologist, Dr. Joseph English, for the wonderful photos included in this section.

Reference

Hepatitis C. PMID: 31631857.

Question 115

A 63-year-old male is evaluated by a local gastroenterologist for "cirrhosis." His chronic liver serological evaluation is notable for an ANA of 1 : 80; the remainder of his blood tests are negative. Imaging reveals a shrunken, cirrhotic-appearing liver with small ascites.

Other notable labs include WBC 4, Hb 9.4, platelets 57K. Normal renal function. TBili 1.3, AST 67, ALT 45, ALP 119. INR is 1.5.

A percutaneous liver biopsy is performed.

Five days later, the patient presents with melena and SOB. He is complaining of RUQ pain with radiation to his right shoulder. Exam reveals HR 110, BP 96, RR 16, 93% RA. Conjunctival pallor and mild scleral icterus. The patient is tender in his RUQ.

Laboratory studies:

TBili 2.6, AST 72, ALT 40, ALP 128. WBC 9, Hb 5.9, platelets 57K. INR 1.5.

The patient undergoes a noncontrast CT scan reveals no free air or hemoperitoneum. There is scant new "ascites." The patient has another melanic stool in the ER. He is administered 2 units of blood with improvement in his vital signs and appropriate response in his hemoglobin. An urgent endoscopy is performed with the following finding:

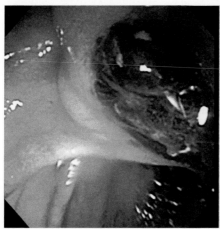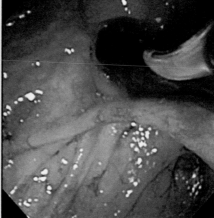

What do you recommend?

A Clipping of the bleeding source
B Band ligation of the bleeding source
C IR consult for angiography and embolization
D Antibiotics and conservative management
E Octreotide and IV antibiotics

C is the correct answer.

Commentary – Liver Biopsy

Clinical Pearls: Liver Biopsy

1. Bleeding with liver biopsy risk is 0.05%; patient should be observed 2–4 hours after biopsy.
   a. Anti-platelet agents should be held ~5 days before liver biopsy. Can be resumed 2–3 days post.
   b. Warfarin also should be held for 5 days and can be resumed the day after.
   c. Heparin 12–24 hours pre biopsy.
   d. Hemobilia presents with classic (Quincke's) triad of GIB, biliary pain, and jaundice. This results from fistulous communication between the portal vein and the biliary tree. Bleeding is usually arterial. Typically presents after 5 days. Clot within the bile duct can rarely lead to cholangitis:
      i. Transcatheter arterial embolization is treatment of choice for significant active bleeding:
         1. Bilhemia, passage of bile into the bloodstream on the other hand is characterized by a rapid rise in total and direct serum bilirubin without other signs of hepatic dysfunction or biliary obstruction. It is typically related to hepatic trauma. The pathophysiology is related to the pressure gradient between the common bile duct (typically ~12 mmHg) and the hepatic vein (~5 mmHg) which results in the direct flow of bile into the hepatic vein.
2. Infectious complications appear to be increased in posttransplant patients with choledochojejunostomy.
3. All patients who undergo liver biopsy should ideally have imaging prebiopsy to evaluate for Chilaiditi syndrome wherein the colon is abnormally positioned between the liver and diaphragm, intrahepatic gallbladder, and focal vascular lesions.
4. Biopsy in setting of thrombocytopenia (i.e. less than 60K) or elevated INR should be based on local practice and expertise. TEG may be helpful for a more accurate bleeding risk assessment in such patients. DDAVP may be considered in patients with renal failure or on HD.
5. Transjugular approach should be considered in patients with:
   a. Small cirrhotic livers
   b. Ascites
   c. Morbidly obese
   d. When HVPG is desired
6. Contraindications to liver biopsy:
   a. Uncooperative patients
   b. High risk of bleeding (see above):

i. Risk of bleeding with liver biopsy in patients with suspected hepatic amyloid has been reported at 5%.
7. Specimen adequacy:
   a. Recommendations are to use 16–18 g caliber needle, specimen length between 2 and 3 cm resulting in >11 portal tracts.

Notes

An endoscopic image of hemobilia post liver biopsy is shown here. This section also allowed me an excuse to use one of my favorite hepatology words: bilhemia; learn what it means and impress your friends, but it is very unlikely to be tested on.

Reference

Liver biopsy. PMID: 19243014.

Question 116

A 68-year-old male with a history of HCV and minimal fibrosis was successfully treated 6 years ago and discharged from the clinic. He presents now to the ER with 4 days of left lower quadrant abdominal pain. He has had low-grade fevers for 2 days, but this morning recorded a temperature of 101.6 F. He endorses anorexia and some night sweats.

The patient acquired his HCV from a blood transfusion many years ago. He has now achieved an SVR. Pretreatment elastography revealed a kPa of 4.2 (IQR 12%). The patient underwent a colonoscopy 2 years ago with good bowel prep revealing moderate left-sided diverticulosis and some small hyperplastic polyps.

On exam the patient is in some distress complaining of abdominal pain. His temperature is 100.1, HR 102, BP 138/60. Abdominal exam: tender diffusely, but especially in left lower quadrant.

Laboratory studies:

WBC of 18K with 92% neutrophils. TBili 1.2, AST 23, ALT 26, ALP 149. BMP normal. A contrast CT scan is obtained in the ER.
What do you recommend?

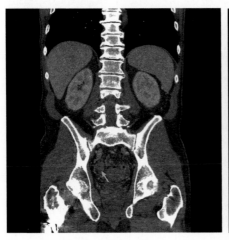 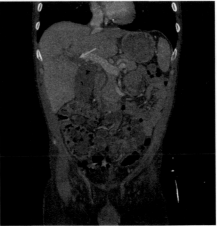

A Colonoscopy
B IV antibiotic and heparin drip
C CT enterography
D Thrombolytics
E IVC filter

B is the correct answer.

Commentary – PVT

Clinical Pearls: Portal Vein Thrombosis (PVT) Non-Cirrhotic

1. All venous thromboses are multifactorial; Virchow's triad: hypercoagulability, endothelial injury, and reduced blood flow.
2. Without cirrhosis?
   a. A systemic hypercoagulable state is often implicated:
      i. Myeloproliferative neoplasms: polycythemia vera (PCV), essential thrombocythemia, primary myelofibrosis, JAK2 V617, Factor V Leiden, *Prothrombin* gene mutation (G20210A), Protein C and S deficiency, Antithrombin deficiency.
      ii. Acquired thrombophilia: antiphospholipid syndrome (APLS), paroxysmal nocturnal hemoglobinuria (PHN).
   b. Other systemic risk factors: autoimmune disease and vasculitis, inflammatory bowel disease, pregnancy, exogenous hormones.
   c. Local factors: intrabdominal infection (pancreatitis, umbilical vein sepsis, cholecystitis, diverticulitis – illustrated in this case example). Trauma, abdominal malignancy, and surgery (splenectomy, Whipple procedure, gastric bypass, liver-related surgery included transplantation).
3. Most common presentation of acute, noncirrhotic PVT is abdominal pain and fever. Extension of PVT into the superior mesenteric vein (SMV) is much more likely to present with bowel ischemia and infarct (rare however in only 2% of cases). LFTs are usually normal. Transient small ascites can be seen.
4. AC should be initiated at diagnosis:
   a. Rates of recanalization are ~40%.
   b. Minimum treatment duration of 6 months (but may vary depending on etiology).
   c. If there is progression of thrombus despite medical therapy, then there may be a role for thrombolysis or surgery.
5. Patients with unrecognized or untreated acute PVT or those who don't respond are at risk of developing portal cavernoma: extrahepatic PV obstruction with or without thrombosis of the intrahepatic branches.
   a. These patients are at high risk of developing varices: ascites and encephalopathy are less common manifestations.

Notes

Coronal images provided here from the same patient show colonic diverticulitis and near-complete portal vein thrombosis. The management approaches for PVT in patients with cirrhosis and those without are slightly different. We discuss both scenarios.

Reference

Diagnosis, development, and treatment of portal vein thrombosis in patients with and without cirrhosis. PMID: 30771355.

Question 117

A 23-year-old college student presents to your hospital with massive hematemesis. After stabilization, an urgent endoscopy reveals multiple columns of large esophageal varices with red wale signs. Five bands are placed, and the patient is placed on combination octreotide and antibiotics. Liver function tests are normal and synthetic parameters are preserved. Imaging reveals a noncirrhotic liver with acute sub occlusive thrombus in the main portal vein and splenic vein with a 15 cm spleen. Hepatic veins are patent.

The patient is diagnosed with G20210A mutation, and hematology is recommending anti-coagulation. What do you recommend?

A Nonselective beta-blocker, serial esophageal band ligation, and continue anti-coagulation.
B TIPS and anticoagulation.
C Surgical devascularization.
D Surgical spleno-renal shunt.
E Splenic artery embolization.

B is the correct answer.

Commentary – PVT in Cirrhosis

Clinical Pearls: Portal Vein Thrombosis in the Setting of Underlying Cirrhosis

1. PVT is related to factors of Virchow's triad. In patients with cirrhosis unique factors include the following:
   a. Static blood flow from PHTN.
   b. Portosystemic shunt leading to "steal."
   c. Malignancy.
   d. Inherited thrombophilia: Factor V Leiden, Prothrombin Gene mutation (G20210A).
   e. Acquired thrombophilia: increased factor VIII, Protein C&S deficiency, antithrombin deficiency.
   f. NASH.
      i. Studies suggest patients with NASH cirrhosis have the highest incidence of PVT at the time of LT.
   g. Local factors: HC, surgery, local regional therapy (trans-arterial chemoembolization, radioembolization), TIPS.
2. Studies have not clearly shown a benefit from genetic thrombophilia testing in all patients with cirrhosis and PVT.
3. Distinguishing between malignant and "bland" PVT is critical. Radiographic features and AFP may be helpful; in some cases, there is role for biopsy.
4. The most recent purposed classification of PVT in cirrhotic relies on anatomic descriptors, the timing of thrombosis, and relationship to clinical sequelae.
5. Annual incidence of PVT in patients with cirrhosis: 10–15%.
6. PVT is typically found incidentally, but should be suspect in any cirrhotic patient with worsening decompensation:
   a. On the flip side a prospective study from Italy showed that preventing the development PVT has been associated with decreased hepatic decompensation and improved survival.
7. Spontaneous resolution of (namely nonocclusive) PVT has been reported in up to 40% of cases.
8. Most experts recommend the use of AC in cirrhotic patients who are candidates for transplantation:
   a. To prevent progression (namely into SMV).
   b. And promote recanalization.
9. Ideally anti-coagulation should be started within six months of diagnosis of clot (increases rates of recanalization by 30%).
   a. Direct oral anticoagulants (DOACs) are now being used more widely in clinical practice due to acceptable safety profile without the need for blood monitoring; however, data are limited at this time to allow full recommendation.

b. EGD is required to assess for varices and appropriate prophylaxis (nonselective beta blockade or endoscopic band ligation) is recommended.
c. In patients presenting with acute PVT and variceal bleed, TIPS and AC is the treatment of choice.
   i. Studies suggest AC does not increase risk of bleeding or mortality.

Reference

Diagnosis, development, and treatment of portal vein thrombosis in patients with and without cirrhosis. PMID: 30771355.

Question 118

A 62-year-old female with rheumatoid arthritis is referred to you for "cirrhosis." The patient was referred to hematology for chronic thrombocytopenia. A bone marrow biopsy revealed tri-lineage hematopoiesis. A CT scan with contrast revealed a mildly nodular liver with splenomegaly (16 cm) and significant portal hypertension with a recanalized umbilical vein and a portal vein measuring 1.9 cm in diameter. Hepatic and portal veins are patent.

Past Medical History: Rheumatoid arthritis. She has a history of deep venous thrombosis many years ago following hip surgery. Medications include Aspirin, Azathioprine, Celecoxib, and a multivitamin. She has no high-risk behavior.

On exam the patient has splenomegaly and caput medusa, but no cutaneous stigmata of liver disease.

Laboratory studies:

WBC 3.2, Hb 10.4, Platelets 52K. TBili 1, AST 22, ALT 33, ALP 187, GGT 74. INR 1. Albumin 4.2

A complete chronic liver workup is negative.

An EGD reveals grade II EV with moderate gastropathy. A colonoscopy is normal.

A transjugular liver biopsy is performed. Free hepatic pressure is 7 mmHg, wedged pressure is 20 mmHg.

The pathologist contacts you after reviewing the electronic medical records and is surprised that there does not appear to be significant fibrosis. She states the biopsy specimen is adequate with 17 portal tracts. What do you recommend helping establish the diagnosis?

A Intraoperative examination of liver with wedge biopsy
B MRI/MRCP with elastography
C Reticulin stain on biopsy specimen
D Ultrasound with Doppler
E Bone marrow Biopsy

C is the correct answer.

Commentary – NRH and NCPHTN

Clinical Pearls: Nodular Regenerative Hyperplasia (NRH) and Noncirrhotic PHTN

1. An uncommon condition characterized by the diffuse transformation of normal hepatic parenchyma into small, regenerative nodules with little to no fibrosis.
2. Believed to be a hyperproliferative response to obstructive portal venopathy.
3. On gross exam of liver, nodules are small 1–3 mm in size. Superficially may resemble cirrhosis and may have a cirrhotic appearance on imaging.
4. NRH is a histological diagnosis; it is most easily made using a reticulin stain demonstrating nodules with expanded liver cell plates surrounded by zones of reticulin compression.

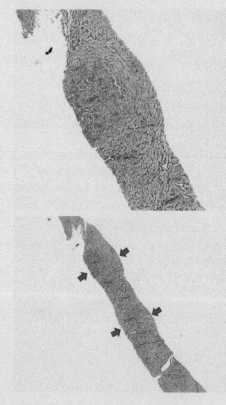

5. NRH has been associated with numerous conditions:
   a. Vascular abnormalities, namely of the portal vein.
   b. Drugs, especially azathioprine.
   c. Polyarteritis nodosa, rheumatoid arthritis
   d. Early PBC
   e. Antiphospholipid syndrome
   f. Posttransplantation, postmajor liver surgery

6. Many patients may be asymptomatic; 25% of patients will have mild elevation in ALP.
7. The most clinically significant clinical complication is the development of portal hypertension:
   a. NRH should be on the differential of patients who present with unexplained PHTN.
   b. TIPS and surgical shunts are good options in NRH patients with complications that can't be medically managed.
8. Infection with parasite schistosomiasis is the most common cause of noncirrhotic PHTN worldwide:
   a. Diagnosis is made by detection of schistosomal eggs in stool:
      i. Anthelminthic treatment (praziquantel) with cure rates of >80%.
9. Idiopathic noncirrhotic portal hypertension (INCPH) is characterized by PHTN in the absence of
   a. Biopsy proven cirrhosis, obstruction of PV or hepatic veins, and other causes of PHTN.

Notes

NRH is another one of my favorite diagnoses to make. It is somewhat underrecognized, especially in patients post solid organ transplant. The biopsy specimen here is a reticulin stain highlighting minimal fibrosis but clear "nodules," highlighted by the blue arrows. When a patient presents posttransplant with PHTN, and all the pieces don't seem to fit? think NRH and pursue a transjugular liver biopsy with gradients.

Reference

Nodular regenerative hyperplasia: Not all nodules are created equal. PMID: 16799965.

Question 119

A 57-year-old male with a history of COPD and CAD is evaluated by his family physician with complaints of severe pain and burning in his right shin. The patient complains of increasing fatigue and unintentional weight loss.

Exam reveals temperature of 100.2 F, HR 94, BP 156/88, RR 14 with O_2 saturation of 96% on room air. BMI is 30 kg/m^2. Examination of his right leg revealed significant hyperalgesia to even light touch. Representative images are shown below.

WBC 14, Hb 14, Platelets 444. Normal renal function. TBili 1, AST 98, ALT 118, ALP 157. HCV Ab negative. HBsAg positive, anti-HBc total positive, anti-HBs negative, HBeAg negative, anti-HBe positive. HBV DNA pending.

What is the most likely diagnosis?

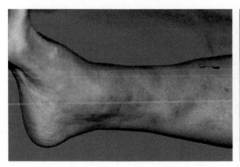 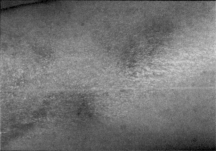

A   Polyarteritis nodosa
B   Lichen planus
C   Non-Hodgkin's lymphoma
D   Porphyria cutanea tards
E   Type II cryoglobulinemia

A is the correct answer.

Commentary – Extrahepatic HBV

Clinical Pearls: Extrahepatic Manifestations of Chronic HBV

1. Most of the extrahepatic manifestations of hepatitis B are viral–antigen driven and associated with immune complex deposition. Extrahepatic manifestations associated with HBV are not as common as HCV.
2. Vasculitides: cryoglobulinemic vasculitis and leukocytoclastic vasculitis; the most severe and well established however is
   a. Polyarteritis nodosa (PAN): systemic necrotizing vasculitis affecting the medium and small arteries. It is not associated with ANCA. HBV infection is now considered one of the criteria for the diagnosis of PAN vasculitis.
   b. Clinical presentation of PAN includes fever, weight loss, and fatigue. All organs can be injured except lungs (distinguishes it from ANCA vasculitis). Rash with palpable usually in the lower limbs (see image above). A body of 40–60% of patients will present with abdominal pain, related to mesenteric ischemia; pancreatitis has also been linked. Mononeuritis multiplex seen in 70% of cases. Febrile polyneuritis is pathognomonic.
   c. Labs may reveal decreased complement, rheumatoid factor, cryoglobulins. Angiography may reveal microaneurysms of medium size vessels. Ultimately, nerve and muscle biopsy may be needed.
   d. Mainstay of treatment is HBV anti-viral therapy
3. Renal
   a. Glomerulonephritis: Membranous glomerulonephritis (MGN), Membranoproliferative glomerulonephritis (MPGN), and rarely IgA nephropathy.
   b. Diagnosis of HBV-associated glomerulonephritis is made by the presence of at least one HBV antigen in the renal tissue.
   c. MGN is the most common associated HBV nephropathy. In most cases, it is self-limited.
   d. Treatment is HBV anti-viral therapy.
4. Juvenile papular acrodermatitis (also known as Gianotti Crosti syndrome):
   a. Syndrome characterized by small, flat, erythematous, popular eruptions – not unique to HBV.
5. Hematologic manifestations
   a. Associated with increased risk of B cell non-Hodgkin lymphoma; OR 2.7 compared to general population.

Reference

The extrahepatic manifestations of hepatitis B virus. PMID: 18760074.

Question 120

In addition to those parameters shared with the MELD score, what two additional parameters are factored into the PELD score?

A Encephalopathy and age
B Etiology of liver disease and age
C Pre-albumin and BMI
D Unconjugated bilirubin and pre-albumin
E Age and growth failure

Question 121

Name the (i) number one indication for pediatric LT, (ii) name the most common malignant indication for pediatric LT, and (iii) name the most common malignancy post pediatric LT

A Urea cycle disorder, HCC, recurrent HCC
B Congenital hepatic fibrosis, fibrolamellar HCC, Skin Cancer
C Alagille syndrome, hemangioendothelioma, genitouretral cancer
D Sclerosing cholangitis, cholangiocarcinoma (in setting of choledochal cyst), colo-rectal cancer
E Biliary atresia, hepatoblastoma, post-transplant lymphoproliferative disorder (PTLD)

120 – E is the correct answer.
121 – E is the correct answer.

Commentary – PELD

Clinical Pearls: Pediatric Liver Transplant and PELD Score

1. Pediatric end stage liver disease (PELD) score was approved by UNOS in November of 2000.
2. The PELD score is based on both laboratory data and growth data:
   a. Labs: INR, TBili, and albumin
   b. Age at listing
      i. Added points if the patient is 12 months or less
   c. Growth failure (based on gender, height, and weight)
      i. Presence of growth failure contributes almost 7 points to PELD score
3. Exceptions to PELD score: urea cycle disorder, organic acidemia, and hepatoblastoma.
4. Number one indication for pediatric LT is biliary atresia (nearly 50%) followed by cholestatic liver disease (progressive familial intrahepatic cholestasis "PFIC", Alagille's, sclerosing cholangitis) and metabolic causes.
5. Between 500–600 pediatric LT are performed per year in the United States (compared to ~8000 adult liver transplants).
   a. 85% long-term survival; nearly 90% of children on waitlist are eventually transplanted.
6. Hepatoblastoma is the most common pediatric primary liver tumor and the most common malignant indication for LT.
   a. The PRETreatment EXTent of disease (PRETEXT) staging system is used to categorize the extent of the disease and potential for tumor resection.
   b. Current practice is usually neo-adjuvant chemo followed by transplant and then 2 cycles of adjuvant chemo.
   c. Children with hepatoblastoma are given priority status on waitlist to decrease wait times.
7. Since size-matched deceased donor organs are a scarce resource in the pediatric population, split liver is a technique that can be utilized.
   a. Consists of left lateral segment (segments 2 and 3)
8. PTLD is the most common malignancy post pediatric transplant (as opposed to skin cancer in the adult population).

Notes

The adult transplant hepatology boards may have a few pediatric questions, these are typically related to PELD score, tumors, and genetic diseases.

Reference

Development of a pediatric end-stage liver disease score to predict poor outcome in children awaiting liver transplantation. PMID: 12151728.

Question 122

A 59-year-old female with autoimmune hepatitis cirrhosis undergoes liver transplant 6 weeks ago. Her course was complicated by severe rejection requiring treatment with thymoglobulin. She is discharged on prednisone and tacrolimus. Her past medical history includes diabetes and recurrent urinary tract infections.

She is admitted now with polydipsia and polyuria. In addition, she has right eye proptosis. A biopsy is performed.

Labs reveal a glucose of 560. She has a gap acidosis of 22 and ketone in her urine.

Representative biopsy images are shown below

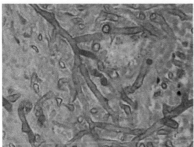 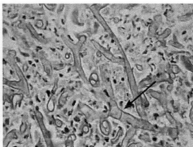

The diagnosis is?

A *Aspergillus fumigatus*
B *Candida glabrata*
C *Cryptococcal gattii*
D Mucormycosis
E Fusarium

D is the correct answer.

Notes
A great set of images provided by transplant infectious disease specialist Dr. Fernanda Silveira demonstrating the classic non-septate hyphae; misshapen with right angular branching (at 90°)

Question 123

What would be the recommended treatment for the patient above?

A Voriconazole
B Amphotericin
C Surgery and amphotericin
D Increase prednisone and FK
E IV Fluconazole

Question 124

Match the fungal infection with the most likely geographic location on the map

Cryptococcus gattii
Coccidioidomycosis
Histoplasmosis
Histoplasmosis and blastomycosis
Blastomycosis

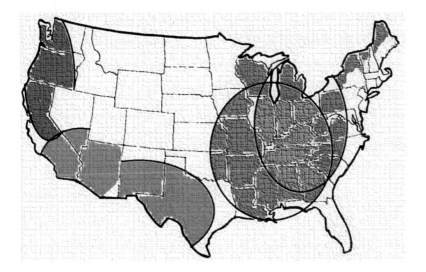

Answers

123 – C is the correct answer.
Answer for *map question* 124:
Cryptococcus gattii: PURPLE
Coccidioidomycosis: RED
Histoplasmosis: GREEN
Histoplasmosis and blastomycosis: GREEN/BROWN
Blastomycosis: BROWN

Commentary – Fungal Infections

Clinical Pearls: Fungal Infections Post Liver Transplantation

1. Incidence of fungal infections post LT is reported between 4% and 40%
   a. >70% caused by Candida species
   b. Second most common is aspergillosis
2. With mortality ranging from 25–67%
3. Anti-fungal prophylaxis should be considered in "high risk" LT patients
   a. Re-transplantation
   b. Reoperation
   c. Dialysis
   d. >40 units of blood products
   e. Choledochojejunostomy
   f. Candida colonization preop
   g. pre LT MELD >30
   h. Biliary leaks
   i. Live donor liver transplant
4. 2–4 weeks or until discharge is general recommendation regarding duration
   a. Fluconazole as first line agent
   b. Aspergillus prophylaxis remains controversial and is generally center specific

Fungus	Risk factors	Diagnosis	Clinical points	Therapy
Candida (albicans, glabrata and emerging pathogen auris)	Anastomotic leak, repeat laparotomy and choledocho-J	Bcx can be negative in 50% of infection Diagnosis requires high index of suspicion	Most common form in tx patients is intrabdominal infection	Empiric therapy with caspo and then Azole therapy is guided by species identification
Aspergillus (fumigatus: 70%, flavus and terreus)	Prolonged surgical time, massive introp blood transfusion, re-tx, steroid resistant rejection, AKI, CMV, DM and broad spectrum abx	CT scan classically shows ground glass opacities, cavities, and nodules with halo sign (80%). Can also infect sinuses. Galactomannan in BAL Biopsy shows septate hyphae, acute angle branching	Majority are pulmonary infection as route is inhalation of mold. Can rapidly disseminate. Overall mortality is 65%	Triazole therapy, specifically voriconazole

Fungus	Risk factors	Diagnosis	Clinical points	Therapy
Cryptococcal (neoformans and gattii)	Soil and Bird droppings. Most infection post tx is reactivation. LTx recipients are much higher risk than other organs, Odds Ratio of 6!	Cryptococcal antigen from serum or CSF	Typically infects lungs and then travels to CNS. Fever, headache, mental status changes, must think Cyrpto	Amphotericin B and flucytosine. High incidence of kidney injury and cytopenia associated with Rx
Scedosporium	Soil dwelling, contaminated water. Donor-derived infection of the recipient after near drowning of the donor has been described.	Culture reveals branching septae hyphae	Typically manifests as pneumonia.	Voriconazole Mortality up to 60%
Mucormycosis	Soil dwelling fungi found near decaying plants and animals DM, neutropenia and high dose steroids are risk factors	On tissue: non-septate hyphae; misshapen with right angular branching (at 90°) (see representative image from question 123).	Rhinosinusitis	Surgery and ampho-B. Mortality with disseminated disease Approaches 100%
Fusarium	Soil dwelling. Usually result of trauma in setting of neutropenia	Appear as fluffy/cottony colonies after 2–5 days of growth	Can lead to disseminated infection in immuno-compromised host	Ampho-B and surgical debridement
Histoplasma	Inhaled spores from disrupted soil Ohio and Mississippi River Valleys	Antigen in urine, serum, or body fluid	Pulmonary infection Disseminated infection 80%	Ampho-B Followed by extended course with azole Mortality 10%
Blastomyces	Inhaled spores from disrupted soil Ohio and Mississippi River Valleys	Antigen in urine, serum, or body fluid	Pulmonary infection Disseminated infection 38%	Ampho-B Followed by extended course with azole Mortality 21%
Coccidioides	Inhaled spores from disrupted soil Southwest states	Antigen in urine, serum, or body fluid Antibodies in cerebrospinal fluid (CSF)	Pulmonary infection Disseminated infection 75%	Ampho-B Followed by extended course with azole Mortality 30-50%

> **Notes**
>
> My only non-multiple choice question. There will not be a matching game on your boards. Enjoy it here.

Reference

Fungal Infections in Liver Transplant Recipients. PMID: 34210106.

Question 125

A 64-year-old African American male presents to your clinic with two months of worsening pruritus. He has no other complaints.

His past medical history includes diet controlled diabetes, chronic sclerosing dacryodenitis, and mild dementia. A colonoscopy 1 year ago was normal other than mild sigmoid diverticulsosis.

Exam is notable for scleral icterus and diffuse excorations.

Laboratory studies:

TBili 7 (conjugated 5.9), AST 130, ALT 174, ALP 918, gGTP 1030
Normal renal function; Albumin 3.6
WBC 6, Hb 14, Platelets 223
The patient undergoes an ultrasound which is followed by an ERC (image A below). He is administered an oral medication and 10 weeks later is labs completely normalized and repeat imaging in the form of an MRCP (image B) is obtained. What medication is most likely to have been administered?

A Acyclovir
B UDCA
C Rituximab
D Plavix
E Prednisone

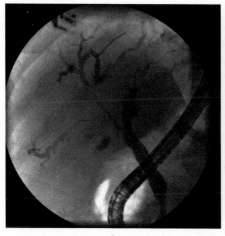

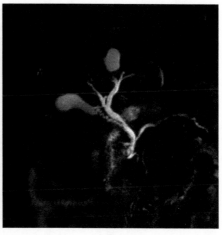

A   B

E is the correct answer.

Commentary – IGG4 Disease

Clinical Pearls: IgG4-Related Hepatobiliary Disease

1. Part of a systemic fibroinflammatory condition termed IgG4-related disease (IgG4-RD) and includes IgG4-related sclerosing cholangitis and IgG4-related hepatopathy (including IgG4-related AIH and inflammatory pseudotumor of the liver and biliary tract). Studies implicate both dysregulation of the immune system and genetic susceptibility in the pathogenesis of the disease.
2. IgG4-sclerosing cholangitis is the most common extra-pancreatic manifestation in patients with autoimmune pancreatitis (AIP) although it can occur without pancreatic involvement.
3. Risk factors and associations: Occupational exposure, allergy/atopy, peripheral eosinophilia, elevated IgE levels and coexistent autoimmune disease.
4. Clinical presentation
   a. Male predominance
   b. Sixth decade of life
   c. 70–80% present with jaundice
   d. Absence of inflammatory bowel disease
5. Labs:
   a. ANA positive 50% of cases; RF in 20%; IgG level are increased in >50% of cases.
   b. Total serum IgG4 are increased in 65–80% of cases at presentation, but can be normal
      i. IgG4 levels can also be elevated in inflammatory, autoimmune, and malignant conditions (and 5% of healthy individuals)
      ii. Use of an IgG:IgG4 ratio >2.4 has sensitivity and specificity of ~90% in distinguishing PSC from IgG4-SC
      iii. Serum IgG4 >5.6 g/L has near PPV of 100% in differentiating IgG4-SC from PSC and cholangiocarcinoma
   c. Imaging findings in IgG4-SC can be impossible to differentiate from PSC. Clues may include long continuous biliary strictures with thickened bile duct walls with associated liver/hilar mass with other organ involvement.
6. Histology: Tissue sampling can support a diagnosis of, but the presence of IgG4-positive cells is nonspecific. Classic features include:
   a. Lymphoplasmacytic infiltration
   b. Storiform pattern of fibrosis
   c. Obliterative phlebitis with a variable presence of eosinophils
   d. >10 IgG4 cells per HPF on biopsy; >50 per HPF on resection specimen
7. Diagnostic criteria, no single test can make the diagnosis
   a. HISORt (Histology, Imaging, Serology, other Organ involvement and Response to therapy) is the most widely used criteria

---

8. Mainstay of treatment is systemic corticosteroids. Typically, 30–40 mg daily for 4 weeks before reducing by 5 mg every 2 weeks
   a. Clinical, biochemical, and cholangiographic improvement should be seen within 4–6 weeks and should be confirmed by repeat imaging.
   b. In the setting of biliary obstruction, stenting is usually indicated even if a response to steroids is expected.
   c. Relapse is seen in >50% of cases and many patients may require a long-term sparing steroid agent (i.e. azathioprine).

Notes

IgG4 is a fascinating disease that can present in a myriad of ways. A favorite subject for GI grand rounds. These images are from a patient with IgG4 sclerosing cholangitis. He initially presented with biliary obstruction necessitating ERC and stent placement. When his bilirubin normalized, we treated him with steroids. A follow-up MRCP showed his disease had essentially "melted away". He has been maintained on azathioprine and will at times have flares in his disease in the setting of medication non-compliance.

Reference

IgG4-related hepatobiliary disease: an overview. PMID: 27625195.

Question 126

All of the following patients should be in an HCC surveillance program except?

A 55-year-old male from Sudan with chronic HBV non cirrhotic on entecavir with normal LFTs and negative HBV DNA; father died of HBV/HCC at 55.
B 57-year-old male with kPa on USE of 17; grade I EV; SVR achieved on DAA therapy 12 months ago.
C 63-year-old with hemochromatosis (C282Y/C282Y) biopsy with 3+ iron, fibrosis 2/4; in phlebotomy program current ferritin 345.
D 38-year-old male with NASH biopsy: 70%, 6/8 and 3-4/4 fibrosis.
E 62-year-old female with PBC cirrhosis on weight-based UDCA; ALP 98.

Question 127

All of the following have been associated as risk factors for the development of HCC EXCEPT

A Metformin
B Dietary aflatoxin
C Alcohol
D Obesity
E Male sex

126 – C is the correct answer.
127 – A is the correct answer.

Commentary – HCC

Clinical Pearls: HCC

1. HCC is the sixth most common cancer worldwide. The incidence in the United States has risen nearly 40% since 2000. HCC is the second most lethal tumor (after pancreatic cancer) with 5-year survival of 20%.
2. Mutations in TERT promoter are the most frequent genetic alterations, accounting for ~60% of cases
   a. Several genes in the chromatin remodeling pathway, particularly ARID1A and ARID2 have been consistently identified as mutation genes in HCC.
3. Risk factors:
   a. Rare in patients without liver disease
      i. 80% of patients with HCC have underlying cirrhosis
   b. Male: female 2 : 1
   c. HBV is the number one cause of HCC worldwide
      i. HBV and dietary exposure to aflatoxin increases risk 60-fold
      ii. Co-infection with Delta
   d. In US incidence of HCC over next 15 years is expected to increase 100%, largely in part due to the epidemic in NAFLD.
   e. Alcohol, smoking, HIV, and evidence to suggest obesity/diabetes are risk factors.
   f. Achievement of SVR through antiviral therapy reduces risk of HCC from 6% to 1.5%
      i. Patients with cirrhosis who achieve SVR should still be surveyed for HCC.
4. Surveillance
   a. All patients with cirrhosis who are eligible for curative treatment and/or are liver transplant candidates.
   b. Patients with chronic HCV and advanced fibrosis (F3 or F4 on Metavir) are at risk of developing HCC and should undergo surveillance.
   c. The major exception to the "cirrhosis" rule is HBV. The following noncirrhotic HBV patients should undergo surveillance
      i. Asian male HBV >40
      ii. Asian female HBV >50
      iii. HBV with family history of HCC
      iv. African or North American blacks with HBV
   d. Ultrasound every 6 months is the recommended method for surveillance +/− AFP

5. Diagnosis
   a. Radiological hallmarks on contrast enhanced CT or MRI in a cirrhotic liver: hyperenhancement in arterial phase and washout in portal venous phase is enough to make diagnosis.
   b. The Liver Imaging Reporting and Data System (LiRADS) uses this and other features to classify lesions based on the likelihood that they represent HCC
      i. LR-1 100% benign
      ii. LR-2 probably benign
      iii. LR-3 intermediate probability for HCC
      iv. LR-5 definite HCC
      v. LR-M malignant, but not compatible with HCC
      vi. LR-NC non-categorizable
      vii. LR-TIV tumor in vein
   c. An inconclusive pattern should prompt liver biopsy
      i. The most common histological grown patter in HCC: Trabecular pattern.
   d. Patients with cirrhosis and lesions that are less than 1 cm should undergo surveillance every 3–4 months and consider for a return to conventional surveillance if the nodule is stable after 12 months.
6. Staging
   a. Barcelona Clinic Liver Cancer (BCLC) algorithm
   b. Eastern Cooperative Oncology Group Performance Status
      0: Fully active without restrictions
      1: Restricted, but ambulatory and able to do light work
      2: Ambulatory but unable to carry out work
      3: Capable of limited selfcare; confined to bed/chair more than 50% of wake hours
      4: Completely disabled; bed-bound

Stage	Liver function	Performance status	Tumor burden	Estimated survival
Very early stage (0)	Preserved liver function	ECOG-PS 0	Solitary tumor ≤2 cm	5+ years
Early stage (A)	Preserved liver function	ECOG-PS 0	Solitary tumor >2 cm or 2–3 tumors all ≤3 cm	5+ years
Intermediate stage (B)	Preserved liver function	ECOG-PS 0	>3 nodules or ≥2 nodules if any >3 cm	2+ years
Advanced stage (C)	Preserved liver function	ECOG-PS 1-2	<Macrovascular invasion or extrahepatic spread	~1 year
Terminal stage (D)	End-stage liver function	ECOG-PS >2	Non-transplantable HCC	3 months

> **Notes**
>
> There is some literature on HCC in non-cirrhotic NAFLD, a scary prospect! That being said, for the boards, other than HBV, only patients with advanced fibrosis should be surveyed for HCC.

Reference

Hepatocellular carcinoma. PMID: 30970190.

Question 128

A 52-year-old male with cirrhosis from alpha-1 antitrypsin deficiency is referred to your center for a liver transplant. Imaging reveals a 6.7 cm LI-RADS 5 lesion with tumor invasion and several pulmonary lesions suspicious for metastases. His AFP is 1245.

He has small esophageal varices, no ascites, and no encephalopathy.

Laboratory studies:

Na 136, Cr 1; TBili 1.1, AST 39, ALT 49, ALP 216; INR 1.1; Albumin 3.5
WBC 9, HB 11, Platelets 154

The patient is presented at tumor board and the decision is to treat with checkpoint inhibitors (CPI) Atezolizumab and Bevacizumab.

The patient presents to the emergency room 4 months later with bloody diarrhea. He reports crampy abdominal pain and ~3–5 loose bowel movements per day × 8 days. He has no fever. His abdominal exam shows no peritoneal signs. Infectious etiology including C. diff is ruled out. CT scan shows moderate thickening of the recto-sigmoid. A colonoscopy is performed with image below; biopsies are obtained.

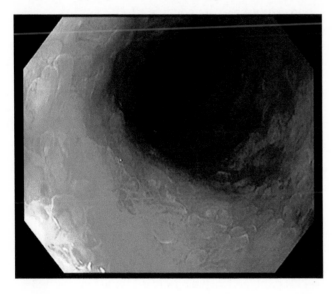

Which of the following do you recommend?

A Discontinue CPI
B Metronidazole
C IVIG and oral corticosteroids 0.5–1 mg/kg/day
D Infliximab
E Stop CPI and start oral corticosteroids 0.5–1 mg/kg/day

E is the correct answer.

Commentary

Clinical Pearls: Systemic Medical Therapy for HCC

1. Molecular targeted agents: First line
   a. **Sorafenib (Nexavar®)** Approved in 2007 based on *SHARP* trial. Oral tyrosine kinase inhibitor that suppresses tumor proliferation. Prolong survival compared to placebo for advanced HCC, but use has been limited given its poor antitumor effects and high toxicity (namely hand-foot skin reaction).
      i. Caution in patients with significant hyperbilirubinemia
   b. **Lenvatinib (Lenvima®)** is an oral kinase inhibitor that selectively inhibits receptor tyrosine kinase involved in tumor angiogenesis and malignant transformation. *REFLECT* trial showed improved survival compared to sorafenib: 13.6 versus 12.3 months. Tumor shrinkage and necrotic effects were excellent in Lenvatinib arm. Lower incidence of subjective adverse events. Approved in 2018.
      i. Contraindicated if GFR <30
      ii. Hypertension (HTN) and diarrhea are common side effects
2. Molecular targeted agents: Second-line drugs
   a. **Regorafenib (Stivarga®):** An oral inhibitor of multiple protein kinases. Molecular structure is very similar to sorafenib. *RESORCE* trial: First drug to show efficacy as second line therapy after progression on sorafenib when compared to placebo. Survival advantage 10.6 months versus 7.8 months in placebo arm. Approved in 2017.
   b. **Cabozantinib (Cabometyx®):** An oral multikinase inhibitor. *CELESTIAL* Trial: When used as a second line drug, it prolongs survival (compared to placebo) in patients with HCC who are refractory or intolerant to sorafenib (10.2 versus 8 months). Approved in 2019.
      i. Adverse reaction 68% and included hand-foot skin syndrome (17%), HTN (16%), diarrhea (10%).
   c. **Ramucirumab (Cyramza®):** Recombinant human immunoglobulin IgG1 monoclonal Ab that inhibits VEGFR02. IV formulation. *REACH* trial demonstrated that it prolonged survival compared to placebo in unresectable advanced HCC who were refractory or intolerant to sorafenib in a subgroup of patients with AFP >400 ng/mL and including gross vascular invasion (8.5 versus 7.3 months). The drug was approved for this subgroup in 2019.
3. Immune checkpoint inhibitors
   a. **Nivolumab (Opdivo®):** The world's first recombinant human IgG4 monoclonal antibody specific for human PD-1. In *CheckMate* trial, patients with advanced HCC, response rate was 20%; updated results revealed overall survival of 28.6 months when used as first line therapy and 15 months as second line. Approved in 2020.

b. **Pembrolizumab (Keytruda®):** Recombinant human IgG4 monoclonal anti-body specific for human PD-1. Approved by FDA as second-line agent after sorafenib failure. *KEYNOTE* trail failed to reach pre-specified p value (clinically positive, but statistically negative). Approved in 2018.

c. Combination immunotherapy: **Atezolizumab (Tecentriq®) and Beva-cizumab (Avastin®).** In the *IMbrave* 150 study, patients with advanced or metastatic and/or unresectable HCC: HR for death with Atezo and Beva was 0.58 compared to sorafenib; overall survival at 1 year was 67% versus 55%. Complete response rates of 33%. Combination was approved in 2020. Now considered standard of care for advanced HCC.

   i. Recommendations are for EGD prior to initiation of Beva to rule out varices and treat appropriately if present given the reported increased risk of gastro-intestinal bleeding.

   ii. Ectopic varices, non-healing wounds and active DVT are contraindications

d. Checkpoint inhibitors are considered a contraindication in patients with a history of organ transplantation given the reported high risk of rejection (up to 40%).

   i. The role of immunotherapy as a *bridge* pre-LT is not well established. Experts recommend discontinuing therapy ~3 months pre-LT.

e. Immune mediated colitis

   i. Typically, pancolitis is seen 3–6 months after initiation. For moderate colitis, therapy should be withheld and if symptoms persist for a week, steroids should be administered. Infliximab can be given in severe cases.

f. Liver injury caused by immune checkpoint inhibitors has been described with histological features showing similarities to autoimmune hepatitis, but serological markers (IgG, ANA) are uncommon.

Notes

HCC medical therapy has exploded in the last few years with new medications and regimens being approved every several months. There is usually a lag of a couple of years when it comes to new medications and the boards, but we anticipate some of these points will be fair game in the near future.

Reference

Systemic therapy for intermediate and advanced hepatocellular carcinoma: Sorafenib and beyond. PMID: 29783126.

Question 129

All of the following have been identified as post-transplant risk factors for bone loss EXCEPT?

A Glucocorticoids
B Azathioprine use
C Tacrolimus
D Cholestatic liver disease
E Immobility

B is the correct answer.

Commentary – Bone Loss After Transplant

Clinical Pearls: Bone Loss Post Liver Transplantation

1. Bone loss post liver transplant is greatest within first 3–6 months; can be as high as 50% within first year
2. Pre-existing factors include cholestatic liver disease, alcoholism, hypogonadism, and abnormal vit-D metabolism
3. Post-transplant factors: High dose steroids, cyclosporine and FK, immobility, advanced age, prior fracture, and poor nutrition
4. Fractures can occur in up to 65% of patients. The most common sites are spine, ribs, hip, and pelvis
5. Patients with normal bone mineral density (BMD) should be tested every 2–3 years post-transplant with DEXA scan; patients at higher risk (on steroids, severe cholestasis) should be tested yearly
   a. Z score is a comparison with controls of the same age
   b. T score is standard deviation less than the mean of a young, healthy individual
      i. T score less than −2.5 SD below mean is consistent with osteoporosis
6. Weight bearing exercise and calcium supplements should be recommended for all LT with or at risk for BMD: 1–1200 mg calcium daily to maintain vit-D levels 30 ng/mL
7. An algorithm to initiate anti-resorptive therapy (namely bisphosphonate therapy: examples: alendronate, zoledronate) assigns points based on risk factors. If 5 points or more, treat:
   a. alcohol/cholestatic disease (2 points)
   b. steroids 5 mg or more per day (3 points)
   c. history of previous fracture (3 points)
   d. T score less than 2.5 (3)
   e. between 1–2.5 (1)
      i. risk of esophagitis/esophageal ulcer with oral bisphosphonate is low if properly administered
8. Patients treated should undergo interval follow-up DEXA scan; improvement may take up to 2 years

Reference

Bone disease and liver transplantation: a review. PMID: 34420781.

Question 130

A 39-year-old male undergoes colonoscopy for anemia and heme positive stool. Images are shown below. Genetic testing reveals a germline mutation is detected in the APC gene.

▶ Question

The risk of what liver tumor is highly increased in this patient's children.

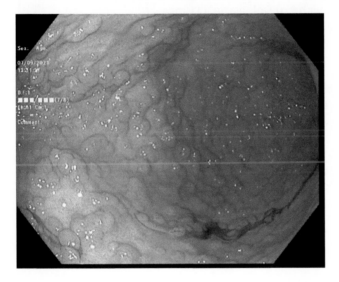

A Fibrolamellar HCC
B Serous cystadenoma
C Cholangiocarcinoma
D Hepatoblastoma
E Hemangioendothelioma

D is the correct answer.

Commentary – FAP and Liver Tumors

> ### Clinical Pearls: Familial Adenomatous Polyposis and Liver Tumors
>
> 1. Familial adenomatous polyposis (FAP) is an AD disease cause by a mutation in the adenomatous polyposis coli (APC) gene
> 2. FAP is characterized by an early onset of multiple colorectal adenomatous polyps with an inevitable progression to carcinoma if left untreated
> 3. FAP has been associated with extracolonic neoplasms
>   a. UGI tract carcinomas
>   i. duodenal
>   ii. periampullary
>   b. desmoid tumors
>   c. jaw osteomas
>   d. papillary thyroid carcinoma
>   e. medulloblastoma
>   f. adrenal adenoma
>   g. pancreatic tumors
> 4. Hepatic tumors have also been described
>   a. hepatoblastoma – develop in young patients with FAP at least 100× more frequently than the general population
>   b. HCC
>   c. rarely adenomas

Reference

Hepatocellular adenoma associated with familial adenomatous polyposis coli. PMID: 23293720.

Question 131

A 14-year-old female presents to your clinic with abnormal liver tests. She is relatively asymptomatic other than occasional pruritus and occasional loose stools. Exam reveals some excoriations.

Laboratory studies:

TBili 1.1, AST 218, ALT 298, ALP 1008, GGT 899
IgG 1940, ANA, and smooth muscle are negative, p-ANCA positive
Viral serologies negative. Alpha one 214, Ceruloplasmin 28.
MRCP reveals findings consistent with "mild" PSC but no dominant strictures
Colonoscopy reveals mild erythema and superficial ulceration in the rectum

▶ Question

What do you recommend?

A ERCP
B UDCA 15–25 mg/kg
C UDCA 15–25 mg/kg and 40 mg daily of prednisone
D Liver biopsy
E CT scan of chest

Question 132

A 26-year-old male follows in your clinic for PSC. He presented 3 years ago with pruritus and elevated liver enzymes. He was placed on UDCA 15 mg/kg with improvement in his symptoms and mild reduction in his liver enzymes.

His other medical history includes ulcerative colitis, which has responded to mesalamine. A colonoscopy 4 months ago revealed relatively quiescent disease. His gallbladder was removed 4 years ago for "stones".

The patient comes in for scheduled follow-up. He has no significant complaints although his girlfriend says he complains of fatigue.

On exam: Thin with a BMI of 20 mg/kg^2, relatively well appearing gentleman. + scleral icterus, otherwise normal exam.

Laboratory studies:

WBC 4, Hb 11, Platelets 132. Normal renal function, INR 1.3. NH3 78. Serum IgG4 is 49. Serum IgG 1600. ANA 1 : 160, smooth muscle negative. ANCA positive, LK-Ab negative.

LFTs over last 3 years are shown below

	TBili	AST	ALT	ALP	GTP
Diagnosis	2.2	118	112	339	462
2 years	1.7	78	49	219	321
Current	10.6	55	88	632	459

Ca 19-9 is 54, CEA is 1.2

An MRCP reveals diffuses intrahepatic PSC with no dominant stricture; a cirrhotic appearing liver with increasing splenomegaly and small periesophageal varices and a moderate sized splenorenal shunt. An EGD reveals no intraluminal varices.

▶ Question

What do you recommend?

A Course of antibiotics
B ERCP
C Embolization of SR shunt
D Prednisone 40 mg PO QD × one month and repeat LFTs
E Referral for liver transplant

131 – D is the correct answer.
132 – E is the correct answer.

Commentary – PSC

Clinical Pearls: PSC

1. Diagnosis:
   a. Cholestatic biochemical profile
   b. Multifocal strictures and segmental dilation on cholangiography
      i. Isolated intrahepatic disease may be associated with better prognosis
   c. Secondary causes of sclerosing cholangitis have been excluded
   d. Patients who have histological features of PSC, but normal cholangiogram are classified as having small duct PSC (5–10%)
      i. Liver biopsy is not required for diagnosis of PSC; periductal concentric ("onion-skin" appearance around the bile duct; see histology image) fibrosis is classic histopathological findings but is infrequent

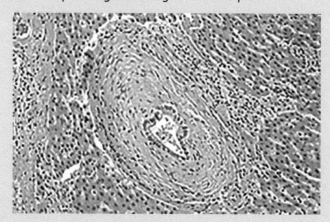

2. ~70% of patients are male with a mean age at diagnosis of 40 years
3. Incidence of colitis ~70% (UC≫Crohn's)
   a. Conversely ~8% of patients with IBD have PSC
4. ANCA most common autoantibody positive 50–80%; elevated IgG ~60%
5. Recommendations are to check IgG4 in all patients with PSC
   a. Elevated in ~9% of patients
6. In patients with disproportionately elevated transaminases, liver biopsy is recommended to rule out AIH/PSC overlap
   a. Rare entity (in the United States reports of less than 3%; much higher in the pediatric population)
7. Dominant strictures occur in up to 50% of patients
   a. Can present with worsening jaundice/pruritus and or cholangitis
   b. Should be brushed or biopsied to rule out malignancy
   c. Should be treated with endoscopic dilation +/– stenting
      i. Emerging evidence on the benefits of "scheduled" dilations
      ii. ERCP should be performed with multi-disciplinary assessment in patients with PSC with cirrhosis and PHTN.

8. There is a role for prophylactic antibiotics in patients with recurrent cholangitis
9. Patients with PSC should undergo baseline DEXA to rule out osteopenia/osteoporosis and then every 2–3 years
10. Full colonoscopy with biopsies should be performed with a new diagnosis of PSC
    a. Surveillance every 1–2 years
11. Annual ultrasound to survey for gallbladder (GB) cancer
    a. GB mass should prompt cholecystectomy regardless of lesion size
    b. GB polyp >8 mm should prompt cholecystectomy
12. Cholangiocarcinoma
    a. 10-year risk ~10%
    b. Now the leading cause of death in patient with PSC
    c. Risk factors: elevated bilirubin, variceal bleeding, proctocolectomy, chronic UC with CRC or dysplasia, duration of IBD and polymorphism of NKG2D gene
       i. Some studies to suggest that ½ of all cholangiocarcinoma is detected within the first year of diagnosis of PSC
    d. AGA expert review recommends US/CT or MRI with or without Ca 19-9 q6-12 months
       i. No surveillance in patients less than 20 years or those with small duct disease
13. High dose UDCA is contraindicated in patients with PSC (>28 mg/kg). Controversy exists regarding "medium" dose, that being said, for the boards: No UDCA for PSC.
14. Indications for LT include progression to end stage disease, recurrent cholangitis (typically requires documented bouts of bacteremia to obtain MELD exception points) and rarely refractory pruritus

Notes

In my opinion, PSC is the most frustrating of all the chronic liver diseases for both patients and providers. There is no approved medical therapy and the literature on the role for UDCA is confusing. That said, for the boards (at least at this time), there is no role for UDCA (high, medium or low dose).

Reference

Primary sclerosing cholangitis – a comprehensive review. PMID: 28802875.

Question 133

Which of the following is FALSE regarding outcomes following liver transplantation for alcoholic cirrhosis?

A Overall survival rates of patients transplant for alcoholic cirrhosis are comparable to the other most common etiologies
B The six-month rule accurately predicts the risk of recidivism post LT
C Heavy alcohol use post LT is associated with increased graft rejection and graft loss
D Lack of a partner is associated with increased risk of recidivism
E De novo malignancy > recurrent malignancy post LT in patients with alcoholic cirrhosis

B is the correct answer.

Commentary – Alcohol Recidivism After Transplant

Clinical Pearls: Alcohol Recidivism Post Liver Transplantation

1. As of 2020, alcohol is the number one indication for LT in the United States
   a. Alcohol as an indication for LT has increased in the US by >100% in the last decade
2. 12–33% of patients transplanted for alcoholic liver disease relapse to harmful amount of drinking
3. Risk factors associated with relapse
   a. Psychiatric diagnosis
   b. Lack of social support
      i. Lack of a partner
   c. Unemployment
   d. Missed clinic visits
   e. Cigarette smoking
   f. 6-month rule is not a reliable predictor
4. Addiction counseling pre and post LT may decrease risk of recidivism
5. Alcohol relapse is associated with increased risk of allograft rejection, likely as a result of medication noncompliance
   a. Harmful alcohol use post LT has been associated with increased graft loss and the development of advanced fibrosis

Notes

As the role for liver transplantation in alcoholic liver disease continues to expand, trying to determine post-transplant recidivism is critical for long-term success of the patient and allograft. You can expect to see this subject tested on your exam.

Reference

Recidivism in liver transplant recipients for alcohol-related liver disease. PMID: 33994719.

Question 134

A 59-year-old male with alcoholic cirrhosis is brought to the clinic by his 26-year-old daughter who is a nurse. She is concerned that he is "not himself" lately although she cannot pinpoint exactly what is wrong. The patient stopped drinking 10 months ago. He continues to work. He has small varices, and no ascites. On exam he is awake, alert, and oriented × 3. He has mild scleral icterus and a few spider angiomata. He has bilateral Dupuytren's contracture and caput medusa but no ascites and no edema. He has no asterixis. He is a Child Pugh Class A with a MELD of 11. You perform the following test in the office (see image below). He completes the testing in 72 seconds.

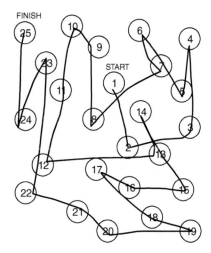

How would you interpret the results?

A Overt encephalopathy, stage I–II
B Moderate encephalopathy, stage III
C Minimal or covert encephalopathy, stage I–II
D Severe encephalopathy with delayed reaction time
E >60 seconds; forced termination, stage III encephalopathy

C is the correct answer.

Commentary – Hepatic Encephalopathy

Clinical Pearls: Hepatic Encephalopathy (HE)

1. A spectrum of potentially reversible neuropsychiatric abnormalities seen in patients with liver dysfunction and or portosystemic shunting
2. Overt HE: Disorientation or asterixis. Affects ~one third of patients with cirrhosis.
3. Minimal HE: Subtle findings that can only be detected using specialized tests; seen in up to 80% of patients with cirrhosis may have minimal HE
4. Categorized based on underlying disease
   a. Type A: Seen with acute liver failure
   b. Type B: Porto-systemic bypass (without intrinsic liver disease)
   c. Type C: Cirrhosis, PHTN, or systemic shunting
5. Severity
   a. Minimal: Abnormal psychometric testing
   b. Grade I: Changes in behavior, mild confusion, changes in sleep wake cycle
      i. Minimal or Grade I are described as having "covert" HE
   c. Grade II: Moderate confusion; typically, will have moderate asterixis
      i. Asterixis is technically not a tremor, but a form of negative myoclonus in which there are irregular abrupt lapses of muscular tone
   d. Grade IIII: Marked confusion, somnolence
   e. Grade IV: Coma, unresponsive to pain
      i. Grade II–IV: "overt" HE
6. Focal neurological deficits may be a manifestation of HE
7. Sarcopenia has been identified as a risk factor for HE (Odds Ratio: 3)
8. Serum ammonia levels should not be used to screen HE in patients who are asymptomatic or have mental status changes in the absence of liver disease or portal-systemic shunt
   a. Serum ammonia levels can be helpful in certain clinical scenarios, but the routine use of this lab test and the monitoring of it remain controversial
9. Psychometric testing
   a. Number connection test (Halstead–Reitan Test; depicted in question above) is the most frequently used in clinical practice.
      i. Test instructions: Scattered across the sheet are numbers 1–25. As quickly as you can, connect the numbers with each other in their correct order, starting with number 1.
         1. Up to 30 sec: no PSE
         2. 31–50 sec 0-I PSE
         3. 51–80 sec 1-II PSE
         4. 81–120 sec II-III
         5. Forced termination III
   b. Stroop test: Psychomotor speed and cognitive flexibility. Available as an "App" on smart phones.

10. Other testing used in clinical practice include EEG, Imaging, and Critical flicker frequency
11. Patients admitted with HE should always undergo investigation for a precipitating cause: Gastro-intestinal bleeding, infection (SBP, urinary infection, pneumonia), electrolyte disturbances, renal failure, sedative, constipation; rarely HCC or PVT.
    a. In patients HE refractory to medical therapy, think of spontaneous shunts
    b. Ornithine transcarbamylase deficiency (OTCD) is an X linked disorder and is the most common urea cycle disorder. It is caused by a defect of the mitochondrial ornithine transcarbamylase. Severe defects lead to hyperammonemic coma in the neonatal period.
    c. Some affected males however exhibit a delayed onset, "late onset OTC". Diagnosis is challenging and requires a high index of suspicion.
    d. Hyperammonemia has been described as a complication in solid organ transplantation (discussed elsewhere in book)
       i. Especially post lung with rates as high as 4% with mortality approaching 75%. Treatment is generally focused on neuroprotective agents and decreasing cerebral edema, hemodialysis, and antibiotics.
    e. Hyperammonemia has also been reported in patients on anti-epileptics, most commonly this has been linked with valproic acid with severe cases reported in 5%. Risk factors include dose of VA, concomitant use phenytoin, phenobarbital, and carbamazepine. L-carnitine supplementation may help.
12. Capacity to drive
    a. Studies evaluating this question have reached disparate conclusions
    b. Reasonable to restrict driving in patients with persistent PSE and where there are historical or clinical findings to suggest increased risk of accidents

Reference

Hepatic encephalopathy. PMID: 28076712.

Question 135

Rifaximin with or without lactulose has been shown to do which of the following?

A Reduce readmission from PSE
B Prevent post TIPS PSE
C Improve QOL in patients with cirrhosis and PSE
D Prevent mortality in patients with cirrhosis
E All the above

E is the correct answer.

Commentary – HE Therapy

Clinical Pearls: Treatment of Hepatic Encephalopathy

1. Always attempt to determine an underlying precipitant and treat accordingly (i.e. infection, electrolyte disturbance, renal failure, upper gastrointestinal bleeding)
2. Nutritional support
   a. 1.2–1.5 g/kg/day; patients should not be "protein restricted"
      i. Some data to suggest benefit of branched-chained amino acids and beneficial effect on HE
3. Lactulose
   a. In the colon, lactulose is catabolized by bacterial flora resulting in acidic pH. Reduction in pH favors the formation of the nonabsorbable NH4+ from NH3, trapping NH4+ in the colon and reducing plasma ammonia
   b. 30–60 mL 2–3×/day titrated to 2–3 soft stools per day
   c. Can also be administered as an enema
4. Polyethylene glycol (PEG)
   a. Studies suggest PEG has beneficial effect on the treatment of HE compared to lactulose with suggestion of more rapid resolution
5. Rifaximin
   a. Typically used in addition to lactulose. Recommended dose of Rifaximin is 550 mg po BID
   b. Has been shown to
      i. Mortality benefit
      ii. Reduction in recurrent PSE
      iii. Reduce readmission
      iv. Improve quality of life (QOL)
6. Other antibiotics have shown some efficacy but are no longer recommended given side effect profile (neomycin, metronidazole)
7. L-ornithine-L-aspartate (LOLA), used commonly outside the United States and does seem to be beneficial and well tolerated
8. Post TIPS HE
   a. Seen in up to 30% of patients
   b. Recent data shows benefit of rifaximin +/− lactulose to prevent post TIPS HE
9. Large spontaneous portosystemic shunts
   a. In selected patients with refractory, HE due to shunts, embolization seems to be effective without a significant increase in worsening complications related to PHTN.

Reference

Overt hepatic encephalopathy: current pharmacologic treatments and improving clinical outcomes. PMID: 34242619.

Question 136

Your hepatology fellow was splashed with blood while performing an endoscopy on a patient with HBV. The patient is treatment naïve and has active viremia. The patient is negative for HIV and HCV. Your fellow immediately comes to your clinic post-procedure and is quite anxious. You check her HBV serologies and they reveal:

HBsAg negative, anti-HBc total negative, anti-HBs 49 mIU/mL

What do you recommend?

A Do nothing and offer reassurance
B Confirm HBV serologies and DNA level of patient
C Administer HBV vaccine and HBIG
D Administer HBIG alone
E Start viral prophylaxis with entecavir for 2 weeks and then repeat blood work

A is the correct answer.

Commentary — HBIG

Clinical Pearls: Hepatitis B Immune Globulin (HBIG)

1. Proposed mechanism of action of HBIG includes binding to the viral particles and HBsAg resulting in neutralization and thereby preventing viral attachment to the hepatocytes.
 2. Post exposure prophylaxis should be administered ideally within 24 hours of needlestick, ocular or mucosal exposure or within 14 days of sexual exposure
    a. Decision to administer to health care personnel should be based on their vaccine history and HBV serologies
    b. Prevention post LT
       i. Anhepatic phase given with the liver transplant (20,000 units)
       ii. Daily for first 7 days
       iii. Every 2 weeks starting day 14 until month 3
       iv. And then monthly thereafter (depending on individual center protocol)
       v. There is no role for HBIG when you are surface antigen negative
    c. Pediatric
       i. Administered intramuscular at dose of 0.5 mL with 12 hours after birth given with HBV vaccine
          1. Vaccine second dose given 1 month, and final dose given at 6 months
             a. Infant should then be tested at 12–15 months

Reference

Post-exposure prophylaxis for Blood-Borne Viral (BBV) Infections. PMID: 33113403.

Question 137

A 27-year-old female presents to the emergency room from her primary care office with a two-day history of intermittent fevers, cephalgia, and vague abdominal discomfort.

The patient is married and lives with her husband and 2-year-old child. She works at a daycare. She has no high-risk behavior. Her medical history is unremarkable.

Exam: Temperature 100.4 F, BMI 24 kg/m². She is lying in bed with a damp cool cloth on her forehead. Neurological exam is negative including meningeal signs. Abdominal exam reveals a palpable spleen tip.

Notable laboratory studies: WBC 10 with 24% neutrophils and 62% lymphocytes with 12% atypical lymphocytes.

TBili 0.8, AST 144, ALT 228, ALP 219, GGT 319. Kidney function is normal. LDH 321

A liver biopsy is obtained:

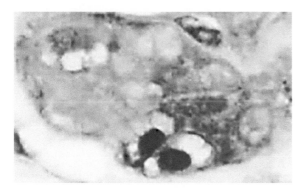

Which of the following blood tests would confirm the diagnosis?

A HEV IgM
B CMV IgM
C Stool test for giardia
D Microscopic agglutination test (MAT) for Leptospirosis
E Parvovirus IgM

B is the correct answer.

Notes
A nice image of an Owl's Eye Nucleus in a patient with CMV provided by my younger brother (a pathologist) Dr. Sajjad M. Malik.

Question 138

Which of the following is the host cell receptor for the SARS-COV-2 virus into the liver?

A NTCP
B CD81
C Human Protein Tim1
D ACE2
E CD4

D is the correct answer.

Commentary

Clinical Pearls: Systemic Viruses (Non-Hepatotropic) that Can Cause "Hepatitis"

1. Herpesviruses
   a. HSV 1 and 2
      i. Rare cause of hepatitis but when it occurs is presents as ALF with mortality upwards of 80%
      ii. In pregnant women usually HSV 2; can also present as ALF
         1. Clinical clue: Serum bilirubin is usually not very high (less than 5)
         2. Up to 50% mortality for mother and child
      iii. HSV hepatitis requires immediate treatment: Acyclovir 5 mg/kg q8 hours × 7 days
   b. Congenital cytomegalovirus (CMV)
      i. In immunocompetent host resemble mononucleosis
      ii. Clinical clues or fever, headache, splenomegaly, normal bilirubin with predominant cholestatic injury profile, atypical lymphocytes
      iii. Typical intranuclear inclusion surrounded by clear halo impart the classic "owl's eye" appearance
      iv. Occasionally causes granulomatous hepatitis
      v. Usually self-limited; supportive care
   c. Epstein-Barr Virus (EBV)
      i. Fever, malaise, fatigue, sore throat, and palpable lymphadenopathy, splenomegaly>hepatomegaly, atypical lymphocytes.
      ii. Elevation in liver tests is very common; LFTs mixed but tendency toward cholestatic; ~5% will develop jaundice, although rare cause of ALF has been reported; most cases are self-limited
      iii. Clinical clue: 80% of patients will develop morbilliform rash following administration of ampicillin
2. Parvovirus
   a. Parvovirus B19 causes erythema infectiosum (Fifth disease also known as "slapped cheek syndrome") in children. Adults with parvovirus B19 may develop transient Aplastic crisis. Severe hepatitis has been reported.
3. Coronavirus
   a. COVID 19 caused by severe acute respiratory syndrome coronavirus-2 (SARS-Co-V-2)
   b. ACE2 is the host cell receptor for SARS-COV-2; it is present in type 2 alveolar cells, the GI tract, and the liver
   c. 2–11% of patients with COVID-19 have underlying chronic liver disease
      i. 14–53% have been reported to develop some form of liver injury
      ii. Liver injury is significantly more frequent in critically ill patients and associated with poor outcome

---

iii. Patient with cirrhosis (especially Childs B and C) infected with COVID-19 have worse outcomes
iv. Scattered reports of COVID-19 vaccine causing liver injury including an autoimmune type of hepatitis. Data is too new and too scant to be fair game for boards at this time.

Reference

Viral infections by nonhepatotropic viruses. clinical hepatology. PMCID: PMC7123179.

Question 139

A 43-year-old male with PSC undergoes a deceased donor liver transplant. The donor is a 57-year-old who died of an anoxic brain injury.

The Donor is CMV IgG positive, IgM negative
The Recipient is CMV IgG negative, IgM negative

Which of the following do you recommend?

A Oral ganciclovir for 3–6 months
B Oral valganciclovir for 3–6 months
C Monitor CMV nucleic acid testing (NAT) monthly and treat if viremia is detected
D IV valganciclovir × 1 week followed by oral ganciclovir for 3–6 months
E IV ganciclovir 1 week post operative followed by monitoring CMV NAT monthly and treat if viremic symptoms

B is the correct answer.

Commentary – CMV

Clinical Pearls: CMV and Liver Transplant; Donor/Recipient Serology

1. Transplant recipients with donor seropositive and recipient seronegative status are at high risk of primary CMV infection
   a. CMV Donor(D) positive/Recipient(R) negative incidence: 44–65%.
   b. R positive: 8–19%.
   c. Only 1–2% among D negative/R negative.
2. Primary infection is defined as CMV viremia in a previously unexposed transplant recipient.
3. CMV disease is evidence of CMV infection with symptoms
   a. Syndrome: fever, malaise, cytopenias.
   b. Tissue invasive disease.
4. CMV reactivation is evidence of CMV replication in patients previously positive for CMV serology.
5. CMV is the most common viral infection in LT recipients, occurring in up to 30% of recipients without antiviral prophylaxis.
6. Clinical presentation is classically fever, cytopenia, and hepatitis within the first 3 most post LT.
7. CMV infection increases risk of acute rejection, chronic allograft dysfunction, hepatic artery thrombus (HAT), post-transplant lymphoproliferative disorder (PTLD), bacterial, fungal, and other viral infections, accelerated HCV course.
8. Universal prophylaxis and pre-emptive therapy are two most employed strategies to prevent CMV infection/reactivation
   a. Prophylactic strategy depends on D/R serological status
      i. CMV D positive/R negative universal prophylaxis is recommended for 3–6 months.
      ii. CMV D positive or D positive/R positive prophylaxis OR pre-emptive therapy, duration 3 months.
      iii. CMV D negative/R negative no prophylaxis recommended.
   b. Pre-emptive therapy: detect presence of early CMV replication prior to onset of symptoms. Pros: cost and drug exposure; Cons requires frequent lab monitoring (which may offset cost benefit)
      i. Once weekly NAT testing × 12 weeks post LT.
      ii. If patient becomes viremic above a defined threshold, antiviral therapy is initiated and continued until two consecutive CMV DNA returns negative.
   c. Universal prophylaxis
      i. Recommended for D positive/R negative.
      ii. Ganciclovir and valganciclovir are two most commonly used drugs (choice is center dependent; some will use IV ganciclovir for a week followed by oral valganciclovir for duration).
         1. Oral ganciclovir should not be used because of poor bioavailability.
      iii. Duration 3–6 months.

Reference

Cytomegalovirus infection in liver transplant recipients: current approach to diagnosis and management. PMID: 28663679.

Question 140

You are contacted by the hospital health department regarding a visiting surgical resident from Turkey. He has never been vaccinated for HBV. His serologies reveal: HBsAg negative, anti-HBc total negative, anti-HBs negative.

You administer HBV vaccination Recombivax (10 mcg HbsAg/mL) at day 1, end of 1 month, and 6 months later.

Repeat serologies 1 year later reveal: HBsAg negative, anti-HBc negative, anti-HBs of 5 IU/L.

▶ Question

What do you recommend?

A Patient is considered immune, nothing further, monitor serologies yearly
B Single dose booster vaccine
C Repeat series with Recombivax 10 mcg
D Repeat series with increased dose (40 mcg)
E Administer immunoglobulin followed by standard dose (10 mcg) vaccine series

D is the correct answer.

Commentary – HBV Vaccine

Clinical Pearls: HBV Vaccine

1. In 1991 the WHO endorsed that all countries should integrate HBV vaccination in their national immunization program.
   a. Global vaccine coverage for infants ~85%
2. Administered at day 0, end of 1 month and 6 months.
3. Minimally accepted immune response is anti-HBs titer of ≥10 IU/L. Overall 90% of healthy adults achieve protective level.
4. Rate of protection decreases with:
   a. Increasing age, smokers, men, diabetes, cirrhosis, chronic renal failure, organ transplant recipients, immunocompromised, celiac disease (possibly related to HLA haplotypes)
5. Vaccine is recommend for following adults:
   a. Household/intimate contacts of those with chronic HBV
   b. High risk sexual or drug behavior
   c. Incarcerated persons
   d. Residents and staff of developmentally disabled persons
   e. Health care and public safety workers
      i. Healthcare workers with chronic HBV should not perform high risk procedures if their DNA is >1000
   f. End stage kidney disease, dialysis patients
   g. Chronic liver disease
   h. HIV
   i. Diabetics
   j. Persons traveling to high risk areas
6. Prevaccination serology screening (as opposed to universal vaccine) in adults is highly cost-effective
7. Most recommend *against* vaccination for US-born individuals who are isolated anti-HBc positive as they likely had prior HBV exposure and are unlikely to respond to vaccination
8. Patients on dialysis and immunocompromised hosts should receive higher dose of conventional HBV vaccine (40 mcg compared to 10–20 mcg).
9. Non-responders should receive a 2nd course of HBV vaccine with an increased dose (40 mcg).
10. Post vaccine testing is not indicated for most healthy adults, but is indicated for
    a. Health care workers, patient on dialysis, sex partners of chronic HBV patients, newborns born to mothers with HBV and immunocompromised patients
11. A single dose "booster" can be administered to HD patients when anti-HBs levels decline to less than 10

Reference

Hepatitis B vaccine and immunoglobulin: key concepts. PMID: 31293917.

Question 141

A 38-year-old female from Taiwan with chronic HBV has been followed in your clinic for nearly 5 years.

Her bloodwork prior to the initiation of antiviral therapy was:

TBili 0.8, AST 108, ALT 47, ALP 118
HBsAg positive, HBeAg positive, anti-HBe negative, anti-HBc total positive
HBV DNA 47,000 IU/mL: genotype B

A liver biopsy showed moderate inflammation and fibrosis of 2/4.
The patient was started on entecavir 0.5 mg and has done well.
Labs and serologies from now and 18 months ago are provided below:

	18 Months ago	Current
AST	18	18
ALT	14	16
HBsAg	Positive	Positive
eAg	Negative	Negative
eAb	Positive	Positive
DNA	Negative	Negative

An elastography reveals a kPa of 2.4 (IQR of 8%)

The patient is interested in coming off therapy.

What do you inform her

A She does not meet any guideline recommendations for discontinuation of therapy

B Chronic HBV patients can be controlled with undetectable DNA, but will never develop surface antigen loss and so therapy should be indefinite

C Improvement in fibrosis on therapy is very rare and the elastography results are likely erroneous

D HBeAg loss, normalization in her LFTs, and negative DNA do not lower her risk of HCC and so she should remain on antivirals indefinitely

E Discontinuation of therapy in her particular case is reasonable and likely safe; however, you would recommend a minimum of 12 months of "consolidation" therapy.

E is the correct answer.

Commentary – HBV Therapy Duration

Clinical Pearls: HBV and Duration of Treatment

1. All major guidelines recommend that patients with chronic HBV (including those with compensated cirrhosis) can stop nucleos(t)ide therapy if they achieve HBsAg loss (with or without the development of anti-HBs) that persists for at least 1 year. This however is quite rare.
2. Non-cirrhotic patients who are HBeAg positive can discontinue NA therapy if they achieve HBeAg seroconversion (loss of HBeAg and development of anti-HBe) and negative HBV DNA and after they complete 12 months of "consolidation" therapy
   a. The probability of durable HBeAg seroconversion in this group is ~90% At 1–2 year follow-up.
   b. There is progressively increasing data on a small but significant number of patients who develop HBsAg loss after NA discontinuation with reports anywhere from 10% to 20%
      i. The best predictor of HBsAg loss following NA discontinuation has been HBsAg level: <100 IU/mL at discontinuation.
3. The reported risk of relapse/flares in this cohort is low; however, most guidelines recommend close monitoring of ALT and HBV DNA levels for the first year.

Reference

Can we stop nucleoside analogues before HBsAg loss? PMID: 30803099.

Question 142

A 28-year-old male is referred to your clinic for "abnormal imaging". The patient underwent a right upper quadrant ultrasound 3 weeks prior to evaluate complaints of nausea and vomiting during an episode of suspected gastroenteritis. Multiple lesions were seen in his liver which prompted the MRI seen below. The official read is "concerning for diffuse metastatic disease".

On exam the patient is accompanied by his wife. They are both quite anxious. Exam is normal.

Past medical, surgical history is unremarkable. He takes no medications. He has no significant family history.

Lab tests including LFTs, CEA, Ca 19-9, and AFP are all normal. Viral serologies are negative.

You review the images with your radiologists who note that the liver is non-cirrhotic with no evidence of portal hypertension. There are "too numerous to count" small lesions, measuring up to 1.5 cm, seen scattered uniformly throughout the liver. The lesions are T2 hyperintense and T1 hypointense, without appreciable enhancement. The lesions did not show evidence of mass effect on hepatic vasculature. There is no communication between the biliary tree and lesions on magnetic resonance cholangiopancreatography.

What do you recommend?

A Liver biopsy and sampling of the lesions
B Reassurance
C Push enteroscopy if negative, cALPsule endoscopy
D Referral to medical oncology
E Referral to surgery for hepatoportoenterostomy

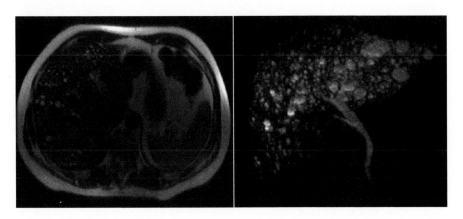

B is the correct answer.

Commentary – Biliary Hamartomas

Clinical Pearls: Biliary Hamartoma

1. Also known as Von Myenburg Complex
2. A benign condition, reportedly occurring in up to 5% of the population
   a. Malignant transformation has been reported, but it is limited to case reports
3. Likely a congenital malformation; potentially related to other diseases such as congenital hepatic fibrosis, polycystic liver disease, and Caroli's disease.
4. Consists of well-circumscribed, small (typically less than 1 cm) round or irregular shaped cystic lesions
   a. Sometimes described as producing a "starry sky" appearance
5. Usually discovered incidentally. Many times mistaken as metastatic disease
6. There are no standard guidelines are screening intervals

Notes

I have a handful of patients with Von Myenburg Complex. Most come from outside institutions with concern for "diffuse metastatic disease. Although there are 1–2 reported cases in the literature of malignancy associated with biliary hamartoma, for the most part, this entity appears to have a benign course.

Reference

Multicystic biliary hamartoma: A report of a rare entity and a review of the literature. PMID: 25460436.

Question 143

A 34-year-old female underwent an emergent TIPS for a massive variceal bleed nine months ago. She has underlying alcoholic cirrhosis but has since stopped drinking and is attending a relapse prevention program regularly. She underwent an upper endoscopy 10 days previously to evaluate some vague abdominal discomfort. EGD revealed medium sized esophageal varices without high risk stigmata. She had mild gastritis. Biopsies were negative for *Helicobacter pylori*. There were no gastric varices. Her abdominal discomfort is not particularly bothersome to her.

She says she feels great and over the last couple of weeks her sleep has improved and her energy level is increasing.

On exam the patient appears well. She has diffuse spider angiomata but believes they are improving. She has no ascites and mild lower extremity edema. Her mentation is good and she has no asterixis.

Laboratory studies:

WBC 6, Hb 12, Platelets 77K; MCV 84. Normal renal function. TBili 1.6, AST 18, ALT 21, ALP 109, gGTP 33. INR 1.3.

Current medications include lactulose 30cc TID, Rifaximin 550 mg po BID, Furosemide 20 mg, Spironolactone 50 mg.

An ultrasound with doppler is obtained. The liver is cirrhotic and there is mild peri-hepatic ascites. Velocities within the TIPS measure roughly 30 cm/s. In addition, there is hepatopedal flow identified within the branches of the right and left portal vein.

▶ Question

What do you recommend?

A Increase diuretics to 40 of lasix and 100 mg of aldactone
B Order a formal TIPS interrogation with venogram
C Arrange repeat EGD for banding of varices
D Order a triphasic CT of the abdomen
E Check serum venous ammonia level

B is the correct answer.

Commentary – TIPS Complications

Clinical Pearls: TIPS Complications

1. Intraperitoneal hemorrhage from transgression of liver capsule occurs 1–2% of cases.
2. Post TIPS PSE reported in ~33% of cases
   a. Risk factors for post-TIPS hepatic encephalopathy (HE): Hyponatremia, Sarcopenia, older age, prior history of HE, larger shunt diameter (>10 mm), alcohol-related cirrhosis
   b. Severe disabling encephalopathy 1–3%
      i. Most experts recommend dilating stent to 8 mm (as opposed to 10 mm) to decrease risk of post TIPS HE
   c. There is evidence now on prophylactic HE treatment pre-TIPS (rifaximin and/or lactulose)
   d. Acute liver injury
      i. Transient ischemic hepatitis is not uncommon immediately post TIPS.
      ii. Acute liver failure is rare but a grave compilation. Ultimately transplant may be only option.
   e. Biliary obstruction is a contraindication to TIPS
      i. Performing TIPS in a patient with dilated bile ducts can increase the risks of creating a biliary-venous fistula. This can lead to bilhemia (bile directly into the blood stream)
      ii. It can also present as TIPS occlusion, anemia, multiorgan failure, and sepsis
   f. TIPS migration: Cephalad into the IVC or heart which can cause arrhythmia
   g. TIPS dysfunction: Defined as occlusion (from thrombosis) or stenosis (from pseudointimal hyperplasia)
      i. Recurrence of symptoms that led to initial indication for TIPS placement should prompt US evaluation +/− formal venogram
         1. Shunt velocities 250 cm/s or higher or 50 cm/s or less are associated with >90% sensitivity and specificity for shunt dysfunction
      ii. Rates of primary patency at 2 years ~75% for covered stent (versus 35% for non-covered stent)
      iii. TIPS US should generally be performed every six months.
   h. Cardiac failure, reported in up to 20% of patients
      i. TTE should be performed to assess cardiac function and right sided pressures before an "elective TIPS" is performed
   i. Bowel hernia incarceration has been reported as high as 25% with a majority of patients requiring surgery. The median time to presentation is ~2 months.

j. Endotipsitis or infection of the TIPS shunt is rare; 1% of cases. Presents with sustained, unexplained bacteremia. Usually presents in conjunction with TIPS thrombosis. Treatment is lifelong antibiotics versus liver transplant.

k. Hemolytic anemia typically occurs 7–14 days post TIPS: increase in unconjugated bili, reticulocystosis, and decrease in serum haptoglobin. Usually spontaneously resolves.

Reference

Transjugular intrahepatic portosystemic shunt complications: prevention and management. PMID: 26038620.

Question 144

A 53-year-old female has been following in your clinic for years. She has autoimmune hepatitis which has been refractory to medical therapy.

Over the last year she has developed worsening ascites. She has required four large volume paracentesis in the last 6 months. Her last was 2 weeks ago for 8 L.

On exam, she is in no distress. She has mild scleral icterus, spider angiomata. She has small ascites with a palpable spleen. She has a moderate-sized umbilical hernia. She has mild lower extremity edema. Afebrile, HR 78, BP 88/42, RR 14, oxygen saturation 96% on room air; Her BMI is 21 kg/m².

An EGD 6 months ago revealed medium sized varices.

Her current medications include tacrolimus 0.5 mg daily, Spironolactone 200 mg, furosemide 80 mg, and Nadolol 20 mg.

An ultrasound shows new subocclusive thrombus in the main portal vein. A shrunken cirrhotic liver with small ascites. No lesions are seen.

Laboratory studies:

Na 131, K 5.1; BUN 21, Cr 1.4. WBC 4, Hb 10, Platelets 47K. TBili 2.3, AST 89, ALT 112, ALP 108; INR 1.4
Urine Na is less than 10
Which of the following do you recommend?

A Discontinue nadolol
B Discontinue diuretics
C Arrange for TIPS
D Refer for LT
E All of the above

E is the correct answer.

Commentary

Clinical Pearls: Refractory Ascites

1. Nearly half of all cirrhotics will develop ascites within 10 years of diagnosis
   a. First line treatment is sodium restriction: <2 g/day
   b. Followed by diuretics in ratio 100 mg spironolactone to 40 mg furosemide
2. Refractory ascites will develop in only 10%
   a. Carries a 2 year mortality of 65%
   b. All appropriate patients should be considered for liver transplantation
3. Definition of refractory ascites
   a. Lack of response to sodium restriction and maximal diuretics (400 mg of spironolactone and 160 mg of furosemide)
      i. If urine sodium is less than 30 mmol/day during diuretic therapy, patient likely has refractory ascites and diuretics should be discontinued
   b. Many patient will not be able to reach these doses of diuretics because of kidney injury, hypotension, and electrolyte disturbances
      i. Diuretics generally should be discontinued when sodium drops below 125
4. Controversy regarding use of non-selective beta-blockers in patients with refractory ascites. Most advocate discontinuation if systolic BP is <90 mmHg.
   a. Carvedilol in particular should not be administered in patients with refractory ascites
5. LVP is the standard first line treatment of tense ascites
   a. Albumin infusion (8 g for every 1 L removed) has shown to decrease post paracentesis circulatory dysfunction (PPCD) and decrease mortality.
6. A randomized control trial showed that TIPS compared to TAPS (repeated LVP) improved transplantation-free survival at 1 year. The selection of patients is critical for good outcomes.
   a. Generally MELD less than 18
7. Some data on the use of automated low-flow ascites pump (alfapump system) which is a subcutaneous implantable and rechargeable device which diverts ascites fluid to the urinary bladde. Generally used with prophylactic antibiotics, AKI is reported in up to 30% of patients.
8. There is some data regarding the long-term beneficial use of albumin administration (~40 g/week) in patients with ascites.
9. Some date on the successful use of midodrine (alpha-1-adrenergic agonist) 7.5 mg po TID (starting dose) in improving control in patients with refractory ascites.

Notes

If you haven't guessed by now, here's a TIP: you should know everything there is to know about TIPS for your exam!

Reference

Management of severe and refractory ascites. PMID: 33838859.

Question 145

A 44-year-old male with schizophrenia is brought to the emergency by his younger brother with increasing abdominal distension. The patient was found at home with multiple empty medicine bottles from the local health and nutrition store. His brother says he has not seen him in over a year.

The patient says he has been bolstering his immune system in order to protect himself from the "killer virus".

On exam the patient was oriented but anxious. He was non icteric. He had moderate to large ascites and splenomegaly. There was no asterixis.

Laboratory studies:

WBC 5, Hb 11, Platelets 98K.
TBili 1.1, AST 39, ALT 34, ALP 88.
INR 1
A full evaluation for chronic liver disease is negative.
Ultrasound reveals a hypoechogenic liver with moderate ascites.
A transjugular liver biopsy reveals a wedged hepatic pressure of 18 mmHg with a free pressure of 4 mmHg. A liver biopsy reveals enlarged, lipden-laden stellate cells. There was sinusoidal fibrosis but no overt cirrhosis.
What investigation would help you to arrive at a diagnosis?

A EGD with small bowel biopsies
B Stool for O&P
C Review of his medications
D Fat pad biopsy
E Quantitative copper measurement on liver tissue

C is the correct answer.

Commentary — Vitamins and Liver Disease

Clinical Pearls: Vitamins and the Liver

1. Fat soluble vitamins: D, A, K, and E are common manifestations of liver disease, especially patients with cholestatic liver disease.
   a. Vitamin A (retinol). Principally stored in hepatic stellate cells. Deficiency leads to xeropthalmia (dryness, fragility and clouding of the cornea) and night blindness; poor bone growth and hyperkeratosis.
      i. Chronic (>3 months) hypervitaminosis A can lead to liver injury. Liver biopsy is diagnostic and shows enlarged, lipid-laden stellate cells (formerly known as Ito cells). Extended use of high-dose Vitamin A can lead to PHTN without frank cirrhosis.
   b. Vitamin D deficiency. Deficiency has been linked to increased mortality in patients with chronic liver disease. Major clinical manifestation of vit D deficiency is bone loss.
   c. Vitamin E deficiency is seen most commonly in alcoholics. Deficiency leads to nerve and muscle damage.
      i. Supplementation with vitamin E (800 IU/day) is commonly employed in patients with NASH based on studies showing a reduction in inflammation and steatosis.
   d. Vitamin K deficiency leads to bleeding, poor bone development, and increased risk of cardiovascular disease.
      i. Rapid correction of PT (INR) with vitamin K supplementation suggests coagulopathy may be more nutritionally related or due to cholestasis as opposed to liver failure.
   e. Vitamin B1 (thiamine) deficiency again seen most commonly in alcoholics. Deficiency can lead to Wernicke's encephalopathy characterized by triad: opthalmoplegia, ataxia, and confusion.
      i. Thiamine replacement should be administered before (or together) with glucose.
   f. Zinc deficiency is common in chronic liver disease. Manifestations include dermatitis and diarrhea.
      i. Zinc supplementation and effects on HE have been marginal.
   g. Niacin (vitamin B3) deficiency: Pellegra leads to the 3 Ds (dermatitis, dementia, and diarrhea), although niacin deficiency has not been linked with liver disease excess niacin supplementation has been associated serious hepatotoxicity.

Notes

My co-author thought this question was too simple. Did you get it right?

Reference

Nutrition in the management of cirrhosis and its neurological complications. PMID: 25755550.

Question 146

A 63-year-male with alcoholic cirrhosis is sent to your clinic. He stopped drinking one month ago and is doing relatively well. Exam reveals spider angiomata, palmar erythema a firm palpable liver without audible bruit. He has bilateral Dupuytren contracture. His BMI is 21 kg/m². HR 92, BP 120/60.

Laboratory studies:

WBC 8, Hb 12, Platelets 110. Na 133, Cr 1; Albumin 3.8. TBili 1.5, AST 88, ALT 61, ALP 108, gGTP 254. INR 1.1

An in clinic transient elastrography reveals a kPa of 16.4 (IQR 9%). A triphasic CT scan reveals a cirrhotic liver with patent vessels, no ascites, and no lesions. There are moderate sized peri-esophageal varices and a recannalized umbilical vein. Spleen measures 14 cm.

With regards to variceal screening +/− management you recommend?

A Surveillance EGD
B Can forgo EGD
C Carvedilol 6.25 mg po BID
D Measure elastrography after an additional 5 months of abstinence and then reassess
E Elastrography lacks accuracy, obtain MRI with PDFF and elastrography.

A is the correct answer.

Commentary – Non-invasive Assessment of Liver Fibrosis

Clinical Pearls: Noninvasive Tests for Evaluation of Liver Disease

1. Liver biopsy remains the gold standard for the assessment of liver fibrosis, however given risks, cost, patient preference, and sampling error (~15% when it comes to fibrosis staging), noninvasive measurements are increasingly being used.
2. Liver stiffness measurement (LSM) can be obtained by different methods. For Shear wave US with elastography or Fibroscan LSM <8 kPa (for MRE <3) can be used to rule out advanced fibrosis; ≥15 kPa (MRE >4.7) is highly suggestive of compensated advanced chronic liver disease; >20–25 clinically significant portal hypertension (CSPH)
   a. Transient elastrography
   b. Point-shear wave elastography (integrated into US)
   c. Bidimensional shear wave elastrography (2D-SWE)
   d. MRE
      i. Meal ingestion, exercise, venous congestion, inflammation, and obstructive cholestasis can overestimate fibrosis.
         1. Testing should be done after minimum of 3 hour fast
      ii. LSM is not recommended to detect fibrosis regression after SVR in HCV patients
3. Controlled attenuation parameter (CAP) is a point of care technique for detection of steatosis
   a. 275 dB/m can be used to diagnose steatosis
4. MRI-PDFF is the most accurate noninvasive method for detecting and quantifying steatosis
5. Serum tests to rule out advanced liver disease in patients
   a. ELF <9.8
   b. FibroMeter <0.45
   c. FiroTest <0.48
   d. FIB-4 <1.3
   e. NFS <−1.455
   f. ALPRI <0.3
6. Serum markers of fibrosis and noninvasive scores are not recommended for fibrosis staging in patients with PBC. LSM however does seem to be accurate. Treatment and risk stratification in PBC include: GLOBE, UK-PBC risk score.
7. In patients with compensated advanced liver disease due to viral hepatitis, HIV-HCV coinfection, alcohol, NAFLD, PBC, and PSC an LSM <20 with a platelet count >150 is validated to rule out high-risk varices and void endoscopic screening.
8. CT should not be used for primary screening for esophageal or gastric varices.

Notes

Liver stiffness measurement (LSM) has become a well-recognized, established, and validated parameter in nearly every form of chronic liver disease. It is highly effective in ruling out advanced disease but in many cases, it should be used as an adjunct to supplement your entire clinical picture.

Reference

Clinical Practice Guidelines on noninvasive tests for evaluation of liver disease severity and prognosis – 2021 update. PMID: 34166721.

Question 147

In regard to the rejection response: the donor antigen-presenting cell (APC) that are found in the graft organ present to T-cell receptor from the recipient. This is termed:

A Signal 1
B Signal 2
C Signal 3
D Signal 4
E Signal 5

Question 148

A 53-year-old male undergoes a liver transplant for HCV cirrhosis. He is treatment naïve. Explant analysis revealed an incidental 1.1 cm HCC. He receives a graft from a 39-year-old deceased donor who is

HCV NAT positive. Post-operative day 3 the patient AST is 3400, INR 2.9 with a lactate of 5.2. All vessels are patent on US. After 6 weeks in the ICU the patient is transferred to the medical floor.

Liver tests reveal: TBili 7.4, AST 328, ALT 444, ALP 403. A liver biopsy is performed. Liver biopsy shows histopathological findings consistent with antibody mediated rejection (AMR) with C4d staining. Serum DSA test is positive.

Which of the following did NOT contribute to the "2nd hit" leading to this patient's AMR

A Recurrent HCV
B Primary Non-Function
C DCD donor
D Incidental HCC
E B&C

Question 149

A 23-year-old male underwent a liver transplant over 10 years ago. He comes in today with his wife to establish care. He admits he has not taken any medications in over 5 years. Exam reveals a well-appearing male with healed chevron surgical scar and a small incisional hernia.

Liver tests: TBili 0.4, AST 18, ALT 20, ALP 98. A RUQ US with elastography reveals a kPa of 3.3 (IQR of 9%). The patient's wife wants to know the status of his graft and so you obtain a liver biopsy. The biopsy is completely normal.

How would you define this patient post-transplant "status"?

A Operational tolerance
B Immunological tolerance
C Prope tolerance
D Subclinical allograft injury
E Silent allograft injury

147 – A is the correct answer.
148 – D is the correct answer.
149 – A is the correct answer.

Commentary – Transplant Immunology

Clinical Pearls: Transplant Immunology

1. Innate immune activation is via antigen presenting cells. It stimulates adaptive immunity (T and B cells) which promote alloreactivity and can lead to rejection.
2. Innate: First line of defense, no memory; same response every time and is nonspecific.
   Innate stimulates the adaptive response. Innate immune cells include:
   a. Polys (PMNs, eosinophils, basophils)
   b. Monocyte/Macrophage
   c. Natural Killer and Natural Killer T cells
   d. Dendritic cells
3. Adaptive: Initial effector response; helper, memory; increase response every time; these are specific
   a. Lymphocytes
      i. Cellular immunity
         1. CD4positive: T helper (class II MHC)
            a. Class II major histocompatibility class (MHC) are expressed on antigen presenting cells (macrophages and dendritic cells), activated T-cells, B cells and Kupffer cells
               i. Proliferating helper T cells that develop into effector T cells differentiate into two major subtypes
                  1. TH1 – dominant in rejection
                  2. TH2 – dominant in long-term graft survival
         2. CD8 positive: T cytotoxic (class I MHC)
            a. Class I major histocompatibility class are expressed on all nucleated cells
   b. Humoral immunity
      i. B cells
      ii. Plasma Cells
4. Types of immune response
   a. Hyperacute (pre-formed ABO antibodies). Pre-existing antibodies exist if graft is not ABO-matched; allo-antibodies can be generated during previous blood transfusions, previous transplantation, or pregnancy
      i. Desensitization protocols (plasmapheresis, IVIG, rituximab +/− splenectomy)
   b. Acute (T cell mediated rejection: TCMR; HLA Antibodies may potentiate injury)
   c. Chronic: Fibrosis and vasculopathy and ductopenia; a mix of TCMR and antibody mediated rejection (AMR)

5. Initial rejection response is via the direct pathway. The donor antigen presenting cells that are in the graft stimulate recipient T cells – these T cells (CD4 and CD8) then cause acute rejection.
   a. APC presents T-cell receptor CD3 (SIGNAL 1). *See illustration below*
   b. SIGNAL 2 is co-stimulation involving CD28 expressed on T-cells binding to B7 on ALPC. Activating T-cells.
   c. Intracellular calcium increases. Which activates calcineurin which dephosphorylates NFAT (nuclear factor of activated T-cells). NFAT stimulates the nucleus and production of inflammatory cytokines. Most important being IL-2.
   d. Stimulation of IL-2 receptor (CD25) is SIGNAL 3. SIGNAL 3 stimulates the synthesis and proliferation of T-cells.
6. Late pathways are involved in chronic rejection. Where recipient APC goes into the donor graft and pick up donor antigens then present them to recipient T cells and causes a low-grade response.
7. Antibody mediated rejection. Two hit hypotheses. Injured graft and donor specific antigen (DSA):
   a. Presence of donor specific antibodies in circulation (one hit)
   b. Injury to graft (2nd hit): DCD, ischemic-reperfusion injury, delayed graft function, viral hepatitis, t-cell-mediated rejection, etc. An injured graft expresses HLA-class II which allows the antibody to bind which then causes further injury.
8. Tolerance
   a. Immunological tolerance: Absence of immune reactivity toward specific antigens but preservation of immunity against foreign antigens, in the absence of ongoing immunosuppression.
   b. Operational tolerance: Clinical circumstance in which graft function is stable without rejection in the absence of IS.
   c. Prope tolerance: Minimal IS with stable graft function (as little as possible without rejection).
   d. Regulatory T Cells (T-regs)
      i. Naturally produced in the thymus and induced in the periphery **to control effector responses** to auto and allo-antigens. Balance of effector and T-regs can determine the outcome on whether you develop a tolerance state.
      ii. Express: high levels of CD 25, FOX P3. T-regs suppress the immune response through IL-10. IL-10 has potent immunosuppressive capacity and is key in development of tolerance.
   e. In very select groups there may be an ability to wean off IS
      i. Pre-weaning biopsy can help predict success. Surveillance biopsy during their course is also critical.

Reference

Transplantation immunology: what the clinician needs to know for immunotherapy. PMID: 18471555.

Question 150

Basiliximab functions by blocking what portion of the antigen presenting cell/T-cell depicted below?

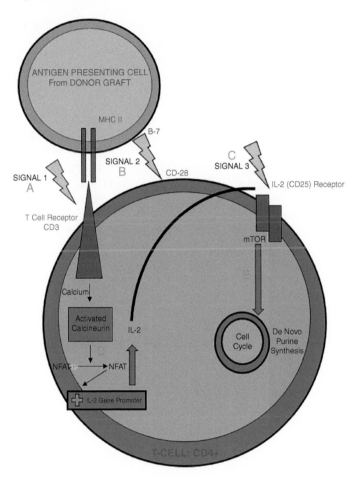

C is the correct answer.

Clinical Pearls: IS and Rejection (refer to illustration on page: 359 with special attention to "red stop signs")

1. OKT-3, Anti-CD3: blocks signal 1 (no longer available in US).
2. Anti-thymocyte globulin (ATG) and Anti-CD52(alemtuzumab or Campath): block signal 1 and 2 (see image)
3. Calcineurin inhibitors (CNI) block calcineurin (part of Signal 1 and 2)
   a. Cyclosporine. forms a complex with cyclophilin and this binds calcineurin. Inhibits Nuclear factor of activated T-cells from entering cells. Excreted in bile. Half-life 8 hours. Nephrotoxicity, DM, HTN, HLD. Hair growth.
      i. Caution drug-drug interaction (DDI): Cyclosporin and statin can lead to an increase in the concentration of statin and subsequent increased risk of rhabdomyolysis
   b. FK-506 (Tacrolimus). Binds to FKBP-12 (immunophilin). Forms a complex that inhibits calcineurin. 25× more potent inhibitor of calcineurin compared to cyclosporin. Nephrotoxicity, Neurotoxicity, DM, HTN, HLD. Hair loss, rare: HUS.
4. Steroids – Pan-immunosuppressant
5. CTLA-4Ig (Belatacept), blocks signal 2
6. SIGNAL 3. T-cell proliferation is blocked by
   a. IL-2 receptor antagonists
      i. Daclizumab
      ii. Basiliximab
   b. mTOR inhibitors Sirolimus and Everolimus
      i. Side effects: Pancytopenia, impaired wound healing, HAT, Hypertriglyceridemia (inhibit lipoprotein lipase and so increase lipids), proteinuria, oral and gi ulcers, pneumonitis; excreted in bile
      ii. Sirolimus
         1. Blackbox warning increased risk of HAT; because of this only used after 30 days
         2. ½ life 63 hours
      iii. Everolimus
         1. indicated in combo with low dose tacrolimus >30 days; combo may spare renal function
         2. ½ life 30 hours
   c. mTOR inhibitors AZA and MMF
      i. Mycophenolate: Noncompetitive inhibitor of Inosine monophosphate dehydrogenase. Interferes with guanine nucleotide synthesis and purine synthesis. Potent inhibitor of B and T cells.
      ii. Side effects: Gastrointestinal, bone marrow suppression. Teratogenic
7. Typical center regimens:
   a. Induction with ATG and IL2-R antagonist
   b. CNI (FK used much more frequently than CSA)
   c. Adjunctive MMF

d. Steroid taper within 3–6 months
e. mTOR-I after 30 days for renal sparing effects (generally should be introduced early, i.e. 1–2 years in those with renal insufficiency as opposed to when renal insufficiency is "established")

Reference

Comprehensive update of the Banff working group on liver allograft pathology: introduction of antibody-mediated rejection. PMID: 27273869.

Question 151

Which of the following is the classic histopathological findings seen in T-cell mediated rejection

A Ductopenia, obliterative arteriopathy, and cholestasis
B Sinusoidal inflammation, peri-portal necrosis, and C4d staining
C Portal inflammation, nonsuppurative destructive cholangitis, reactive hyperplasia
D Cytolysis, necrosis particular in zone 3 (centrilobular)
E Endotheliitis, ductulitis, and mixed portal inflammation

Question 152

A 26-year-old male with a history of end stage liver disease secondary to Wilson disease underwent a liver transplant 4 years ago. The donor was his 31-year-old sister. The patient's post operative course was unremarkable.

The patient has had two bouts of ACR treated in the past with steroids.

The patient returns to the clinic for the first time in 18 months. Other than itching and dark urine, he is feeling great. Exam is notable for scleral icterus and excoriations. His abdomen reveals a healed surgical scar but is otherwise benign. His medication list includes tacrolimus 2 bid, mycophenolate 500 mg BID, Paroxetine, and Mag-oxide.

Laboratory studies:

TBili 10.2 (conjugated 7.2), AST 53, ALT 61, ALP 302, GGT 340; Albumin 4
WBC 4, Hb 14, Platelets 176
Na 140, K 4; BUN 8, Cr 0.7; FK level is pending.
A cholangiogram is normal.
A liver biopsy reveals: obliterative arteriopathy and intrahepatic cholangiopathy, pyknosis and bile duct atrophy with ductopenia involving >50% of bile ducts.
Which of the following is consistent with the diagnosis:

A ERC revealing beaded appearing bile ducts
B ERC revealing narrowing at the biliary anastomosis with upstream dilation
C Predominant increase in hepatocellular enzymes
D Supratherapeutic levels of FK
E Positive CK-19 staining

151 – E is the correct answer.
152 – E is the correct answer.

Clinical Pearls: Rejection

1. Classic/acute/T-cell mediated rejection
   a. lymphocytes are the dominant cell type in TCMR. CD 4 and CD 8.
   b. generally seen within the first 5–30 days, 10–20% patients; symptoms are rare, usually picked up on labs
   c. higher incidence in patients transplanted for AIH; females and younger age
   d. Triad for TCMR:
      i. Endotheliitis
      ii. Ductulitis
      iii. Mixed portal inflammation
         1. direct correlation between eosinophils and rejection; macrophages and plasma cells are also present
   e. mild <50% of portal tracts
      i. treated with increase in maintenance IS without steroids
   f. moderate >50%
      i. treat with steroids and increase in baseline IS
   g. severe >50% of portal tracts and central vein involvement and necrosis
      i. treated with steroids and increase in baseline IS and consider ATG in refractory cases and consider AMR (C4d staining and DSA testing)
   h. if already optimized at time of TCMR add second line agent
   i. consider long-term prednisone in patients transplanted for AIH and those with at least two episodes of severe TCMR
2. Chronic rejection
   a. Indolent, progressive obliterative arteriopathy and intrahepatic cholangiopathy, bile duct atrophy/pyknosis and ductopenia (at least 50%)
   b. Rise in cholestatic enzymes
   c. CK-19 stain
   d. Occurs typically in patients with:
      i. Multiple TCMR
      ii. Non-compliance (transition of child to adult hood)
      iii. Underdosed immunosuppression
3. AMR
   a. See section on AMR
   b. Consider in refractory rejection
   c. C4d staining in venules and DSA in blood with accompanying histology
   d. Sinusoidal inflammation, peri-portal necrosis, and C4d staining in the portal venules and sinusoidal venules
   e. Management of AMR:
      i. Plasmapheresis (remove the antibody)
      ii. IVIG (block the antibody)
      iii. Rituximab and Bortezomib (inhibit antibody production)
      iv. Eculizumab (inhibit the antibody injury)
4. Plasma cell hepatitis more commonly now referred to as 'de novo' autoimmune hepatitis. The de novo prefix distinguishes this entity from a pre-transplant primary AIH. Characterized by a) liver necroinflammation that is plasma cell rich

b) interface hepatitis c) elevated LFTs and d) elevated IgG and autoantibodies. Typically responsive to steroids and seen most commonly in patients transplant for HCV with IFN based regimens hypothesized as a potential trigger

Notes

The immunology section is what gives fellows preparing for the transplant hepatology boards the most anxiety. We have two separate immunology sections to help you. We have taken slightly different approaches. Hopefully, by studying both, the major points will become clear (as mud). This section is dense. It will take a few reads! Please reference the illustration below especially the drugs highlighted in "stop signs" that block the corresponding pathways.

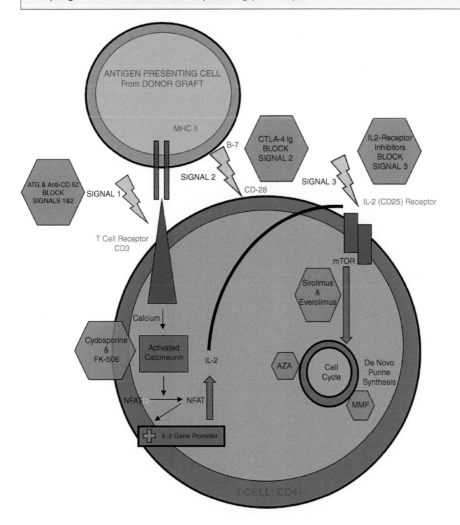

Reference

International liver transplantation society consensus statement on immunosuppression in liver transplant recipients. PMID: 29485508.

Question 153

A 42-year-old male presents with 1 week of nausea, diarrhea, and jaundice. He denies fever or weight loss. He has no past medical history and denies any regular medications. He works as a policeman and takes several dietary supplements including green tea extract. Examination shows normal vital signs and scleral icterus.

Laboratory studies:

ALT 908 U/L
AST 1073 U/L
ALP 94 U/L
Tbili 8.6 mg/dL
INR 1.3
Creatinine 0.8 mg/dL
Acetaminophen level undetectable
CT scan abdomen – normal liver and biliary tree, normal pancreas
HBsAg, anti-Hbc IgM, anti-HAV IgM, anti-HCV all negative
ANA 1:40, SMA negative, quantitative immunoglobulins normal
Anti-HBs positive

▶ Question

Which of the following statements is TRUE

A A liver biopsy will be diagnostic
B This will likely transition to cirrhosis
C He is likely to make a full recovery
D The patient should be started on steroids
E The patient should be started on ursodeoxycholic acid

C is the correct answer.

Commentary – Drug Induced Liver Injury

This patient has an acute liver injury with jaundice but normal liver synthetic function. The differential diagnosis is wide, but an appropriate workup was performed to exclude the common causes. The clue here is in the history. He is taking dietary supplements making idiosyncratic drug-induced liver injury (DILI) a possibility. The acetaminophen level is undetectable and although this does not exclude acetaminophen liver injury it would be unlikely, particularly as jaundice to this degree is unusual. Acute hepatitis A and B are unlikely due to the negative serology, and he appears to have been vaccinated against hepatitis B. The hepatitis C antibody is negative and to be complete, HCV RNA should be checked (even without an obvious risk factor) and even HEV serology would not be unreasonable. His autoimmune serology is also normal, making autoimmune hepatitis unlikely. There is no evidence of biliary disease on imaging and acute cholangitis typically would have more symptomatology.

A liver biopsy is not necessary to make a diagnosis of DILI but characteristic changes can occasionally be seen with certain drugs but in general in a case like this there will be an acute nonspecific hepatitis.

Steroids have been used in DILI but there is no good evidence of effectiveness except in cases of drug-induced autoimmune hepatitis. Ursodeoxycholic acid anecdotally can be used in cholestatic liver injury but without evidence.

The lack of a reliable biomarker makes the diagnosis of idiosyncratic DILI a diagnosis of exclusion. The RUCAM (Roussel Uclaf Causality Assessment Method) can be used which assigns points based on several domains including timing of injury, improvement after the drug is discontinued and exclusion of other causes. Several DILI registries exist including the DILI Network (DILIN) in the United States that use expert opinion to assign causality in cases of suspected DILI. Herbal and dietary supplements (HDS) are an increasingly recognized cause of DILI and making a diagnosis can be even more difficult as this industry has limited regulation and the contents of HDS products are frequently mislabeled. A recent study demonstrated that green tea extract was responsible for 3% of DILIN cases.

In the DILIN, recovery from the acute injury is typical although chronic injury (more than 6 months after onset) can occur in up to 18% of patients.

Clinical Pearls: Drug-Induced Liver Injury

1. No diagnostic finding for DILI – not even biopsy
2. For the boards, usually an antibiotic or herbal and dietary supplement is the culprit
3. If it is HDS, it will be a well-known hepatotoxin
4. Hepatocellular injury with jaundice has significant mortality (Hy's Law)

Reference

ACG Clinical Guideline: the diagnosis and management of idiosyncratic drug-induced liver injury. PMID: 24935270.

Question 154

A 62-year-old male presents for follow-up in the office 6 months after orthotopic liver transplant for alcoholic cirrhosis and HCC. His MELD score at the time of transplant was 8 and he had been downstaged before transplant with multiple locoregional therapies. His explanted liver showed partially treated cancers with invasion of thick-walled vessels. He is feeling well except for some reflux symptoms and discomfort during swallowing.

His medications include tacrolimus 3 mg bid, mycophenolate mofetil 1 g bid, prednisone 5 mg daily.

Examination shows BMI 23 kg/m², BP 150/100 and some oral thrush.

Laboratory studies:

ALT 17 U/L
AST 21 U/L
ALP 67 U/L
Tbili 0.7 mg/dL
Creatinine 1.8 mg/dL
HBV DNA negative
Urinalysis – No proteinuria
Tacrolimus trough level 9.2 ng/mL

▶ Question

What is the best management option?

A Change the tacrolimus to sirolimus
B Increase the tacrolimus dose if he is started on an antifungal such as fluconazole
C Stop the mycophenolate mofetil
D Increase the prednisone
E Stop the tacrolimus and increase the mycophenolate mofetil dose

A is the correct answer.

Commentary – Post Liver Transplant Medication Side Effects

This man is at risk of his HCC recurring given the findings on the explant. He has developed oral (and probably esophageal candidiasis) that needs to be treated and has developed hypertension and some renal dysfunction without proteinuria. We are told the MELD was 8 at the time of the transplant so this is a new elevation of creatinine. His liver function is normal with a therapeutic tacrolimus level for someone at this point after liver transplant and his HBV DNA is negative on oral antivirals.

Immunosuppressive medication works very well but has a variety of potential side effects. Tacrolimus is a calcineurin inhibitor (CNI) and is the main immunosuppressive drug used after liver transplant and has multiple dose-dependent side effects. It is metabolized by CYP450-3A enzymes so multiple drug interactions are possible. Antifungals such as fluconazole increase the tacrolimus level while anticonvulsants are among a group of drugs that can decrease the level. CNIs are also associated with hypertension, diabetes, and hyperlipidemia. This patient's elevated blood pressure is likely related to the tacrolimus and needs to be treated.

Mycophenolate mofetil is used as an adjunct with CNIs to lower their dose. It inhibits purine synthesis and acts on inosine monophosphate dehydrogenase, an important enzyme in T and B lymphocyte function. It cannot be used as an immunosuppressive agent after transplant by itself. The most common side effect is gastro-intestinal, typically diarrhea which can necessitate dose reduction or discontinuation, but it does not affect renal function.

The main alternative to CNIs is MTOR inhibitors such as sirolimus or everolimus. They are less nephrotoxic but also have an anti-angiogenic effect and so are useful in patients with CNI related renal dysfunction and patients with HCC at high risk of recurrence, although the latter is controversial and would likely not be a board question.

Prednisone is used in the early stages after liver transplant and could be stopped at this stage rather than increase the dose.

Clinical Pearls: Immunosuppression Side Effects

1. Immunosuppressive medications and their side effects and interactions will definitely be on the boards
2. Remember the main side effects of CNIs – renal, metabolic, neurological, cancer risk
3. Multiple drug-drug interactions but the following are most likely to come up on the boards:
   a. Increase CNI level – Azoles, Macrolides, Verapamil, HIV protease inhibitors, Grapefruit
   b. Decrease CNI level – Anticonvulsants, Rifampin, St. John's Wort
4. Review the mechanism of action of CNIs
5. MTORs are renal-sparing and anti-angiogenic

Reference

International liver transplantation society consensus statement on immunosuppression in liver transplant recipients. PMID: 29485508.

Question 155

A 19-year-old male presents for routine evaluation. He is originally from Taiwan and says he has "dormant" hepatitis B. His older sister was told the same thing and their father died in his 50s with liver cancer.

He has no other medical problems and is on no prescribed medication. Physical examination is normal.

Laboratory studies:

Normal CBC and renal function
ALT 72 U/L
AST 63 U/L
ALP 78 U/L
Tbili 0.5 mg/dL
HBsAg positive
Anti-HBs negative
HBeAg positive
Anti-HBe negative
HBV DNA 250,000 IU/mL
AFP 3 ng/mL
Ultrasound abdomen shows normal liver contour, mild increased echogenicity

▶ Question

Which statement is TRUE regarding management of chronic hepatitis B in this patient?

A   His ethnicity mandates he should be started on therapy
B   His ALT and HBV DNA levels are the most important factors in deciding to treat him
C   His family history mandates he should be started on therapy
D   His HBeAg is positive so he should be treated
E   He should get a contrast enhanced MRI scan every 6 months to screen for HCC

B is the correct answer.

Commentary – Treatment and Medication Side Effects of HBV

Chronic hepatitis B (CHB) is defined by the persistence of HBsAg in serum for at least 6 months, but HBV DNA can range from undetectable to several billion IU/mL. Once CHB is identified, it is important to know if the patient is HBeAg positive or negative, the ALT level, and assessment of liver histology and fibrosis by biopsy or elastography if available, as these are the factors that influence treatment decision. Classification of CHB is still used but it is difficult as patients can move between categories and do not always fit neatly into them. Immune-tolerant CHB has very high HBV DNA levels but minimally elevated or normal ALT and normal biopsy. Immune-active CHB has elevated ALT with HBV DNA >20,000 IU/mL in HBeAg positive and >2,000 IU/mL in HBeAg negative patients with chronic hepatitis on biopsy. Inactive CHB has DNA <2000 IU/mL, normal ALT, and anti-HBe positive without inflammation on biopsy.

AASLD guidelines on treatment of CHB are very lengthy as they cover multiple special populations. In the typical CHB patient, documentation of persistently elevated ALT and HBV DNA (>20,000 IU/mL in HBeAg positive and >2000 IU/mL in HBeAg negative) over several months is an indication for treatment.

Several drugs are approved for the treatment of CHB:

1. Pegylated interferon alpha-2a and interferon alpha-2b (in children).
2. Entecavir.
3. Tenofovir (disoproxil fumarate or alafenamide).
4. Others include lamivudine and adefovir but these are associated with viral resistance and telbivudine is associated with myopathy and elevated creatine kinase.

Entecavir and tenofovir are the preferred oral agents. Pegylated interferon alpha has the disadvantage of requiring a subcutaneous injection, but studies suggest it has a higher rate of HBeAg seroconversion and can also induce HBsAg loss in a minority of patients compared to oral antivirals. Tenofovir disoproxil fumarate has been associated with mild renal dysfunction and loss of bone density but these changes were not seen with tenofovir alafenamide in a large recent study so is the preferred drug.

The patient's ethnicity and family history do not influence treatment decisions but do affect the risk of HCC development so guidelines for when to start HCC surveillance in CHB patients reflect this. Ultrasound every 6 months is the preferred imaging modality. The age at which to start screening is based on the ethnicity, age of the patient, presence of cirrhosis, and family history. This patient has a family history, but it is too early to start screening.

Clinical Pearls: HBV

1. In HBV, degree of ALT elevation and DNA level determine the need for treatment
2. HBeAg status affects the DNA level to start treatment (>2,000 IU/mL in HBeAg negative, >20,000 IU/mL in HBeAg positive)
3. HBV treatment guidelines change every few years

Notes

HBV is confusing because of the numerous acronyms used, constant changing of the guidelines and differences in clinical practice and what is recommended. For the boards, it will be non-controversial and straightforward. Remember that observation is not a bad option with repeating labs in a few months.

Reference

Update on prevention, diagnosis, and treatment of chronic hepatitis B: AASLD 2018 Hepatitis B Guidance. https://www.aasld.org/sites/default/files/2019-06/HBVGuidance_Terrault_et_al-2018-Hepatology.pdf.

Question 156

A 53-year-old female presents with a week of dark urine, pale stool, and jaundice. She has a history of primary biliary cholangitis (PBC) and has been maintained on ursodiol for several years.

Examination shows stable vitals, normal temperature, scleral icterus, and a non-tender abdomen with a liver edge just palpable below the costal margin but no ascites.

Laboratory studies:

ALT 648 U/L
AST 584 U/L
ALP 376 U/L
Tbili 7.6 mg/dL
INR 1.2
Creatinine 0.5 mg/dL
Viral serology for HAV/HBV/HCV/HEV all negative
AMA 67 (ULN 20)
ANA 1 : 1280
SMA 81 (ULN 19)
Quantitative immunoglobulins 3900 mg/dL
CT scan abdomen – Hepatomegaly, normal liver contour, normal biliary tree, moderate retroperitoneal lymphadenopathy

▶ Question

What is the most appropriate management of this patient?

A Start liver transplant evaluation
B CT guided biopsy of abdominal lymphadenopathy
C Liver biopsy and consider oral steroids
D Start obeticholic acid
E Add azathioprine

C is the correct answer.

Commentary – AIH//PBC Overlap

This lady has PBC with a strongly positive anti-mitochondrial antibody. However, her ALT and AST are very elevated. Her viral hepatitis studies are negative, and her abdominal imaging shows an enlarged liver with retroperitoneal lymphadenopathy. The autoimmune serology is strongly positive with high titers of smooth muscle antibody, antinuclear antibody, and high levels of gamma-globulins. The most likely explanation for these findings is an overlap syndrome of PBC and autoimmune hepatitis (AIH). Although typically considered separate entities, these two immune-mediated diseases can occur simultaneously or consecutively in a surprisingly high number of patients (5–19%) and diagnostic criteria (Paris criteria) have been established based on the degree of elevation of ALP, ALT, autoimmune markers and biopsy findings. At least 2 of the 3 criteria are required for both PBC and AIH and interface hepatitis is required.

Paris criteria.

PBC criteria	1. ALP $\geq$2×ULN or GGT $\geq$5× ULN
	2. Positive AMA $\geq$1 : 40
	3. Liver biopsy with florid duct lesion
AIH criteria	1. ALT >5× ULN
	2. IgG >2× ULN or positive SMA
	3. **Liver biopsy with interface hepatitis/piecemeal necrosis**

Treatment of PBC/AIH overlap syndrome with ursodeoxycholic acid (UDCA) and immunosuppressive agents is associated with good long-term outcomes so prednisone should be used in this patient. She meets the criteria for diagnosis and steroids should be considered.

Her liver synthetic function and creatinine are normal, so liver transplant evaluation is not needed at this time. Abdominal lymphadenopathy is very common in PBC patients and is not indicative of lymphoma. Obeticholic acid is approved as a treatment for PBC in combination with UDCA in patients without normalization of ALP or in patients who are intolerant of UDCA. Azathioprine is used as a steroid-sparing agent in patients with AIH and could be considered here, but only after the diagnosis is made and the liver enzymes have improved/normalized.

Reference

Primary biliary cirrhosis-autoimmune hepatitis overlap syndrome: clinical features and response to therapy. PMID: 9695990.

Question 157

A 54-year-old male with a history NASH cirrhosis presents for liver transplant evaluation. His liver disease has been complicated by ascites and encephalopathy. He works in construction and is having difficulty with work due to poor exercise tolerance and some shortness of breath.

Vital signs show BP 110/50, pulse 96. Physical examination is notable for multiple spider nevi, palmar erythema, clear lung fields, no ascites, and trace ankle edema.

Laboratory studies:

AST 43 U/L
ALT 57 U/L
Tbili 1.7 mg/dL
INR 1.4
Albumin 2.3 g/dL
Hb 12.8 g/dL
EKG normal sinus rhythm
CXR normal
Contrast MRI abdomen – Cirrhotic liver, no HCC, splenomegaly, patent vessels, mild perihepatic ascites
Cardiac stress test- negative for ischemia
Echocardiogram – EF 70%, normal right sided pressures

▶ Question

What is the next most appropriate test to perform to explain his symptoms?

A Doppler ultrasound
B Liver biopsy
C Cardiac catheterization
D EGD/colonoscopy
E Arterial blood gas

E is the correct answer.

Commentary – Pulmonary Disease in Patients with Liver Disease

This patient describes shortness of breath and decreased exercise tolerance, but his physical examination shows a normal heart and lungs, and his cardiac workup was normal, as was his chest X-ray. The most likely diagnosis is hepatopulmonary syndrome (HPS) which is present in many patients with cirrhosis and often undiagnosed. A cirrhotic patient with a low O_2 saturation on room air in the absence of heart and lung disease is suggestive of HPS.

In fact, his O_2 saturation on room air was 86% with an arterial blood gas showing pH 7.39, PaO_2 54 mmHg, $PaCO_2$ 28 mmHg with an Aa gradient (on room air) of 61 mmHg $((150-5/4(PaCO_2)) - PaO_2)$.

The definition of HPS includes an increased Aa gradient on room air with evidence of intrapulmonary vascular abnormalities or dilatations (IPVDs) in patients with liver disease in the absence of intrinsic lung disease. The IPVDs are thought to arise due to an imbalance of pulmonary vasodilators and circulating vasoconstrictors in cirrhotic patients leading to right to left shunting in the pulmonary vasculature. These are not true anatomical shunts as they partially respond to increased FiO_2. The diagnosis can be confirmed by demonstrating the shunting using agitated saline (bubble) or contrast echocardiogram, labeled macro-aggregated albumin scanning or in rare cases pulmonary angiography.

The other main considerations to explain shortness of breath in cirrhosis would be hepatic hydrothorax and porto-pulmonary hypertension (PPHTN). The physical exam and chest X-ray in this patient excluded hepatic hydrothorax. In patients with PPHTN, the echocardiogram is a good screening test, and the elevated pulmonary pressure can be confirmed on a right heart catheterization.

It is important to make the diagnosis of HPS (and PPHTN) as these patients are granted a MELD exception for listing for liver transplantation. In addition, severe HPS (PaO_2 <50 mmHg) and uncontrolled PPHTN are associated with poor outcome after liver transplantation.

A Doppler ultrasound is used to assess hepatic vasculature, but the patient already had a contrast MRI that was normal. Cardiac catheterization is typically reserved for patients with a positive cardiac stress test. This patient had a normal cardiac stress test. Endoscopic examination is unlikely to show a reason for his symptoms as his hemoglobin was near normal.

There are several other questions on HPS and PPHTN in this book that expand on some of the points above.

Clinical Pearls: HPS/PPHTN

1. HPS is underdiagnosed
2. O_2 saturation <92% should prompt ABG
3. Elevated pulmonary artery pressure (>30–35 mmHg) on echo should prompt a right heart catheterization
4. Important to make a diagnosis of HPS/PPHTN as a MELD exception is available

Notes

A lung/liver case will likely come up on the boards and is important in clinical practice because of the MELD exception. Think of HPS if the oxygen saturation is low. For PPHTN, the right sided pressures will usually be shown.

Reference

International Liver Transplant Society Practice Guidelines: Diagnosis and management of hepatopulmonary syndrome and portopulmonary hypertension. PMID: 27326810.

Question 158

A 58-year-old male with a history of hepatocellular carcinoma and chronic hepatitis B underwent live donor liver transplantation one month ago. He presents for the first outpatient visit after discharge complaining of low-grade fever and diffuse abdominal pain.

His medications include tacrolimus 3 mg bid, mycophenolate mofetil 1 g bid, prednisone 10 mg daily, tenofovir alafenamide 25 mg daily.

Examination shows mild distress, temperature 100.3 °F, BP 130/80, HR 104/min

Laboratory studies:

WBC count 12,000
ALT 25 U/L
AST 32 U/L
ALP 108 U/L
Tbili 0.9 mg/dL
Creatinine 1.1 mg/dL
Tacrolimus trough level 10.2 ng/mL
He is admitted and undergoes abdominal imaging and an ERCP. A representative image is shown below

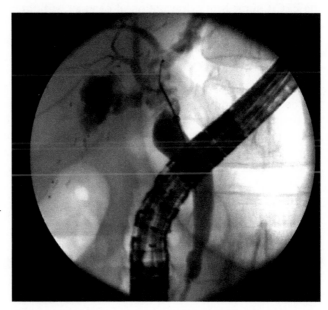

▶ Question

Which of the following statements is true?

A This is a rare complication of live donor liver transplant
B This will require immediate surgical repair
C This can be managed endoscopically
D His tacrolimus should be converted to sirolimus
E This can be managed by percutaneous drainage

C is the correct answer.

Commentary – LDLT Leak

This patient presents with fever, abdominal pain, and leukocytosis a month after liver transplant. An infectious cause is likely. The usual approach would be to get abdominal imaging with an ultrasound or CT scan. In this case, it showed a perihepatic collection but no biliary dilation. An MRI could be considered to get a better idea of the biliary tree. We performed a CT and the collection was drained percutaneously and noted to be bilious. By definition he has a leak if there is bile in the drain. When I did the ERCP, immediate extravasation of contrast was noted at the biliary anastomosis. The cholangiogram demonstrates a cannula with a wire, an 8–9 mm recipient duct (the duodenoscope is 12 mm), filling of some normal-looking intrahepatic ducts consistent with right lobe transplant and contrast extravasating from both sides of the anastomosis indicative of a bile leak.

Biliary complications are common after liver transplantation, but particularly after live donor liver transplant with reports of up to 40%. The management depends on the timing. Unlike a stricture, leaks can often have normal or only mildly elevated liver biochemical tests. If a leak is detected within the first few days after transplant, surgical repair is generally undertaken. However, this patient is a month post-op so surgery should be avoided. Percutaneous drainage alone will not fix a leak this size.

Endoscopic therapy with stenting is highly successful in treating biliary complications after liver transplantation with success rates of 80–90%.

There would be no utility in converting the tacrolimus to sirolimus and in fact may be harmful as sirolimus can impair wound healing.

Notes

I make no apologies for the number of biliary cases in this book. After transplant, at least 10–15% of patients will have biliary issues (double that number if live donor) and most of the time it is fixable in capable hands.

Reference

Endoscopic management of biliary issues in the liver transplant patient. PMID: 30846151.

Question 159

A 39-year-old male presents for follow-up in the office 8 months after orthotopic liver transplant for alcoholic liver disease. His postoperative course was prolonged due to infected abdominal collections and complicated by mental status changes. He has recovered and has been doing well with a good appetite, no fever, and no pain. His only complaint is pain and bleeding when he brushes his teeth.

His medications include cyclosporine 150 mg bid, and mycophenolate mofetil 1 g bid
Examination shows normal vital signs.

Laboratory studies:

ALT 23 U/L
AST 19 U/L
ALP 61 U/L
Tbili 0.4 mg/dL
Creatinine 1.2 mg/dL
Cyclosporine trough level 205 ng/mL
A representative image is shown below

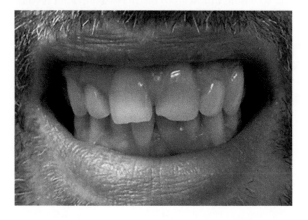

▶ Question

Which of the following statements is true?

A His mycophenolate mofetil should be stopped
B Consideration should be given to converting the cyclosporine to tacrolimus
C Prednisone should be added to his immunosuppression regimen
D His cyclosporine should be increased
E His cyclosporine should be stopped and mycophenolate mofetil should be used as single agent immunosuppression

B is the correct answer.

Commentary – Gingival Hyperplasia from Cyclosporine

This man is doing well but he has developed gingival hyperplasia from cyclosporine which is a relatively common side effect occurring in 25–80% of patients. Cyclosporine is not commonly used after transplant as the other calcineurin inhibitor (CNI) – tacrolimus, has superseded it. Both drugs can cause nephrotoxicity with long-term use as well as metabolic effects, but cyclosporine is associated with hirsutism and gingival hyperplasia. In this patient, the cyclosporine was used after the patient developed mental status changes early after transplant that can be associated with tacrolimus. Now that he has recovered, it would be reasonable to replace the cyclosporine with tacrolimus.

Mycophenolate mofetil is used as an adjunct with CNIs to lower their dose. It inhibits purine synthesis and acts on inosine monophosphate dehydrogenase, an important enzyme in T and B lymphocyte function. The most common side effect is gastro-intestinal, typically diarrhea which can necessitate dose reduction or discontinuation. It can occasionally cause oral ulcers but not gingival hyperplasia.

Prednisone is used early after liver transplantation but has no role in helping gingival hyperplasia.

His cyclosporine level is therapeutic so would not need to be increased even if he did not have gingival hyperplasia.

Notes

Fortunately, we use tacrolimus much more than cyclosporine. Young female patients were not too keen on the hirsutism with the latter! Interestingly, tacrolimus can cause hair loss – I doubt this will be tested on the boards.

Reference

Open prospective multicenter study of conversion to tacrolimus therapy in renal transplant patients experiencing ciclosporin-related side-effects. PMID: 15948861.

Question 160

A 63-year-old male presented with low-grade fever, dark urine, and itching 7 months after simultaneous liver and kidney transplant for hepatocellular carcinoma and end-stage renal disease. His course was complicated by acute cellular rejection of the kidney at 3 months requiring high-dose methylprednisolone and an increase in immunosuppression. He had been on prophylaxis with fluconazole, trimethoprim-sulfamethoxazole, and valganciclovir but these were stopped a month ago.

Examination shows stable vitals, normal temperature, mild scleral icterus, and a non-tender abdomen.

Laboratory studies:

ALT 214 U/L
AST 265 U/L
ALP 501 U/L
Tbili 4.7 mg/dL
INR 1.3
Creatinine 2.1 mg/dL
Tacrolimus level 12.6 ng/mL
Viral serology for HAV/HBV/HCV/HEV all negative
Ultrasound showed a mildly dilated biliary tree
ERCP showed a mildly dilated bile duct, patent anastomosis, and no filling defects. Endoscopic images and biopsy of the major papilla are shown here.

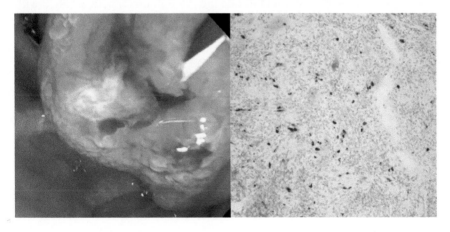

▶ Question

What is the next best test to make a diagnosis?

A Liver biopsy
B ERCP with cholangioscopy
C Bone marrow biopsy
D Quantitative CMV by PCR
E Quantitative EBV by PCR

D is the correct answer.

Commentary – CMV Infection (Papillitis)

This man has developed fever and elevated liver biochemical tests with a dilated biliary tree on imaging. This suggests biliary obstruction and cholangitis. A biliary stricture or stone disease would be the obvious cause but there was no evidence of this on cholangiogram. Malignant biliary obstruction is in the differential diagnosis but he presumably had contrast-enhanced abdominal imaging prior to the transplant.

The recent kidney rejection with an increase in immunosuppression is relevant here, particularly as the prophylaxis was stopped recently. At ERCP, I was concerned about the appearance of the ampulla. The endoscopic image shows an ulcerated papilla which could be due to recent stone passage but is concerning for an infectious or malignant process. Post-transplant lympho-proliferative disorder (PTLD) (which more than half the time is associated with EBV infection) could cause this but surprisingly, the biopsy shows numerous CMV inclusions on immunohistochemical staining making the diagnosis of CMV papillitis. The patient was CMV negative at the time of transplant and the donor was CMV positive. His whole blood quantitative CMV DNA titer was 25,000 IU/L having been negative 2 months prior (while on prophylaxis).

A biliary stent was placed at ERCP and he was treated with ganciclovir with improvement in his liver biochemical tests and resolution of the ulceration at repeat ERCP 2 months later.

CMV reactivation can be seen after liver transplantation, especially in donor positive/recipient negative situations. It can lead to tissue-invasive disease with involvement of any organ, particularly the GI tract.

A liver or bone marrow biopsy would not be indicated in this situation. ERCP with cholangioscopy might be helpful if the cholangiogram had shown pathology in the duct, but that was not the case here.

Notes

This was a great case that I had not seen before. I thought he had passed a stone. It confirms higher dose immunosuppression treats rejection but leaves you at risk for infection, even if it is incredibly localized.

Reference

An unusual finding on endoscopy… A diagnosis of inclusion? PMID: 32602993.
The third international consensus guidelines on the management of cytomegalovirus in solid-organ transplantation. PMID: 29596116.

Question 161

A 61-year-old male presents to the ER with chest pain, shortness of breath, and weakness. He has a history of NASH cirrhosis with a low MELD score and recent imaging that showed no evidence of HCC. His last EGD was 6 months ago that showed small esophageal varices.

Examination shows HR 110/min, normal BP, and oxygen saturation. There is no scleral icterus and a non-tender abdomen with no ascites.

Laboratory studies:

ALT 32 U/L
AST 38 U/L
ALP 98 U/L
Tbili 1.3 mg/dL
INR 1.2
Creatinine 1.1 mg/dL
Hb 6.1 g/dL
Platelets 85,000
EKG sinus tachycardia, no ischemic changes
After red cell transfusion, EGD was performed and a representative image is shown:

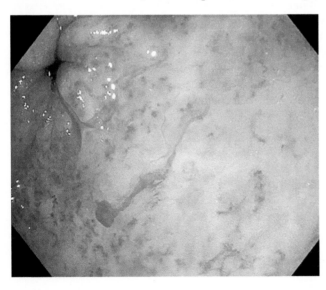

▶ Question

What is the most appropriate management of this patient?

A TIPS
B Argon plasma coagulation (APC) treatment and oral iron
C High dose proton pump inhibitor
D Oral iron
E Surgical antrectomy

B is the correct answer.

Commentary – Gastric Antral Vascular Ectasia

This man presents with symptomatic anemia. The image shows active bleeding from the gastric antrum and despite the absence of the typical "watermelon" appearance this is most consistent with gastric antral vascular ectasia (GAVE).

GAVE is associated with cirrhosis and portal hypertension but can occur in other conditions such as systemic sclerosis. It typically presents with anemia as opposed to brisk GI bleeding. It can have a classic "watermelon" appearance of red stripes in the antrum but can be punctate as in this case. It is a distinct entity separate from portal hypertensive gastropathy.

Characteristic biopsy findings are:

1. Vascular ectasia
2. Spindle cell proliferation
3. Fibrohyalinosis

Treatment is with cautery using APC or other endoscopic coagulation techniques but usually needs to be repeated regularly as it recurs. Recent studies have suggested that radiofrequency ablation and band ligation may have a role to play in treating GAVE. Iron supplementation is required in some cases as iron deficiency can occur.

In this patient, I used APC with a very good response but I had to repeat the procedure every 3–4 months to prevent him needing a transfusion.

Although it is associated with cirrhosis and portal hypertension it does not reliably improve with TIPS. A proton pump inhibitor is useful after coagulation treatment but does not prevent bleeding. Oral iron alone is unlikely to improve the anemia. Surgical antrectomy would be reserved for carefully selected patients with recalcitrant symptoms, well-compensated cirrhosis, and no (or minimal portal hypertension). This patient has varices and a platelet count below 100 so would not be a good candidate.

> **Notes**
>
> In general, portal hypertensive gastropathy affects the proximal stomach while GAVE affects the distal stomach (antrum). APC or RFA can treat GAVE but not gastropathy.

Reference

Gastric vascular abnormalities: diagnosis and management. PMID: 32925176.

Question 162

A 71-year-old Hispanic male underwent liver transplantation 7 months ago for HCC and HCV cirrhosis. His HCV was treated prior to transplant and his HCV RNA has remained negative. There has been no recurrence of HCC on recent chest and abdominal imaging.

He feels well and his diabetes and hypertension are well controlled. His appetite is good, and he is gaining weight. His only complaint is bilateral foot pain when walking his dog.

He is on tacrolimus 6 mg bid and mycophenolate mofetil 1 g bid. Antiviral and anti-fungal prophylaxis were stopped several months ago.

Examination shows a comfortable-looking man with normal vital signs, and he is afebrile. There is no scleral icterus and a non-tender abdomen with a well-healed scar. He has normal pedal pulses.

Laboratory studies:

ALT 12 U/L
AST 15 U/L
ALP 63 U/L
Tbili 0.5 mg/dL
Creatinine 1.1 mg/dL
Tacrolimus trough level 8.3 ng/mL

His right foot is shown below:

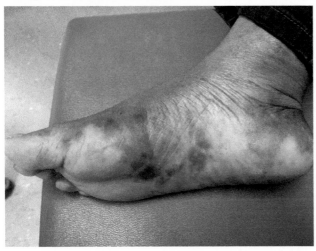

▶ Question

Which of the following statements is **TRUE** about this condition?

A His tacrolimus needs to be increased
B CMV antiviral prophylaxis should be restarted
C Antifungal prophylaxis should be restarted
D His tacrolimus should be switched to an mTOR such as sirolimus
E EBV antiviral prophylaxis should be restarted

D is the correct answer.

Commentary – Kaposi Sarcoma After Solid Organ Transplant

This man is doing well after liver transplant with normal liver function. His tacrolimus level is acceptable and since he is 7 months out his antiviral and antifungal prophylaxis has been stopped. The image shows multiple brownish papular lesions on his foot that were minimally tender. The appearance is classic for Kaposi's sarcoma (KS).

KS is a vascular tumor that is endemic in sub-Saharan Africa and seen in old men of Mediterranean and Jewish origin. In the US, it was really recognized in the 1980s as one of the AIDS defining illnesses. It is associated with human herpesvirus 8 (HHV8) and has an increased incidence with immunosuppression after solid organ transplant. The main differential diagnosis is with bacillary angiomatosis, a cutaneous infection due to Bartonella that is treated with antibiotics. This patient underwent a skin biopsy that showed classic KS changes with a positive HHV8 immunohistochemical stain.

Treatment involves reduction of immunosuppression if possible, but this man is only 7 months out, and reducing immunosuppression may increase the risk of graft rejection. Restarting the CMV/EBV antiviral or antifungal prophylaxis is not required and will not help in any case. Switching the tacrolimus to sirolimus is the best option. The m-TOR drugs have antitumor and anti-angiogenic effects by impairing the production of vascular endothelial growth factor. In some cases, adjuvant chemotherapy with liposomal doxorubicin is required.

Clinical Pearls: Kaposi Sarcoma and Transplant

1. KS is associated with HHV8
2. Bacillary angiomatosis is the main differential diagnosis
3. Immunosuppression should be reduced in KS
4. Converting to sirolimus (or other mTOR) is helpful in KS

Reference

Decreased incidence of Kaposi sarcoma after kidney transplant in Italy and role of mTOR-inhibitors. PMID: 30613958.

Question 163

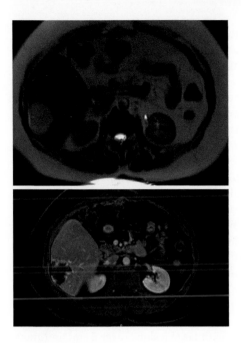

▶ Question

Which of the following statements is TRUE regarding the MRI shown above?

A This study is diagnostic
B If the patient has cirrhosis a liver biopsy is required to make a diagnosis
C There is a risk of malignant transformation in a cirrhotic patient
D This requires surveillance imaging in a pregnant patient
E Surgical resection has poor outcome for large lesions (>5 cm)

A is the correct answer.

Commentary – Hepatic Hemangioma

The MRI shows a lesion in segment 6 of the right lobe measuring 3.8 cm by 4.3 cm that demonstrates peripheral nodular enhancement of variable thickness while the central area remains hypodense after intravenous contrast. This is diagnostic of a hepatic hemangioma.

Hepatic hemangioma is a very common benign liver lesion, usually asymptomatic and picked up as an incidental finding on abdominal imaging. There is a female predominance and typically picked up in the 4th to 6th decades of life. There is a weak relationship with estrogen as they can increase in size during pregnancy, but enlargement has been noted in the absence of estrogen and in post-menopausal women.

Symptoms can occur with large lesions, but liver tests are usually normal. Diagnosis is made on abdominal imaging with the addition of contrast improving the sensitivity and specificity. Since patients with cirrhosis are at risk for HCC, contrast imaging should be performed to differentiate hepatic hemangioma from HCC. A liver biopsy is not required as imaging is very accurate and biopsy runs the risk of bleeding. Microscopically, hepatic hemangiomas are composed of a vascular space lined by a single epithelial layer, and they are not at risk of malignant transformation in cirrhotic or non-cirrhotic individuals.

The risk of enlargement during pregnancy is unclear and does not warrant surveillance as the risk of rupture does not appear to change.

Surveillance should be reserved for patients with large lesions (over 5 cm) and then subsequent imaging should be based on a demonstration of continued growth (3 mm or more per year). Treatment decisions are based on size and symptoms, but surgical resection has very good outcomes. Acute bleeding from hepatic hemangiomas is rare but can be treated with arterial embolization +/− surgery.

There will almost certainly be at least one image of a liver lesion on the boards and it will be relatively straightforward with classic findings as in the above case. You can find examples of other liver lesions in this book such as focal nodular hyperplasia, hepatic adenoma, HCC, and fibrolamellar HCC.

Clinical Pearls: Hepatic Hemangioma

1. Peripheral nodular enhancement with hypodense central area after IV contrast is DIAGNOSTIC for hepatic hemangioma
2. There is a WEAK relationship with estrogen
3. Hepatic hemangiomas do NOT become malignant
4. Lesions over 5 cm should undergo surveillance
5. Acute bleeding is rare but can be treated with embolization and/or surgery

> **Notes**
>
> I see a few of these cases every year and MRI has become so good that they rarely are a diagnostic dilemma but need ++reassurance to the patient.

Reference

EASL Clinical Practice Guidelines on the management of benign liver tumors. PMID: 27085809.

Question 164

A 64-year-old man develops low-grade fever and abdominal pain. He underwent liver transplantation one month ago for HCC and alcoholic cirrhosis. He was outside Milan criteria and required multiple rounds of locoregional therapy to control his tumor burden prior to transplant.

He had a prolonged postoperative course and still feels weak with poor appetite.

His medications include tacrolimus 4 mg bid, mycophenolate mofetil 1 g bid and prednisone 10 mg qd. He is still taking antiviral and antifungal prophylaxis.

Examination shows an uncomfortable looking man with normal BP but mild tachycardia and temperature of 100 °F. There is no scleral icterus and a diffusely tender abdomen.

Laboratory studies:

ALT 103 U/L
AST 85 U/L
ALP 299 U/L
Tbili 2.4 mg/dL
Creatinine 1.4 mg/dL
Tacrolimus trough level 10.1 ng/mL
Doppler ultrasound shows a patent hepatic artery

He undergoes ERCP and his cholangiogram is shown below:

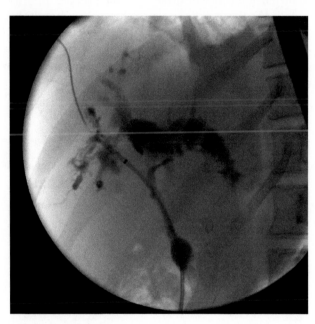

▶ Question

What is the most appropriate management option?

A The portal venous anastomosis should be investigated
B The hepatic venous outflow should be investigated
C Serial endoscopic dilation and stenting of the biliary tree
D Conversion of the biliary duct-to-duct anastomosis to hepaticojejunostomy
E He should be relisted for transplant

E is the correct answer.

Commentary – Ischemic Cholangiopathy

My heart sank when I did this ERCP as it always does when I see ischemic cholangiopathy. The cholangiogram shows dilated and irregular intrahepatic ducts and a long-complicated stricture in the hilar area. This is the typical appearance of ischemic cholangiopathy – a diagnosis that typically carries a bad prognosis. The patient is only a month out from transplant and this appearance of the biliary tree means this graft will not last long and the patient should be relisted for transplant. The hepatic artery could be better visualized with a CT angiogram despite being patent on the Doppler ultrasound, as it may well be stenosed or suffered damage during prior HCC treatment. Remember, the hepatic artery and bile duct are intimately related as the biliary tree is supplied by the peribiliary plexus that comes from the hepatic artery and not the portal vein. As well as interruption to hepatic arterial flow, a DCD allograft can lead to similar changes. There is also a "critical care" cholangiopathy that has been described.

This appearance of the biliary tree would not be seen with problems with the portal vein or hepatic vein. Converting the biliary anastomosis does not fix ischemic cholangiopathy but would be a consideration in an anastomotic stricture that could not be treated endoscopically or radiologically.

Clinical Pearls: Ischemic Cholangiopathy

1. The bile duct is supplied by the hepatic artery (HA).
2. HA stenosis or thrombosis and donation after cardiac death are risk factors for ischemic cholangiopathy.
3. Even if the Doppler ultrasound shows a patent artery, this cholangiogram requires further investigation of the vasculature.
4. This usually needs retransplant.

Notes

After placing a stent, the drainage from the biliary tree in these cases is a combination of bile, pus, sludge, and cast material. Not surprising as the biliary epithelium is sloughing off, a bit like a snake shedding its skin.

Reference

Endoscopic management of biliary issues in the liver transplant patient. PMID: 30846151.

Question 165

A 58-year-old male presents with 2 days of melena to the emergency room. He underwent liver transplantation 10 months ago for NASH cirrhosis. He has been feeling unwell for several weeks with anorexia, occasional sweats, and has lost 10 pounds. His postoperative course has been normal otherwise. He has diabetes and hypertension that are well controlled. He underwent colonoscopy prior to the transplant that was normal.

He is on tacrolimus 3 mg bid, mycophenolate mofetil 500 mg bid, metformin 850 mg bid, amlodipine 5 mg qd.

Examination shows a slightly uncomfortable-looking man with normal vital signs and he is afebrile. There is no scleral icterus, and he has mild diffuse abdominal tenderness, more in the left upper quadrant with a well-healed scar.

Laboratory studies:

ALT 37 U/L
AST 27 U/L
ALP 89 U/L
Tbili 0.8 mg/dL
Creatinine 1.0 mg/dL
Hb 8.7 g/dL
Tacrolimus trough level 6.8 ng/mL
CMV DNA negative
He undergoes EGD with biopsy and an abdominal CT scan and representative images are shown below:

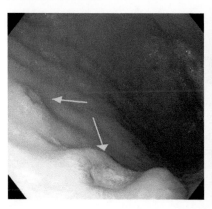 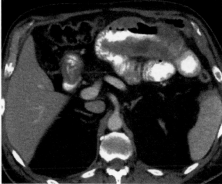

▶ Question

What is the most appropriate management strategy for this patient?

A Increase the immunosuppression and consider immunotherapy/chemotherapy
B Decrease the immunosuppression and consider immunotherapy/chemotherapy
C Start immunotherapy/chemotherapy
D Stop the immunosuppression and start immunotherapy/chemotherapy
E Decrease the immunosuppression and start valganciclovir

B is the correct answer.

Commentary – Post Transplant Lymphoproliferative Disorder (PTLD)

This man has developed gastrointestinal bleeding with evidence of gastric ulceration and a very thickened small bowel on CT scan (seen as narrowing of the oral contrast as it runs through the duodenum). He has lost weight and has sweats while his liver function is normal with an acceptable tacrolimus level. There is no CMV viremia, so this is not due to CMV infection. Post-transplant lymphoproliferative disorder (PTLD) is the most likely diagnosis. The term PTLD encompasses lymphoid and plasma cell proliferations after transplant due to immunosuppression.

PTLD is not uncommon after solid organ transplant and the incidence varies depending on the type of organ. The highest incidence is seen in intestinal or multivisceral transplants (10–30% over 5 years) with less incidence in renal transplant (1–3%) and less still in liver transplant recipients (1–2%).

The pathogenesis in most patients is related to EBV infected B-cells (usually host-derived but occasionally donor-derived) that escape T-cell mediated immune surveillance due to immunosuppression. Up to a third of cases of PTLD are EBV-negative and maybe related to other viruses.

There is no uniform management strategy for treating PTLD as it can vary depending on the type of organ transplant and center preference. However, reduction of immunosuppression if possible is paramount. Hence, choices A and C are incorrect. Stopping the immunosuppression (choice D) would not be appropriate. Other treatment options include rituximab (anti-CD20 monoclonal antibody) in patients that express CD-20, chemotherapy, radiation, or a combination. Immunotherapy with EBV-specific cytotoxic T cells is available for recalcitrant cases.

The prognosis of PTLD is variable and depends on several factors, particularly the burden of disease but has improved since the introduction of rituximab.

Clinical Pearls: PTLD

1. Highest risk of PTLD is in intestinal and multivisceral transplants
2. PTLD is mainly related to EBV infected host B-cells
3. Up to a third of PTLD cases will be EBV negative
4. Treatment of PTLD requires reduction of immunosuppression

Notes

You may not see this often after liver transplant but in a big transplant center you will see it several times a year after other organ transplants. Another reason why hepatologists should cover GI procedures on all the transplant patients, not just liver transplant.

Reference

Multicenter analysis of 80 solid organ transplantation recipients with post-transplantation lymphoproliferative disease: outcomes and prognostic factors in the modern era. PMID: 20085936.

Question 166

A 23-year-old female presents with abnormal LFTs 2 years after undergoing a live donor liver transplant for PSC. She received a right lobe graft from her father. She is doing well in school, exercises daily, and denies fever, abdominal pain or pruritis. She has had a colectomy and has a J-pouch. Her postoperative course was uncomplicated with a normal pouchoscopy last year. She undergoes an MRI as shown below.

Laboratory studies:

ALT 53 U/L
AST 61 U/L
ALP 287 U/L
Tbili 1.1 mg/dL
Creatinine 0.8 mg/dL
Hb 13.2 g/dL
Tacrolimus trough level 5.7 ng/mL

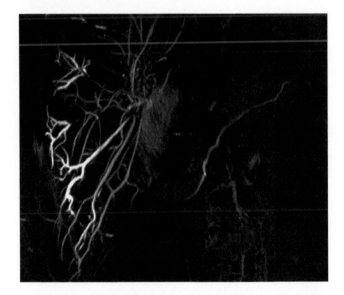

▶ Question

Which of the following is a risk factor for this condition?

A Prior colectomy
B Live donor liver transplant
C Female sex
D Short cold ischemia time
E Tacrolimus based immunosuppression

B is the correct answer.

Commentary – Recurrent PSC (After LDLT)

The MRI shows the biliary tree of a right lobe transplant with evidence of a hepatico-jejunostomy. There are areas of dilation and stricturing compatible with a sclerosing cholangitis type picture. This occurs in up to 15–20% of patients after transplant and there is no effective treatment. Since the presentation is usually with cholestatic LFTs, the main differential diagnoses are chronic rejection, particularly if the imaging findings are subtle, and stenosis of the hepaticojejunostomy (with or without secondary sclerosing cholangitis). This is an important distinction to make as chronic rejection is treatable with high dose tacrolimus and a stenotic hepaticojejunostomy can be dilated at ERCP or PTC. There are multiple large series looking at outcomes after transplant for PSC and several risk factors for recurrence have been identified.

These include:

1. Younger age
2. Sex mismatch
3. Male sex
4. Coexistent IBD
5. Presence of an intact colon after transplantation (so colectomy is protective)
6. CMV infection
7. Recurrent acute cellular rejection and steroid-resistant cellular rejection
8. Cholangiocarcinoma
9. Live donor transplant

Notes

Some of the risk factors listed here for recurrent PSC are based on smaller series so I doubt they will be asked on the board exam with the possible exception of the presence of an intact colon.

Reference

Risk factors for recurrent primary sclerosing cholangitis after liver transplantation.
PMID: 26186988.

Question 167

A 55-year-old homeless male presents with fever, right upper quadrant pain, and diarrhea. He has had multiple ER visits over the last few months for similar complaints.

Exam reveals stable vital signs, temporal wasting and several purplish, non-tender papules on the forehead and nose.

Laboratory studies:

ALT 99 U/L
AST 83 U/L
ALP 723 U/L
Tbili 2.9 mg/dL
Creatinine 1.1 mg/dL
CT scan shows a heterogeneous liver but no obvious ductal dilation.
He undergoes ERCP as shown below:

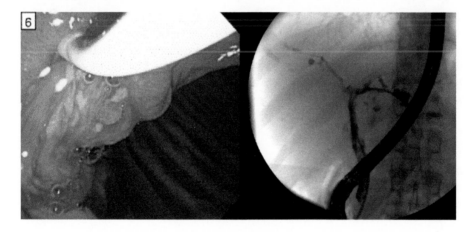

▶ Question

All of the following are associated with this entity EXCEPT?

A Cytomegalovirus (CMV)
B Mycobacterium avium-intracellulare (MAI)
C Cryptosporidia
D Herpes simplex virus (HSV)
E Cyclospora

D is the correct answer.

Commentary – AIDS/HIV Cholangiopathy

I saw this case many years ago and I anticipated what this cholangiogram would look like based on the presentation. The endoscopic image shows sludge draining from the ampulla and the cholangiogram shows a sclerosing cholangitis-like picture. The patient was a wasted, homeless male with purplish papules on the face (Kaposi sarcoma), very suggestive that he has AIDS, making the diagnosis likely to be AIDS/HIV cholangiopathy.

This entity is thought to be due to infection-related strictures of the biliary tree that occurs in patients with a CD4 count less than 100 (although can occur in patients with higher CD4 counts). Organisms that are associated include Cryptosporidia (most common), CMV, MAI, Microsporidium, Cyclospora, Isospora, Giardia, and Histoplasma.

Management involves treating the cholangitis and infection but mainly antiretroviral drugs to treat the HIV.

Notes

This type of cholangiogram has an ever-expanding differential diagnosis: AIDS cholangiopathy, PSC or secondary sclerosing cholangitis, ischemic cholangiopathy, IgG4 sclerosing cholangitis, recurrent pyogenic cholangiopathy and recently even drug-induced liver injury and COVID cholangiopathy! As always with the boards, the stem gives you the clues.

Reference

Cryptosporidiosis and the pathogenesis of AIDS-cholangiopathy. PMID: 12360421.

Question 168

A 42-year-old male presents for routine follow-up. He has a history of ulcerative colitis and underwent total colectomy and a J-pouch 5 years ago for long-standing disease. He was diagnosed with primary sclerosing cholangitis at that time based on elevated liver enzymes and an MRCP. He has no fever, abdominal pain and his weight is stable. His only medication is PRN loperamide.

Examination shows normal vital signs and he is afebrile. There is no scleral icterus, and he has a non-tender abdomen.

Laboratory studies:

ALT 89 U/L
AST 97 U/L
ALP 548 U/L
Tbili 1.1 mg/dL
Albumin 3.9 mg/dL
INR 1.0
Platelets 230
CA19-9 24 U/mL
He undergoes MRI and MRCP with two contrast enhancing lesions measuring 9 and 10 mm are seen as shown below:

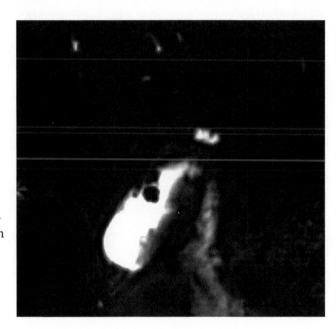

▶ Question

What is the most appropriate management strategy for this patient?

A Repeat MRI in 6 months
B Perform percutaneous biopsy
C Refer for surgery
D ERCP
E US to determine gallstones versus polyps

C is the correct answer.

Commentary – Gallbladder Cancer in PSC

This man has at least two enhancing lesions in the gallbladder. We are not told how long they have been there or what they looked like on a prior scan. We are told they are 9–10 mm and he has well maintained liver synthetic function and a normal platelet count.

Guidelines for cancer screening in PSC are based on very little data but there is an increased risk of cholangiocarcinoma, gallbladder cancer, and colon cancer. Most centers advocate imaging every 6–12 months, but the modality can vary. We would use MRI/MRCP (and tumor markers) as it has better sensitivity for detecting cholangiocarcinoma.

This patient has lesions >8 mm which is an indication for cholecystectomy. Repeating an MRI or getting an USS or ERCP is not necessary, and a biopsy would be technically challenging.

Gallbladder cancer is an uncommon cancer in general but has a dismal prognosis due to advanced disease at diagnosis. There are several notable risk factors apart from PSC including porcelain gallbladder, Salmonella infection, and gallstone disease. The latter likely explains the geographic variation in incidence with high rates seen in South America (particularly Chile), parts of South Asia, and Japan.

Clinical Pearls: HIV Cholangiopathy

1. PSC increases the risk of several cancers – CCA and HCC but also colorectal ca, pancreatic ca, and gallbladder ca.

Reference

AGA clinical practice update on surveillance for hepatobiliary cancers in patients with primary sclerosing cholangitis: expert review. PMID: 31306801.

Question 169

This image is from a 7-year-old female who presented with intermittent abdominal pain, nausea, and vomiting. Liver function tests are normal.

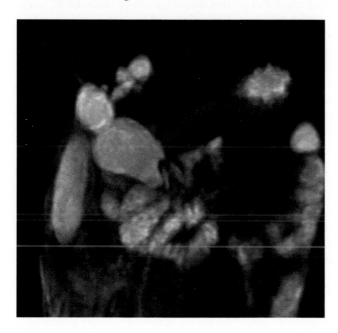

▶ Question

Which is the most appropriate management?

A Perform ERCP to confirm the diagnosis
B Begin annual surveillance MRI
C Defer surgery until she turns 18 years old
D Perform surgical resection now
E Refer for liver transplantation

D is the correct answer.

Commentary – Choledochal Cyst

The scan is an MR cholangiogram showing a markedly dilated biliary tree with cystic changes, in other words, a choledochal cyst. This diagnosis can be made on imaging, so ERCP is not required. Choledochal cysts can be classified based on the location of the cysts and the presence of an abnormal pancreaticobiliary junction (which occurs in up to 70%). The Todani classification divides choledochal cysts into 5 types. You would not be expected to know the specifics for the boards but essentially type 1 (and subtypes) affects the extrahepatic bile duct, type 4 involves intra- and extra-hepatic ducts, and type 5 is Caroli's disease which is characterized by saccular dilations of the intra-hepatic ducts (described elsewhere in this book). In this case, it would be a type 4A choledochal cyst – both intra- and extra-hepatic cystic dilations. Choledochal cysts are uncommon in the Western world but are more common in Japan. Cysts can be congenital or acquired and can be associated with a variety of developmental anomalies. This girl fits the typical presentation – age less than 10 years, abdominal pain, nausea, and vomiting. Liver tests are often normal but can be elevated with jaundice.

The most important thing to remember with choledochal cysts is the increased risk of cholangiocarcinoma (up to a third of patients), particularly type 1 and 4 cysts, that increases with age. The recommendation is to remove the cyst completely and perform hepaticojejunostomy, although this does not completely eliminate the risk of cancer, particularly in patients with intrahepatic cysts that cannot be fully removed. Hence, deferring surgery until she turns 18 years old or annual surveillance imaging would be inappropriate. Liver transplantation would be an option for Caroli's disease.

Clinical Pearls

1. Choledochal cysts can be congenital or acquired
2. There is an increased risk of cholangiocarcinoma (type 1 and type 4 choledochal cysts)
3. Surgical resection is recommended (at time of diagnosis) due to the risk of CCA

Notes

With better imaging these cases are picked up in children but I still see an adult case every couple of years.

Reference

Bile duct cyst as a precursor to biliary tract cancer. PMID: 17187167.

Question 170

A 27-year-old male presents to the ER with low-grade fever and jaundice. He has a history of primary sclerosing cholangitis (PSC) diagnosed last year when he presented with abnormal liver tests on routine testing. He had a normal colonoscopy recently. He has no pain, and his weight is stable. He takes no medication.

Examination shows normal vital signs and temperature 99.7 °F. There is scleral icterus, and he has a non-tender abdomen.

Laboratory studies:

ALT 96 U/L
ALP 473 U/L
Tbili 7.3 mg/dL
INR 1.0
CA19-9 1503 U/mL

He undergoes abdominal imaging and then ERCP as shown below:

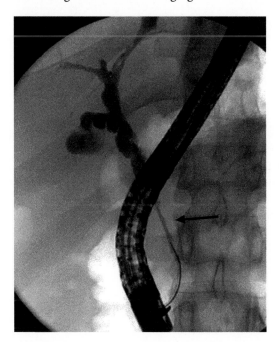

▶ Question

Which method is most likely to make a diagnosis?

A Brush cytology and intraductal biopsy
B Brush cytology is not required – the elevated CA19-9 is diagnostic for cholangiocarcinoma
C Brush cytology combined with cholangioscopy directed biopsy
D Brush cytology combined with molecular/genetic analysis
E Brush cytology alone

D is the correct answer.

Commentary – A Dominant Stricture in PSC and Making a Diagnosis of Cholangiocarcinoma (CCA)

This is a situation that I have encountered many times and up until recently, I struggled with.

This young man presents with a common issue in PSC – new onset jaundice. The ERCP image shows a distal stricture with upstream dilation of the bile duct and cystic duct with evidence of intrahepatic PSC. Is it benign or malignant?!

We use the term "dominant" stricture but this does not have a universally accepted definition. I usually reserve the term for a stricture in the extra-hepatic duct (or left or right common hepatic duct) that has pre-stenotic dilation – so the duct above (proximal) is dilated. There have been some consensus conferences on PSC to try to come up with a definition that will be important in clinical trials.

An elevated CA19-9 can often be seen in a jaundiced patient and is not diagnostic of CCA. Making a diagnosis of CCA in PSC is notoriously difficult as brush cytology and biopsy have low sensitivity, not really improved much with cholangioscopic directed biopsies.

Recent molecular and genetic techniques such as fluorescent in-situ hybridization (FISH) and next-generation sequencing (NGS) have increased the diagnostic yield. I doubt any detailed knowledge of FISH and NGS will be required for board purposes.

Just remember that a new stricture in a jaundiced PSC patient requires some sort of intervention and sampling. In this case it was benign.

Notes

PSC is a frustrating disease on several levels, mainly due to the lack of effective treatment. Diagnosis should be based on imaging in the majority of cases. The first time you do an ERCP you are colonizing the biliary tree so you need to have a good reason to do it. I can think of 3 good reasons (and several other reasons) – cholangitis, a change in the labs- especially new jaundice or a significant increase in CA19-9 (especially if not jaundiced) or a change in the imaging — a new stricture or maybe stones/sludge.

Reference

Long-term outcomes of positive fluorescence in situ hybridization tests in primary sclerosing cholangitis. PMID: 19877179.

Question 171

A 57-year-old male presents to the office with a history of neuroendocrine tumor, metastatic to the liver. He feels well and has been on several different chemotherapy regimens.

On exam he is alert in no distress without scleral icterus. He has an enlarged nodular liver.

Laboratory studies:

ALT 34 U/L
ALP 289 U/L
Tbili 1.3 mg/dL
INR 1.0
Creatinine 0.9 mg/dL

His last PET-CT is shown below (unchanged from 1 year prior):

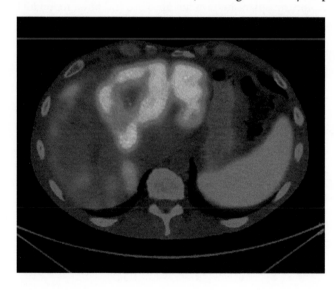

▶ Question

All of the following are associated with good outcome after liver transplantation for this disease EXCEPT?

A Histologic grade G1 or G2
B Hepatic tumor involvement of 75%
C Pre-transplant resection of all extra-hepatic lesions
D Duration of stable disease over 6 months

B is the correct answer.

Commentary – Liver Transplantation for Metastatic Neuroendocrine Tumor (NET)

The PET CT scan shows active disease, mainly in the left lobe and we are told that the disease has been stable for a year. Liver transplantation for metastatic NET is possible as typically the tumor is slow growing, even in the presence of immunosuppression, and as long as the histologic grade is favorable. The histologic grade is based on the mitotic and proliferative (Ki-67) index, with a KI-index over 10% considered a poor prognostic marker. Oncologic treatments have improved over the last decade such that even if the disease is not cured there is a significant survival benefit. Guidelines have been developed for listing and transplanting metastatic NET but are based on retrospective data. Milan criteria exist for NET and include grade 1 or 2 disease, portal drainage of the primary tumor, resection of extra-hepatic disease, hepatic tumor burden of less than 50%, and stable duration of disease for more than 6 months. If patients fit these criteria, 5-year survival of approaching 90% has been reported.

UNOS uses the Milan criteria and includes age under 60 years. These criteria apply to patients listed for deceased donor transplant but are not absolute and often individual centers will consider NET patients for transplant on a case-by case basis.

Clinical Pearls: LT for NET

1. NET with liver metastases is an indication for liver transplantation basically if histologic grade is acceptable and disease is confined to the liver (and primary lesion).
2. The aim is acceptable 5-year survival, even if cure of the NET is not possible.

Notes

I did not include the worst case I saw with this disease. A young patient weighing 120 pounds, 30 pounds of which was the liver with metastatic NET. Demonstrates that these are indolent and can take years to present.

Reference

Liver transplantation for colorectal and neuroendocrine liver metastases and hepatoblastoma. Working Group Report From the ILTS Transplant Oncology Consensus Conference. PMID: 32217939.

Question 172

A 64-year-old male presents to the ER with abdominal pain, nausea, and vomiting and 2 days of melena. He has a history of HCV cirrhosis and a 3 cm HCC treated with Yttrium 90 (Y90) microspheres 3 months ago. His initial AFP was 450 ng/mL. He is undergoing treatment for HCV and is currently listed for a liver transplant. He takes occasional ibuprofen for headaches that he attributes to his HCV medication.

On exam he is alert in no distress without scleral icterus. He has mild epigastric tenderness but no rebound.

Laboratory studies:

Hb 8.7 g/dL
ALT 232 U/L
ALP 405 U/L
Tbili 1.1 mg/dL
INR 1.2
Creatinine 1.1 mg/dL
AFP 2.3 ng/mL
He undergoes imaging with Doppler US that shows patent vessels and MRI that shows cirrhosis and a 100% necrotic HCC. Intrahepatic biliary dilation is noted with an abrupt cutoff in the extrahepatic duct. EGD with an image of the duodenal bulb and a representative cholangiogram is shown below. A month later repeat EGD/ERCP shows no change.

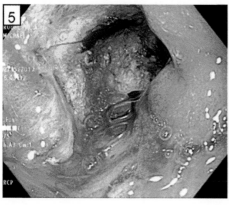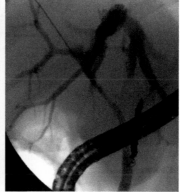

▶ Question

What is the most likely diagnosis?

A HCC infiltration in the duodenum
B NSAID related duodenal ulcer
C Hepatic artery thrombosis
D Ischemia due to Y90 microsphere deposition
E Intestinal lymphoma

D is the correct answer.

Commentary – Complications of Y90 Treatment

The EGD shows a larger ulcer in the duodenal bulb and the cholangiogram shows a long extra-hepatic bile duct stricture. I had difficulty getting the scope to pass to the ampulla. We are told the HCC is well treated with a normal AFP so this is unlikely to be due to HCC. A duodenal ulcer from NSAIDs is possible but should not cause a biliary stricture and should show some evidence of healing within a month. Hepatic artery injury is possible with Y90 and hepatic artery thrombosis can lead to biliary strictures but the Doppler was normal and duodenal ulceration is not associated. Aberrant Y90 microsphere deposition is not uncommon and can lead to intestinal ulceration. Biopsy of the ulcer edge, in this case, demonstrated inflammation with Y90 microbeads seen on pathology. This can take a long time to heal.

Y90 has multiple potential complications including post-embolization syndrome, gastrointestinal ulceration, hepatitis, biliary necrosis and bilomas, pancreatitis, radiation-related complications such as pneumonitis and dermatitis.

The specifics of Y90 are unlikely to show up on the boards but complications from locoregional therapies for HCC in general would be fair game. Remember that Y90 and chemoembolization involve gaining access to the hepatic artery so biliary complications are not uncommon.

Notes

I used this case as it has a differential diagnosis that makes you think a little. HCC metastasizes to the lung and bones but can cause intraperitoneal spread if it ruptures. I have not seen it invade into the bowel. Lymphoma and NSAIDs can cause ulcers but should not lead to a biliary stricture (although lymphoma could infiltrate the ampulla). Injury to the biliary tree from hepatic artery manipulation during chemotherapy (or due to the chemotherapy) is well recognized.

Reference

An unusual cause of abdominal pain and biliary obstruction in a patient with hepatocellular carcinoma. PMID: 28865732.

Question 173

A 34-year-old female with a long history of Crohn's disease and PSC is seen for abdominal pain, pruritis, weight loss, and dark urine. She has undergone ERCP with stents in the past for a dominant stricture and a remote cholecystectomy. She takes mesalamine and 5 mg prednisone.

On exam she is alert in no distress without scleral icterus with a soft abdomen

Laboratory studies:

ALT 63 U/L
ALP 573 U/L
Tbili 1.7 mg/dL
Platelet count 83
INR 1.1
Creatinine 0.7 mg/dL
CA19-9 353 U/L
MRI is shown below:

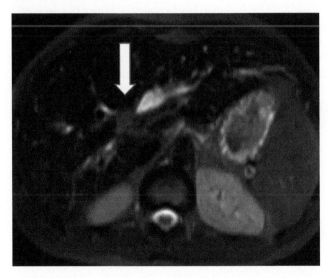

▶ Question

If she is being referred for liver transplantation what is the next most appropriate management step?

A Percutaneous biopsy of liver lesion
B ERCP with brushing/biopsy
C Laparoscopic exploration and biopsy
D Open surgical exploration and biopsy
E EUS guided biopsy

B is the correct answer.

Commentary – Liver Transplantation for Cholangiocarcinoma (CCA)

The MRI shows an enhancing mass in the caudate lobe close to the bifurcation leading to intrahepatic ductal dilation in the left system. Together with the history of PSC, presentation and elevated CA 19-9 is very concerning for CCA.

CCA is a relative contra-indication for liver transplantation, but several centers have a protocol for unresectable hilar (perihilar) CCA in the setting of PSC that can lead to 70–75% 5-year post-transplant survival. Diagnosis should be made by intraluminal brushing or biopsy. Transperitoneal or EUS biopsy is a contra-indication as there is a high risk of tumor seeding. If a diagnosis cannot be made at ERCP and sampling, a malignant-looking stricture with elevated CA19-9 or positive molecular/genetic testing such as fluorescent in-situ hybridization or next-generation sequencing is sufficient. This means choices A, C, and D are incorrect; this patient had a malignant looking mass and elevated CA19-9 and so did not need an extra-luminal biopsy. The protocol includes neoadjuvant radiation and chemotherapy followed by staging laparotomy prior to transplantation. Unfortunately, many patients do not make it to transplant and even those that do may not get an adequate MELD exception to have a realistic chance of a deceased donor, as is the case in regions of the country where a high MELD score is required to get transplanted (for blood type A and O). In our center, despite having a CCA transplant protocol, we try and perform surgical resection in patients with well-maintained synthetic function and minimal portal hypertension or try and find a live donor.

Clinical Pearls: LT for CCA

1. Avoid percutaneous or trans-peritoneal biopsy in suspected CCA
2. Transplant is an option in selected patients under protocol, so CCA is only a relative contra-indication to transplant

---

Notes

CCA, along with GB cancer, are the two diagnoses I really hate making. In some ways, it is much better to make the diagnosis on the explant after the patient has been transplanted and hope the patient does not develop recurrent disease.

Reference

Liver transplant for cholangiocarcinoma. PMID: 29735023.

Question 174

A 46-year-old female presents to the clinic for routine follow-up. She underwent a liver transplant for fulminant liver failure 20 years ago and is maintained on tacrolimus. She has hypertension and diabetes controlled on medications but has not been seen in the office for 5 years. She is asking about weight loss surgery as she has gained more than 100 pounds since the surgery. Fibroscan shows advanced fibrosis.

On exam she is alert in no distress without scleral icterus with a soft, obese abdomen. BMI is 39 kg/m²

Laboratory studies:

ALT 52 U/L
ALP 89 U/L
Tbili 1.1 mg/dL
Creatinine 0.9 mg/dL
A triple phase CT scan is shown below:

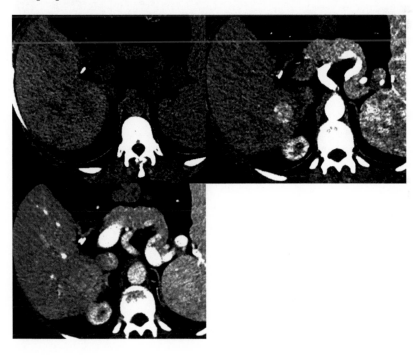

▶ Question

What is the most appropriate management strategy?

A Proceed with surgical weight loss surgery
B Get abdominal MRI scan
C Get liver biopsy
D Refer for liver transplantation
E Repeat scan in 6 months

D is the correct answer.

Commentary – De Novo Hepatocellular Carcinoma (HCC) After Liver Transplantation

The CT scan shows a 2 cm enhancing mass in segment 6 with venous washout diagnostic for HCC. No additional testing is required to make the diagnosis. This patient has developed de novo HCC after liver transplantation – a rare complication. Her best option is redo liver transplantation. She should not be referred for weight loss surgery.

Transplanted patients are at risk for developing de novo NASH, particularly in the setting of weight gain, diabetes and hypertension. This lady has not been seen for several years and likely developed NASH cirrhosis and then HCC. If patients develop allograft cirrhosis, they should be surveyed for HCC with 6 monthly imaging as in the pre-transplant population. She qualifies for the MELD exception as the tumor is 2 cm and she should be referred for liver transplantation and the tumor can be treated with locoregional therapy while waiting.

> **Notes**
>
> Weight gain after transplant is a common problem so de novo NASH is not surprising. I suspect we will see more of these types of cases in the future.

Reference

De-novo hepatocellular carcinoma after pediatric living donor liver transplantation.
PMID: 29359020.

Question 175

A 59-year-old female presents to the clinic for routine follow-up. She underwent a liver transplant for alcohol-related liver disease and hepatocellular carcinoma 18 months ago. She has done well on tacrolimus. She has remained sober and managed to quit smoking. Her hypertension is controlled on amlodipine. Her only complaint is reflux symptoms and a persistent sore throat.

On exam she is alert in no distress without scleral icterus with a soft abdomen.

Laboratory studies:

ALT 12 U/L
ALP 77 U/L
Tbili 0.6 mg/dL
Creatinine 0.5 mg/dL
An EGD is performed and the lesion below was seen in the oropharynx just above the vocal cords.

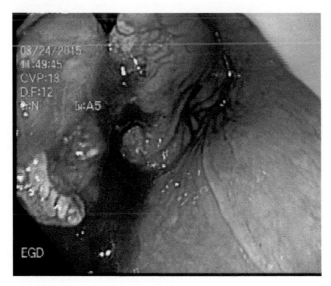

▶ Question

Biopsy is most likely to show?

A Post transplant lymphoproliferative disorder (PTLD)
B Squamous cell carcinoma
C Adenocarcinoma
D Metastatic thyroid cancer
E Metastatic hepatocellular carcinoma

B is the correct answer.

Commentary – Head and Neck Cancer After Liver Transplantation

The image shows a friable mass and biopsy confirmed invasive squamous cell carcinoma. The incidence of thyroid cancer is not increased after transplantation and hepatocellular carcinoma metastasizes to lungs and bone. Adenocarcinoma is unlikely in the oropharynx. PTLD is a possibility but typically presents as ulcerated lesions in the gastrointestinal tract or with lymphadenopathy.

This patient's tobacco, alcohol use, and immunosuppression put her at considerable risk for head and neck cancer. There is also data that human papillomavirus and hepatitis C also increase the risk of head and neck cancer after solid organ transplantation.

Screening for skin cancer is recommended annually in transplant recipients but there are no recommendations for head and neck cancer. However, there should be a low threshold to investigate oral symptoms in transplant patients with smoking and alcohol history.

Notes
I am not surprised at how often I see this. Smoking and drinking are not a good combination in transplant recipients.

Reference

Risk factors and incidence of de novo malignancy in liver transplant recipients: a systematic review. PMID: 20602682.

Question 176

A 33-year-old male underwent a deceased donor liver transplant for acute alcoholic hepatitis 10 days ago. His postoperative course has been complicated by poor urine output. Yesterday he developed a fever and an elevated white count. Imaging showed a patent hepatic artery with residual ascites and several perihepatic collections.

His medications include tacrolimus 6 mg bid, mycophenolate mofetil 1 g bid, and prednisone 15 mg daily.

Examination shows an ill looking male, temperature 101.3 °F, BP 100/70, HR 112/min

Laboratory studies:

WBC count 28,000
ALT 78 U/L
AST 62 U/L
ALP 89 U/L
Tbili 4.6 mg/dL
Creatinine 3.7 mg/dL
Lactate 3.6 mmol/L (normal <2)
Tacrolimus trough level
10.2 ng/mL
He undergoes ERCP as shown below:

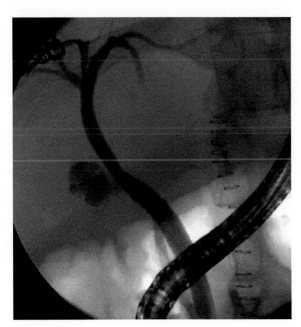

▶ Question

Which is the best management option?

A Operative intervention with bile duct reconstruction
B Operative intervention with conversion to a Roux-en-Y hepaticojejunostomy
C Re-transplantation
D Radiologic intervention
E Endoscopic intervention

E is the correct answer.

Commentary – Early Bile Leak After Liver Transplantation

The image shows extravasation of contrast from the mid-extra-hepatic bile duct- a bile leak likely from the duct-to-duct anastomosis (or less likely the cystic duct). Since access has been achieved, placing a stent into the bile duct across the anastomosis will heal the leak in the vast majority of cases (as was the case here). Operative intervention is rarely needed unless the leak is very large or does not heal. Interventional radiology will be difficult to perform in this setting where the proximal duct will not be dilated.

Leaks are almost always a technical issue and occur early in the postoperative period. Risk factors for biliary leaks are not as well defined as they are for bile duct strictures. In historical terms, late bile leaks occurred after the removal of a t-tube which is rarely used today.

Leaks occur up to 10–15% after deceased donor transplant and are more common after live donor transplant where the ducts and anastomosis are smaller and there is the potential for a cut surface leak.

Leaks can lead to subsequent bile duct strictures.

> **Notes**
>
> Despite the 40-year history of liver transplant, biliary complications remain a frequent problem after transplant. Fortunately, they are relatively easy to fix. It seems that we are seeing more cases now than ever, perhaps a consequence of increasing utilization of extended criteria organs in the MELD era – a fact we published on 10 years ago (see reference below).

Reference

Post-transplant biliary complications in the pre- and post-model for end-stage liver disease era. PMID: 21445926.

Question 177

A 55-year-old male presents with abnormal liver enzymes for several years. He does not drink significantly, and his only relevant family history is myeloma in his father.

His only complaint is several months of shortness of breath on exertion and nonproductive cough. His weight has been stable with normal appetite and bowel movements. He denies any fever, chills, or abdominal pain

Physical exam reveals normal vitals. His BMI is 29 kg/m^2

There is no scleral icterus or spider nevi. Heart and lungs are normal. Abdomen reveals a smooth liver felt 3 cm below the right costal margin. There is no splenomegaly, ascites, or ankle edema.

Ultrasound abdomen is normal.

Laboratory studies:

Tbili 0.5 mg/dL
AST 73 U/L
ALT 96 U/L
ALP 479 U/L
GGTP 452 U/L
A liver biopsy is performed and a representative image is shown below (H&E 250X)

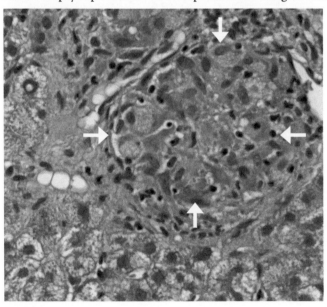

▶ Question

Which of the following is NOT required to make a diagnosis?
A A medication history
B Special staining of the liver biopsy
C Autoimmune serology
D Chest imaging
E Bone marrow biopsy

E is the correct answer.

Commentary – Hepatic Sarcoid

The histology shows a well-circumscribed hepatic granuloma. There is a clue that he has pulmonary symptoms so hepatic sarcoid is high on the differential. Autoimmune studies, (especially anti-mitochondrial antibody) should be checked as primary biliary and autoimmune cholangitis are on the differential.

Granulomatous hepatitis is a diagnosis of exclusion where the liver is infiltrated by granulomas. This can be seen in PBC but also in TB and with a variety of bacterial and fungal infections, hence the need to exclude these entities with serology and special staining on the biopsy before making a diagnosis.

Several drugs are associated with hepatic granulomas including allopurinol, quinidine, sulfa drugs, and intravesical BCG for bladder cancer.

This patient had a serum ACE level twice the upper limit of normal and had had a chest X-ray several months previously that demonstrated hilar prominence.

A bone marrow biopsy typically would not be necessary.

Hepatic sarcoid is typically an indolent disease and the development of cirrhosis and portal hypertension are uncommon. Most patients with hepatic sarcoid do well with just periodic assessment.

Notes

Sarcoid is like syphilis and lupus – can do pretty much anything to any organ. I have never transplanted a patient for hepatic sarcoid. All the patients that had sarcoid were transplanted for concomitant disease (usually NASH).

Reference

Granulomatous liver disease. PMID: 22541705.

Question 178

As the transplant medicine consultant, you are asked to see a 57-year-old female for altered mental status.

She underwent bilateral cadaveric lung transplant 10 days ago for idiopathic pulmonary hypertension. There has been difficulty weaning her off the ventilator and she has become lethargic and unresponsive. She was not known to have underlying liver disease and had no significant alcohol consumption.

On exam she is intubated and unresponsive, afebrile with normal vital signs and has 98% O_2 saturation on 2 L nasal cannula. There are no localizing neurological signs with a soft, non-tender abdomen without hepatosplenomegaly and no ascites.

Ultrasound shows a normal looking liver and spleen.

Laboratory studies:

Hb 8.7 g/dL
WBC 6.2
Creatinine 0.6 mg/dL
Tbili 0.7 mg/dL
AST 25 U/L
ALT 27 U/L
ALP 93 U/L
Albumin 1.9 g/dL

▶ Question

Which of the following is the most appropriate next test to obtain?

A Abdominal MRI scan
B CMV serology
C Arterial ammonia level
D HSV serology
E Chest CT scan

C is the correct answer.

Commentary – Idiopathic Hyperammonemia Post Lung Transplant

Making this diagnosis can make you look very smart but this is not a diagnosis you want to make. This patient has developed idiopathic hyperammonemia after a lung transplant and the prognosis is typically very poor and usually fatal. It can occur in up to 4% of lung transplant recipients and usually presents within the first few weeks after transplant. It appears to be associated with the development of major gastrointestinal complications, use of total parenteral nutrition and lung transplantation for primary pulmonary hypertension. One study suggested that deficiency of liver glutamine synthetase may be responsible, but the exact mechanism is unclear and importantly can occur in the absence of liver disease.

Ammonia levels can be elevated if there is overproduction but typically if there is impaired clearance through hepatic dysfunction or porto-systemic shunting. Ammonia readily crosses the blood-brain barrier leading to functional and structural abnormalities, which are manifested as neuropsychiatric dysfunction.

Viral infection is unlikely without fever and elevated WBC. Abdominal MRI is not necessary with a normal ultrasound already and the oxygen saturation is normal, so chest imaging is unlikely to be helpful.

Reference

Fatal hyperammonemia after orthotopic lung transplantation. PMID: 10681283.

Question 179

A 60-year-old male presents with several episodes of hematemesis and melena. He has a history of cirrhosis secondary to alcohol that has been complicated in the past by multiple admissions for variceal hemorrhage, encephalopathy, and ascites. He has undergone esophageal variceal band ligation, most recently 4 months ago.

He has not taken any prescribed medication for more than a month after his prescriptions ran out.

Exam demonstrates a wasted looking man with a BP of 120/80 and pulse 104 beats per minute, regular.

He is alert and oriented and his abdomen is mildly distended. Melena is noted on rectal exam.

Laboratory studies:

Hb 7.7 g/dL
Plts 53,000
INR 1.6
Creat 0.7 mg/dL
Tbili 2.5 mg/dL
He undergoes EGD and imaging:

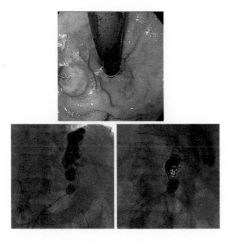

▶ Question

Which is the most accurate statement?

A This procedure will increase his portal hypertension
B This procedure requires a transjugular porto-systemic shunt (TIPS)
C This procedure requires trans-splenic access
D This procedure requires trans-hepatic access
E This procedure will decrease his portal hypertension

A is the correct answer.

Commentary – Balloon Occluded Retrograde Trans-Venous Obliteration (BRTO) of Gastric Varices

The endoscopy shows gastric varices in the fundus on a retroflexed view with stigmata of recent bleeding. The radiologic images show a balloon being inflated and contrast/sclerosant injected into gastric varices and in the second image, coils have been placed. The BRTO procedure involves passing a catheter into the inferior vena cava through the femoral vein. The catheter is passed into the left renal vein and then the splenic vein through a splenorenal shunt. The gastric varices can be identified coming off the splenic vein and a balloon is inflated, and foam or coils can be deployed to prevent retrograde flow. In most cases, access to the splenic vein can be achieved through the left renal vein. Transhepatic, trans-splenic, or TIPS are not required but are occasionally necessary. Since the gastric varices are decompressing the portal system, obliteration will worsen portal hypertension.

Complications of BRTO include balloon rupture such that sclerosant can leak into the systemic circulation and can cause pulmonary embolism or recurrent gastric variceal bleeding due to the sclerosant not obliterating the varices. Coils can also migrate. We recently saw a case with amazing images where coils had migrated into the stomach (and were confused for a migrated feeding tube) and we had to use a variety of devices to remove them (PMID 33915170).

Clinical Pearls: BRTO

1. BRTO increases portal hypertension
2. Sclerosant and/or coils can leak or migrate leading to complications such as pulmonary embolism

---

Notes

I have been fortunate to have had amazing interventional radiology departments wherever I have worked. In addition to bleeding cases, I have worked alongside my IR colleagues and performed rendezvous cases for tough biliary cases. The types of cases they can do will only increase. TIPS started when I was in medical school. BRTO has only become mainstream in the last decade.

Reference

Balloon-occluded retrograde transvenous obliteration for treatment of gastric varices. PMID: 34239700.

Question 180

A 66-year-old male presents with bleeding from his colostomy. He had undergone colonic resection for colorectal cancer 3 years ago complicated by liver metastases requiring a liver resection and multiple cycles of chemotherapy and radiation.

Exam demonstrates a thin man with a BP of 142/73 and pulse 92 beats per minute.

He is alert and oriented and his abdomen mildly distended. Maroon stool is noted in the colostomy bag.

Laboratory studies:

Hb 6.9 g/dL
Plts 68,000
INR 1.8
Creat 0.7 mg/dL
Tbili 1.5 mg/dL
Albumin 2.1 mg/dL
CT scan demonstrates ascites, patent portal and hepatic vessels, and splenomegaly. EGD shows small non-bleeding esophageal varices but no blood in the upper GI tract.
He undergoes additional studies as shown below:

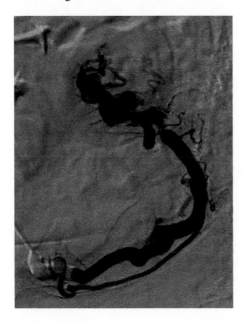

▶ Question

All of the following are reasonable management options EXCEPT?

A Cyanoacrylate injection
B Transjugular porto-systemic shunt (TIPS)
C Balloon retrograde transvenous obliteration (BRTO)
D Coil embolization
E Surgical distal spleno-renal shunt

E is the correct answer.

Commentary – Ectopic (Stomal Varices)

The image shows injection of a vessel coming off a tributary of the superior mesenteric vein and filling of stomal varices (you can see the faint outline of the stoma in the top half of the image). Ectopic varices are relatively uncommon but can present a management dilemma. They are often very distant to the portal vein or splenic vein making radiologic access difficult and porto-systemic shunting less effective. Choices A–D are reasonable approaches depending on local expertise. A surgical shunt would not be a good option as there is significant portal hypertension, a platelet count of less than 100, and evidence of liver synthetic dysfunction. This patient underwent coil embolization with good hemostasis (as shown below with minimal filling of the varices beyond the coils).

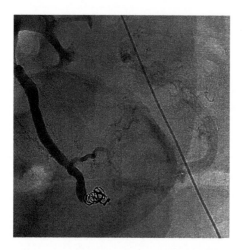

Notes

If ectopic varices come up on the boards it will be straightforward and non-controversial as there are no recognized guidelines. For practical purposes, good interventional radiology will usually be required. Remember if you encounter a bleeding ectopic varix during a scope, it is not wrong to perform endoscopic therapy, but the patient must then immediately be sent for something more definitive (TIPS, embolization, surgery, etc.).

Reference

Portal hypertensive bleeding in cirrhosis: Risk stratification, diagnosis, and management: 2016 practice guidance by the American Association for the study of liver diseases. PMID: 27786365.

Question 181

A 57-year-old female presents with abnormal liver enzymes. She underwent an ortho-topic liver transplant 3 months earlier for end-stage liver disease secondary to hepatitis C complicated by hepatocellular carcinoma. The cancer was treated with transarte-rial chemoembolization prior to transplant. She received a 35 year-old allograft from a HCV-positive donor with 20–30% macrosteatosis. Her postoperative course had been uneventful and symptomatically she felt well.

Her immunosuppression consists of tacrolimus, mycophenolate mofetil, and a taper-ing dose of prednisone. Her exam is remarkable for mild icterus.

Ultrasound and MRI/MRCP of the abdomen show a patent hepatic artery and no duc-tal dilation.

Laboratory studies:

Hb 11.9 g/dL
Plts 173,000
INR 1.1
Tbili 6.6 mg/dL
AST 213 U/L
ALT 277 U/L
ALP 376 U/L
Creatinine 1.2 mg/dL
Tacrolimus level 12.8 ng/mL
A liver biopsy is performed:

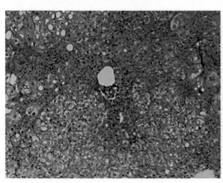 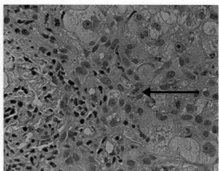

▶ Question

What is the most likely diagnosis?

A Acute cellular rejection
B Chronic rejection
C Bile duct problem
D Fibrosing cholestatic hepatitis C
E Hepatic artery thrombosis

D is the correct answer.

Commentary – Fibrosing Cholestatic Hepatitis C

The liver biopsy shows lobules with hepatocytic cholestasis (high power image – arrowed) with feathery degeneration. The portal tracts are expanded by proliferating bile ductules accompanied by neutrophils. Occasional acidophilic bodies and scattered chronic inflammatory cells are seen. The trichrome stain in the low power image shows periportal fibrosis. There is no evidence of acute cellular rejection, bile duct loss, or ischemic change.

This patient has developed fibrosing cholestatic hepatitis C. This is a rare condition characterized by cholestasis, fibrosis, and a very elevated HCV RNA typically occurring early after liver transplant. It has a very aggressive course without treatment and can lead to early graft loss. The HCV RNA is typically very elevated as it was in this case (38 million IU/mL).

The main differential diagnosis of this pattern of LFTs can be divided into biliary problems due to hepatic artery thrombosis/stenosis, acute rejection, or recurrent hepatitis C. Other possibilities do exist including a drug reaction or acute hepatitis from atypical viruses including CMV. The imaging suggests that the hepatic artery is open, and it would be unusual to get acute rejection with her therapeutic tacrolimus level. Chronic rejection would not occur 3 months after transplant.

This was much more common in the pre-direct acting antiviral drugs for HCV era. It still can occur today as the use of HCV-positive allografts increases but treatment with DAAs will treat this condition.

Notes

Fibrosing cholestatic hepatitis can be seen with other hepatitis viruses and the viral load will be extremely high. Graft loss is swift without treatment.

Reference

Early histologic changes in fibrosing cholestatic hepatitis C. PMID: 17205558.

Question 182

A 35-year-old male presents to the ER with nausea, vomiting, and diarrhea that has been going on for several days. He denies fever or abdominal pain. His girlfriend noticed his eyes looked yellow.

He underwent liver transplant 4 years ago for alcoholic hepatitis. He was maintained on tacrolimus and mycophenolate with prednisone tapered over several months. His postoperative course was significant for an episode of acute rejection 6 months after transplant.

He denies other medical problems. He states he is taking his tacrolimus.

Exam demonstrates an anxious man. His vital signs show a weight of 155 pounds, BP 140/90, pulse 110 and he is afebrile.

He is icteric and has a palpable liver edge. No ascites is noted.

Laboratory studies:

Tbili 13.7 mg/dL
Direct bili 9.8 mg/dL
AST 179 U/L
ALT 194 U/L
ALP 349 U/L
Creatinine 1.2 mg/dL
Tacrolimus level 10.9 ng/mL
Ultrasound shows no biliary dilation. Hepatic artery has normal resistive indices.
Liver biopsy is performed as shown below:

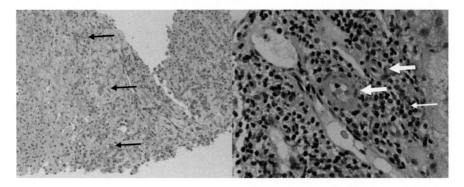

▶ Question

What is the best management option

A Increase the tacrolimus dose
B Add 1 g bid of mycophenolate mofetil to his immunosuppression
C Switch the tacrolimus to sirolimus
D Add 30 mg prednisone to his immunosuppression
E Add 30 mg prednisone and 1 g of MMF to his immunosuppression

A is the correct answer.

Commentary – Chronic (Ductopenic) Rejection

This gentleman has developed chronic rejection likely due to noncompliance. The liver biopsy at low power demonstrates a mild chronic nonspecific inflammatory infiltrate in the portal tract and the lobules are remarkable for severe canalicular and hepatocytic cholestasis (arrows). On higher power it is apparent that bile ducts are either damaged or missing. The two thicker arrows in the second image point to hepatic artery branches. The thinner arrow points to an area where the bile duct used to be and all that is left is some inflammatory cells. This is a very important fact about liver pathology – in the portal tract the bile duct and hepatic artery should be adjacent to one another. A CK7 (cytokeratin 7) stain is usually done in this situation to stain for bile ducts. In this patient, 5 out of 7 portal tracts were missing bile ducts, indicative of ductopenia. Other features of chronic rejection include a foam cell (obliterative) arteriopathy and biliary epithelial atrophy.

The elevated tacrolimus level may indicate that he decided to take more than the prescribed dose when he became jaundiced.

The current incidence of chronic rejection of 3–4% in adults has decreased over the last 15–20 years due to the introduction of stronger immunosuppressive drugs. In children, the incidence of 8–12% has not changed, perhaps related in part due to noncompliance. Several factors are associated with the development of chronic rejection including the number of acute rejection episodes and the histological severity of acute rejection episodes, underlying liver disease, HLA donor-recipient matching, positive lymphocytotoxic crossmatch, CMV infection, recipient age, donor-recipient ethnic origin, and male donor into female recipient. Obviously, not taking the immunosuppression (evidenced by a low tacrolimus or cyclosporine level) is also a risk factor.

Unlike acute rejection, the chronic variety can lead to graft failure. The only effective treatment is to increase the tacrolimus that may lead to improvement in histology and occasionally complete reversibility. Tacrolimus can be used as rescue therapy in patients previously on cyclosporine, particularly if chronic rejection is diagnosed before the bilirubin gets to 10 mg/dL.

Clinical Pearls: Chronic Rejection

1. Histological features of chronic rejection include:
   a. ductopenia (CK 7 stain)
   b. foam cell arteriopathy
   c. biliary epithelial atrophy
2. (High dose) tacrolimus is the only effective treatment

Notes

This is an important differential diagnosis to make in a patient with cholestatic enzymes, particularly in cases where there is no treatment for other conditions such as recurrent PSC or ischemia. I usually have a low threshold for liver biopsy if chronic rejection is on the differential.

Reference

Efficacy of tacrolimus as rescue therapy for chronic rejection in orthotopic liver transplantation: a report of the U.S. Multicenter Liver Study Group. PMID: 9256184.

Question 183

A 22-year-old female presents with acute onset of abdominal pain, nausea, and vomiting. There is no fever, but she has felt cold and had some chills. She denies diarrhea.

She has a history of orthotopic liver transplant for acute liver failure secondary to autoimmune hepatitis three months ago. She had an uneventful postoperative recovery and has been taking tacrolimus, mycophenolate, and prednisone.

She has no past medical history other than depression and denies any change in her medications. She does not smoke or drink and there have been no sick contacts at home.

Examination reveals mild scleral icterus. There is mild epigastric tenderness, but no rebound tenderness and bowel sounds are normal. There is no ascites or splenomegaly. Extremities reveal no edema.

Laboratory studies:

pH 7.4
Lipase normal
Hb 11.6 g/dL
WBC 11.3
Tbili 3.1 mg/dL
AST 436 U/L
ALT 475 U/L
ALP 289 U/L
FK level 9.9 ng/mL
She undergoes imaging and a radiological procedure as shown

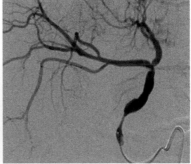

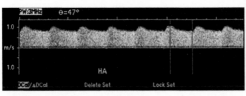

▶ Question

What is the most likely diagnosis?

A Hepatic artery thrombosis
B Hepatic artery stenosis
C Portal vein thrombosis
D Hepatic venous stenosis
E Inferior vena cava stenosis

B is the correct answer.

Commentary – Hepatic Artery Stenosis (HAS)

This lady has an acute onset of abdominal pain and fever 3 months after transplant and a significant rise in her transaminases. Diagnostic considerations include acute rejection, infection (CMV), biliary obstruction, or hepatic artery obstruction. Rejection is unlikely given the therapeutic FK level. Infection is a definite possibility as she is febrile and within the first few months of transplant when immunosuppression is still high. She needs blood cultures to be sent and empiric antibiotics should be started. She needs imaging which should include an ultrasound to look at the biliary tree and the hepatic vessels. She should have a CMV DNA test sent. The markedly elevated transaminases might suggest an ischemic insult and indeed this lady has developed HAS, a relatively common complication after liver transplant.

The first image is an ultrasound with Doppler study that demonstrates a patent hepatic artery but a classic tardus parvus waveform with a low resistive index (RI) of 0.24. The hepatic artery had a more normal waveform on a prior study with an RI measuring 0.58 a month previously. The portal vein and hepatic veins were patent with normal Doppler color flow and direction. The tardus parvus refers to the Doppler linear flow velocity versus time spectrum obtained in an arterial flow system in which there is proximal occlusive disease with a post-stenotic pressure drop. The RI is an indicator of resistance of an organ to perfusion. In ultrasonography, it can be calculated from the peak systolic velocity and the end-diastolic velocity of blood flow (1-end-diastolic velocity divided by peak systolic velocity), and a value of 0.6–0.8 is considered normal.

The angiogram (second image) demonstrates the hepatic artery with a proximal segment of severe stenosis/stricture and a second stricture at the level of the bifurcation of the right and left hepatic arteries. These strictures underwent balloon angioplasty with improved flow noted immediately afterward.

The incidence of HAS after OLT is 5–6% and it is a risk factor for hepatic artery thrombosis. Treatment initially was surgical but there are several case series describing the results of interventional radiology.

Risk factors for HAS include poor hepatic artery flow at the time of OLT but this presents early. Later HAS has no apparent risk factor. Surgical treatment results in initial patency rates of 70–80% but biliary strictures can develop in 25–30% of patients and retransplantation can be required.

Angioplasty and stenting of the hepatic artery can be effective in about 50% of patients but there is a significant restenosis rate and a risk of hepatic artery thrombosis (although lower than if HAS is not treated).

In this patient, there was initial improvement but she subsequently developed biliary strictures and was relisted for liver transplant.

Clinical Pearls: Hepatic Artery Stenosis

1. Incidence is 5–6%
2. Tardus parvus waveform with low resistive index on Doppler
3. Angioplasty can be used to treat but only 50% effective
4. Risk of ischemic cholangiopathy in 25–30%

Reference

Clinical outcomes from hepatic artery stenting in liver transplantation. PMID: 16498642.

Question 184

A 38-year-old female presents for evaluation of a liver mass. She has a history of chronic hepatitis C that was successfully treated 4 years ago. FibroScan suggested stage 2 fibrosis prior to treatment. She has been essentially well but had experienced some dyspepsia for a few days a month ago and underwent an upper GI endoscopy and CT scan which were both normal.

She does not drink alcohol or smoke. She is originally from Mexico and had a blood transfusion at the time of an ectopic pregnancy as a teenager that required a hysterectomy. She has been on hormone replacement therapy as a result.

She denies any prescribed or over the counter medications.

On exam she is very anxious. Her sclerae are anicteric and her abdomen is soft without masses.

Laboratory studies:

Hb 13.0 g/dL
Plts 203,000
INR 1.1
Tbili 0.3 mg/dL
AST 23 U/L
ALT 20 U/L
ALP 87 U/L
Albumin 3.5 g/dL
Creatinine 0.6 mg/dL
HCV RNA negative
AFP 26 ng/mL
CT scan is shown below:

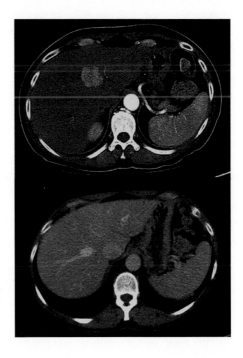

▶ Question

What is the next best step in management?

A Stop hormone replacement therapy
B Perform liver biopsy
C Perform MRI
D Surgical resection
E Reassurance

E is the correct answer.

Commentary – Focal Nodular Hyperplasia

The differential diagnosis in a patient presenting with a contrast enhancing liver mass is wide. In patients with cirrhosis or chronic hepatitis B infection, one should be vigilant about hepatocellular carcinoma. In females with no obvious liver disease, hepatic adenoma, or focal nodular hyperplasia should be considered in the differential diagnosis. In this case she has hepatitis C but mild fibrosis so should not be at risk for hepatocellular carcinoma. The liver enzymes and AFP were normal. The CT scan showed a mass measuring 3.1 cm in segment 4 of the liver. The mass demonstrated lobular contour with arterial enhancement that equilibrates on delayed images. There was a thin linear vascular scar within the mass. All of these are classic characteristics of focal nodular hyperplasia.

Focal nodular hyperplasia (FNH) is the most common benign hepatic tumor that is not of vascular origin. It is usually a solitary lesion found predominantly in women between the ages of 20 and 50 years. The characteristic finding is the presence of a central stellate scar containing a large vessel with multiple branches radiating through the fibrous septae to the periphery. One-third of patients may have nonspecific abdominal pain. The remainder of patients often have no symptoms. A confident diagnosis can usually be made through an imaging modality and tissue diagnosis is usually not required. Based on CT scan, the lesion becomes hyperdense during the hepatic arterial phase and becomes isodense during the portal venous phase with the central scar. In an ambiguous case, a second imaging modality such as an MRI scan can be helpful differentiating FNH from others. The MRI scan with gadolinium infusion produces a hyperintense mass in early contrast images which later becomes isointense with respect to normal liver in delayed images. FNH may be responsive to estrogens. It is generally believed that oral contraceptive pills or hormone replacement therapy are not related to FNH. However, it is reasonable to obtain a follow-up imaging study in 6–12 months to ensure the stability of FNH in women who continue taking these drugs.

Clinical Pearls: FNH

1. FNH enhances on contrast scan and has a central stellate scar
2. Mainly female
3. Younger population – usually age 20–50 years

Reference

On the pathogenesis of focal nodular hyperplasia of the liver. PMID: 4065824.

Question 185

An 84-year-old male presents with painless jaundice and weight loss. CT scan of abdomen shows dilated intra- and extra-hepatic bile ducts down to the level of ampulla.

Laboratory studies:

Normal CBC
INR 1.0
Tbili 5.2 mg/dL
ALP 800 U/L
AST 125 U/L
ALT 137 U/L
Creatinine 1.0 mg/dL
AFP 2.4 mg/dL
Ca 19-9 113 μ/mL
ERCP images are shown below:

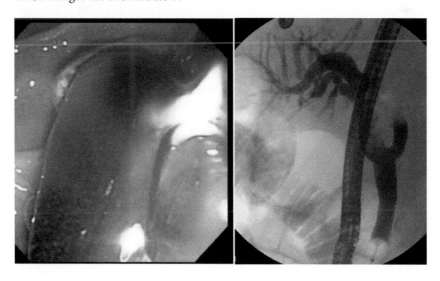

▶ Question

What is the most likely diagnosis?

A Intraductal hepatocellular carcinoma
B Cholangiocarcinoma
C Hepatoblastoma
D Mucinous cystic neoplasm of the liver
E Intraductal papillary neoplasm of the bile duct

E is the correct answer.

Commentary – Intraductal Papillary Neoplasm of Bile Duct (IPNB)

This was a shock for the interventional fellow when we did this case – mucus pouring out of the ampulla. IPNB is a rare tumor that closely resembles the intraductal papillary mucinous neoplasm (IPMN) of the pancreas. IPNB is characterized by intraluminal growth, sometimes in papillary masses with bile duct obstruction and dilatation. Papillary tumors generally produce a large amount of mucin and when the mucin flow obstructs the duodenal papilla, both proximal and distal to the tumor bile ducts become diffusely dilated. The symptoms may mimic obstructive jaundice, sometimes complicated by cholangitis or stone formation. Endoscopy showing mucin draining from the ampulla is diagnostic as seen on the endoscopic image. The cholangiogram shows an occlusion image with the balloon inflated in the very distal duct and a diffusely dilated biliary tree with heterogeneous filling defects representing mucin (near the cystic duct take-off). Occasionally, papillary tumor is seen as fine irregularities of the bile duct wall with a velvety or serrated contour. Several different histological types of IPNB have been described and are associated with invasive cancer. Surgical resection with hepaticojejunostomy is often indicated. In nonsurgical patients, a generous biliary sphincterotomy can relieve biliary obstruction but can require often needs repeating.

Intraductal spread of HCC is rare and does not lead to mucin production and neither does CCA. Hepatoblastoma is a malignancy of early childhood and presents with a liver mass. Mucinous cystic neoplasm of the liver encompasses biliary cystadenoma and cystadenocarcinoma. They present as a large avascular cystic mass that does not connect to the biliary tree.

Reference

Characterization of Intraductal Papillary Neoplasm of the Bile Duct with Respect to the Histopathologic Similarities to Pancreatic Intraductal Papillary Mucinous Neoplasm. PMID: 30982236.

Question 186

This CT scan is from a 44-year-old female from Lebanon presenting with mild upper abdominal fullness and occasional pain. Weight has been stable.

Laboratory studies were normal.

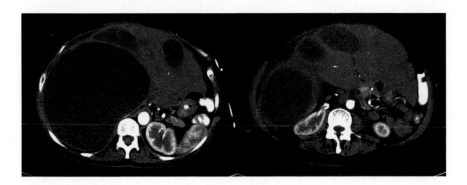

▶ Question

All the following are appropriate management EXCEPT

A Percutaneous aspiration, injection, and re-aspiration
B Surgical resection
C Observation
D Serological testing for *Echinococcus granulosus* and *Echinococcus multilocularis*
E Albendazole

C is the correct answer.

Commentary – Echinococcal (Hydatid) Cyst

Echinococcal (hydatid) cysts of the liver are caused by the larval form of the tapeworm, *Echinococcus granulosus* or *Echinococcus multilocularis*, which is usually acquired from infected dogs or foxes. *E. granulosus* leads to cystic echinococcosis and *E. multilocularis* causes alveolar echinococcosis (more severe disease) although both cause liver (hydatid) cysts. Echinococcal disease is reported throughout the Middle East, South America, Eastern Europe, and China. After the primary infection, the patients usually remain asymptomatic for many years. The cysts are fluid-filled structures limited by a parasite-derived membrane. Patients are often asymptomatic until the cyst reaches at least 10 cm in diameter. Cysts greater than this size (as in this case) have a higher risk of complications and should be treated. The right lobe of the liver is affected most commonly. When symptoms do occur, the patients may have hepatomegaly, nausea, vomiting, intraperitoneal leakage, or biliary obstruction. The combination of imaging and serological testing usually makes the diagnosis of echinococcal cysts in the liver. When CT scan or ultrasound reveals separation of the hydatid membrane from the cyst wall and nearby daughter cysts, a diagnosis of hydatid disease is highly likely. Surgical resection is indicated for complications or when cysts are larger than 10 cm. Percutaneous aspiration, injection (of scolicidal agent), and re-aspiration (PAIR) is useful for large cysts without daughter cysts but there is a potential risk for anaphylaxis that is mitigated by using adjunctive albendazole. In most cases of hydatid liver disease, treatment consists of medical therapy with albendazole. In the patients with severe symptoms, surgery is should be also considered.

Although you often only read about these cases rather than see them in the flesh, exotic infectious diseases with good images that require intervention are common on the boards.

Reference

Clinical management of cystic echinococcosis: state of the art and perspectives.
PMID: 30124496.

Question 187

A 63-year-old Chinese male is brought in by his family to the ER with abdominal pain and fever. History is difficult to obtain but he has had similar symptoms multiple times over many years and has undergone surgery and several procedures.

Laboratory studies:

WBC 13.6
Hemoglobin 10.7 g/dL
Tbili 4.2 mg/dL
AST 103 U/L
ALT 116 U/L
ALP 357 U/L
Creatinine 0.7 mg/dL
CT scan:

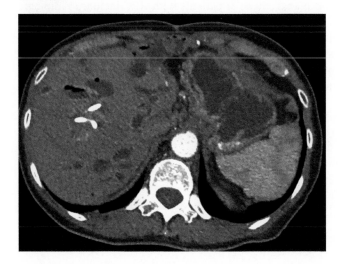

▶ Question

This disease is associated with all the following EXCEPT

A *Echinococcus multilocularis*
B *Clonorchis sinensis*
C Opisthorchis
D *Fasciola hepatica*
E *Ascaris lumbricoides*

A is the correct answer.

Commentary – Recurrent Pyogenic Cholangitis

The CT scan reveals a prior left sided liver resection, dilated intrahepatic ducts with filling defects, pneumobilia, and the proximal end of a pigtail stent in the right lobe. The patient had undergone an ERCP where many pigmented stones in the bile ducts were removed after sphincterotomy and a stent had been placed several years ago.

Recurrent pyogenic cholangitis (RPC) (previously called Oriental cholangiohepatitis) is a disease characterized by intrahepatic pigment stone formation resulting in biliary obstruction with recurrent cholangitis, dilatation, and stricturing of the biliary tree. Patients typically present with recurrent bouts of pain, fever with or without jaundice. It occurs exclusively in people who live or who have lived in Southeast Asia. RPC most commonly affects the left hepatic ducts possibly due to the more acute angle compared with the right hepatic ducts. Biliary parasites such as *Clonorchis sinensis*, Opisthorchis and *Fasciola hepatica*, and the roundworm Ascaris have been implicated in the pathogenesis of RPC. The organisms are thought to initiate the disease by damaging the biliary epithelium. The diagnosis and management of patients with RPC includes radiologic (percutaneous transhepatic cholangiogram [PTC]), endoscopic (ERCP), and surgical interventions. In patients with acute complications such as cholangitis, ERCP, or PTC is warranted to remove stones and provide drainage. Resection of the left hepatic system can be considered in patients where the disease is confined to the left liver lobe. The disease is associated with the development of cholangiocarcinoma.

Clinical Pearls: Recurrent Pyogenic Cholangitis

1. Exclusively in Asian patients
2. Initial infectious etiology
3. Associated with cholangiocarcinoma

Notes

These cases can be very difficult to manage and I would say of all the cases I have seen, half either have already had surgery or will end up in the OR.

Reference

Current management of recurrent pyogenic cholangitis. PMID: 10515539.

Question 188

The MRI of the right upper quadrant below is from a 33-year-old male who is admitted with fever and pain. He has had multiple prior episodes.

Laboratory studies:

Tbili 1.7 mg/dL
AST 99 U/L
ALT 125 U/L
ALP 563 U/L

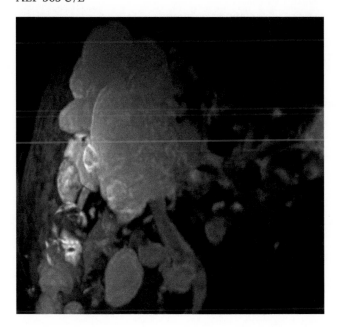

▶ Question

All of the following are associated with this condition EXCEPT?

A Cholangiocarcinoma
B Autosomal recessive polycystic kidney disease
C Congenital hepatic fibrosis
D Hepaticolithiasis
E Choledochal cyst

E is the correct answer.

Commentary – Caroli Disease

The MRCP image shows massively dilated intrahepatic ducts with relative preservation of the extrahepatic duct.

Caroli disease is:

1. Congenital, usually autosomal recessive
2. Characterized by ectatic INTRAhepatic bile ducts with saccular dilation leading to bile stasis and intrahepatic lithiasis and repeated cholangitis
3. Associated with a risk of secondary biliary cirrhosis
4. Associated with polycystic kidney disease
5. Associated with an increased risk of cholangiocarcinoma

Caroli syndrome is Caroli disease associated with congenital hepatic fibrosis and the development of portal hypertension.

Caroli is not associated with choledochal cysts, which involve the EXTRAhepatic duct.

Treatment is supportive and liver transplant is an option for advanced disease.

There is another question in this book that discusses choledochal cysts.

Reference

Pathobiology of inherited biliary diseases: a roadmap to understand acquired liver diseases. PMID: 31165788.

Question 189

A 45-year-old female who underwent liver transplant 8 months ago presents with several days of right upper quadrant pain, dark urine, and pruritis. She has been taking tacrolimus and mycophenolate and had normal liver and renal function a month ago.

Laboratory studies:

Tbili 1.9 mg/dL
AST 75 U/L
ALT 87 U/L
ALP 203 U/L
GGT 273 U/L
Ultrasound shows an 11 mm bile duct and mild intrahepatic duct dilation. Hepatic artery is patent.
ERCP is performed:

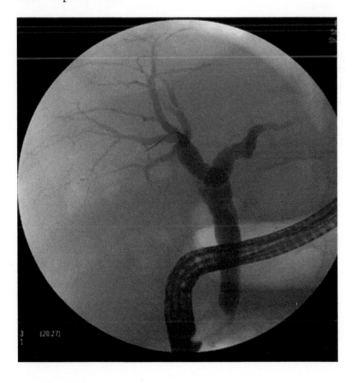

▶ Question

What is the most likely diagnosis?

A Anastomotic stricture
B Non-anastomotic stricture
C Hepatic artery stenosis
D Sphincter dysfunction
E Duct-to-duct mismatch

D is the correct answer.

Commentary – Sphincter Dysfunction

The ERCP image demonstrates a post OLT cholangiogram. The scope measures 12 mm in diameter and hence the extrahepatic duct is dilated to 12–14 mm and the right and left intrahepatic ducts are also dilated. The dilation extends all the way to the ampulla. No filling defects are seen and the anastomosis is barely seen. The cystic duct is seen superimposed over the extra-hepatic duct. A wire has been inserted through a catheter and the tip is seen in the right intrahepatics.

The differential diagnosis is that of cholestatic enzymes after transplant. The hepatic artery is patent which is reassuring, and the appearance does not fit with ischemic cholangiopathy or duct-to-duct mismatch. There still must be concern for biliary obstruction so an anastomotic stricture is the obvious cause. The cholangiogram demonstrates findings consistent with sphincter dysfunction with dilation all the way down to the ampulla. The contrast did not drain well even after I watched for several minutes and hence the treatment of choice should be a sphincterotomy. She did well with normal liver tests afterward.

Sphincter dysfunction is thought to have an incidence of 2–7% after transplant, significantly more common than in the normal population. The pathogenesis is unclear but may be related to denervation of the sphincter muscle around the biliary orifice at the time of transplant leading to sphincter hypertension. This will lead to biliary stasis and cholestatic liver enzymes. In fact, I am surprised it does not occur more commonly and likely partially explains why post-transplant ERCP and cannulation of the bile duct seems to be more difficult.

Reference

Endoscopic management of biliary issues in the liver transplant patient. PMID: 30846151.

Question 190

A 62-year-old male presents with elevated liver enzymes 5 months after liver transplant. He received a 27-year-old allograft with 30% steatosis with a duct-to-duct anastomosis. He takes cyclosporine, mycophenolate, and prednisone. His post-transplant course was complicated by bilious drainage output immediately after transplant and he was taken back to the operating room for a washout 1-week post-transplant. He had mental status changes after surgery and required a switch from tacrolimus to cyclosporine. There was an episode of acute rejection 2 months after transplant that responded completely to a steroid recycle.

Ultrasound-patent vessels, normal arterial resistive indices. No masses and mild intra-hepatic biliary dilation.

Laboratory studies:

Tbili 4.2 mg/dL
AST 122 U/L
ALT 181 U/L
GGTP 853 U/L
ALP 522 U/L
FK level
7.9 ng/mL
Creatinine 1.1 mg/dL
ERCP as below:

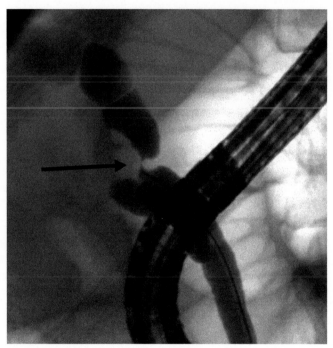

All of the following are risk factors for this condition EXCEPT

A Use of cyclosporine
B Donor steatosis
C Bile leak
D Donor/recipient duct mismatch
E Donation after cardiac death

A is the correct answer.

Commentary – Anastomotic Stricture After Orthotopic Liver Transplant

The bile duct anastomosis remains the Achilles Heel of liver transplant and I have seen the above image on hundreds of patients.

The ERCP image shows a tight stricture (arrowed) at the anastomosis with a dilated donor duct. Biliary strictures can occur in up to 15% of patients following LT. Anastomotic strictures are the most common, accounting for 80% of strictures. These are defined as strictures occurring within 5 mm of the duct-to-duct anastomosis, and they typically occur within the first 6–12 months following LT. Risk factors for anastomotic strictures are numerous and include those attributable to the donor and/or to surgical technique.

Donor Risk Factors Include

1. Advanced age
2. High BMI
3. Donation after cardiac death
4. Prolonged cold ischemia time
5. Macrovascular steatosis >25% in the graft

Surgical Risk Factors Include

1. Surgical technique
2. Disruption of the bile duct blood supply via excessive dissection or use of cautery
3. Size mismatch between the donor and recipient.

In the very early post-transplant period (<1 month), technical issues related to surgical technique predominate, while later, anastomotic strictures occur related to relative ischemia at the site of anastomosis. There are currently few data to suggest that one particular method of duct-to-duct anastomosis is beneficial over another (e.g. end-to-end versus end-to-side or side-to-side). Furthermore, the available data suggests equivalent outcomes when utilizing continuous versus interrupted suturing technique, although a bile leak at the anastomosis predisposes to a stricture. The choice of immunosuppression is not associated with anastomotic strictures.

Treatment is with dilation and stenting (plastic or metal) and is very effective in experienced hands (>90%) such that radiologic or surgical intervention is rarely required.

Reference

Endoscopic management of biliary issues in the liver transplant patient. PMID: 30846151.

Questions 191–200: Immunology Questions

▶ Question 191

Components of the natural (innate) immune system include all the following EXCEPT?

A Macrophages
B T cells
C Natural killer cells
D Neutrophils
E Mast cells

▶ Question 192

Which statement about adaptive immunity is TRUE?

A B cells recognize antigens bound to major histocompatibility complex (MHC) proteins
B T cells have immunoglobulin receptors
C The natural and adaptive immune systems act independently
D Adaptive immunity has a specificity and memory effect
E CD4+ cells recognize MHC class I

▶ Question 193

T cell activation and its effects involve:

A Signals 1, 2, and 3
B Interleukin 4 and 8 induced clonal expansion of activated T cells
C Induction of CD8-positive T-cell mediated toxicity
D Induction of CD4-positive T cell antibody production
E Natural killer cell induction of delayed type hypersensitivity

▶ Question 194

Regarding the major histocompatibility complex (MHC):

A It is located on the long arm of chromosome 6
B Most somatic cells express MHC class I
C Antigen presenting cells include dendritic cells, macrophages, and monocytes
D MHC class I and II molecules have variable beta-pleated and polymorphic alpha-helical regions
E An epitope is part of the T cell that binds to antigen

▶ **Question 195**

MHC class I molecules:

A Have a MHC-encoded alpha chain and non-MHC encoded beta chain (beta-2 microglobulin)
B The alpha chain has 4 domains (a1–a4)
C The a3 and a4 domains interact with peptide antigen
D Present antigen to CD4 positive T cells
E Are expressed on almost all cells in the blood stream including white cells, platelets, and red cells

▶ **Question 196**

MHC class II molecules:

A Are expressed on the surface of T cells
B Are expressed on the surface of neutrophils
C Expression is downregulated by exposure to interferon gamma
D Expression is upregulated by exposure to interleukin-2
E MHC class II/peptide complex presents to CD8-positive T cells

▶ **Question 197**

T cell activation and allorecognition pathways involve all of the following EXCEPT:

A A direct pathway where host T cells recognize allo-MHC molecules on the surface of donor cells
B An indirect pathway where host T cells recognize alloantigen presented by host antigen presenting cells
C The indirect pathway is the major pathway of acute rejection
D Two separate signals are required for T cell activation

▶ **Question 198**

The following are true regarding T helper cells and cytokines EXCEPT:

A Type I helper T (Th1) cells produce IL-2, IFN-gamma and induce macrophages and are associated with delayed type hypersensitivity
B Type II helper T (Th2) cells produced IL-4, IL-5, IL-10, IL-13
C Acute rejection is associated with a Th1 immune response
D IL-4 is a growth factor for B cells
E Allograft tolerance is associated with a switch from Th2 to Th1 cytokine expression

▶ Question 199

T cell activation leads to:

A Membrane bound phosphatidylinositol 4,5-biphosphate (PIP) being hydrolyzed to inositol triphosphate (IP3) and diacylglycerol (DAG)

B IP3 causes increased calcium uptake in the endoplasmic reticulum

C Calcineurin phosphorylates cytoplasmic nuclear factor of activate T cells (NFAT) that then can be translocated to the nucleus and inhibit IL-2 production

D Cyclosporine binds to cyclophilin and tacrolimus binds to the FK506 binding protein (FKBP) leading to upregulation of calcineurin phosphatase activity

E NFkB is activated by several cytokines including TNF and IL-1 leading to transcription of multiple immune modulators- an effect that is inhibited by mycophenolate

▶ Question 200

Mechanisms involved in allograft rejection include:

A CD8 positive T cell-mediated cytotoxicity leading to chronic rejection

B Expression of Il-6, TNF-alpha, TGF-beta, platelet derived growth factor and endothelin is associated with chronic rejection

C CD4 positive T cells initiate B-cell mediated delayed type hypersensitivity

D Activated macrophages cause apoptosis and cell lysis

191 – B is the correct answer.
192 – D is the correct answer.
193 – C is the correct answer.
194 – C is the correct answer.
195 – A is the correct answer.
196 – D is the correct answer.
197 – C is the correct answer.
198 – E is the correct answer.
199 – A is the correct answer.
200 – B is the correct answer.

Questions 191–200

Commentary – Transplant Immunology

This is a huge topic, and a rudimentary understanding is critical, even for us non-immunologist physicians so far removed from medical school that knowing the difference between a T cell and B cell is an achievement.

I will try to stick to the basics but there are plenty of them. You can also refer to the diagrams my co-author put together to add some clarity.

There are two components in the immune system – natural (innate) (a nonspecific response) and adaptive (response to a specific antigen), which act together. For transplant immunology, you need to understand the adaptive system as this is where immunosuppressive drugs act.

Natural Immunity

1. Does NOT recognize specific antigens but rather is nonspecific, involving macrophages, neutrophils, natural killer (NK) cells, multiple cytokines, and complement.

Adaptive Immunity

1. Recognizes a SPECIFIC antigen (on the donor) and is mediated by T and B lymphocytes, and has MEMORY.
2. T cells recognize antigen bound to the major histocompatibility complex (MHC) proteins – this is the initiating event of the adaptive response so remember that rejection (and therefore the action of immunosuppressive drugs) is a T cell phenomenon.
3. B cells are involved in antibody production and have immunoglobulin receptors.
4. Activation of T cells involves two signals where the T cell and antigen interact:
   a. SIGNAL 1 where the T cell receptor (TCR) interacts with antigen on the antigen-presenting cell (APC).
   b. SIGNAL 2 where there is a costimulatory receptor/ligand interaction on the surface of the T cell and APC.
5. Activated T cells potentiate CD-8-positive T cell cytotoxicity, B-cell mediated antibody production and macrophage mediated delayed type hypersensitivity (DTH). Interleukin-2 is an important cytokine in this process.

6. MHC is on the short arm of chromosome 6.
7. MHC proteins are expressed on many cells and are critical in graft rejection as they are the conduit for T cells to recognize antigen (since it is bound to MHC on cell surfaces) rather than free floating foreign proteins, as T cells do not recognize antigen unless it is bound to MHC.
8. MHC has two types – class I and II
9. MHC class I and II have a conserved beta-pleated sheet and two variable (polymorphic) alpha-helical regions that provide the platform for the antigen to sit in.
10. An epitope is a defined amino acid sequence on the antigen (not the T cell).
11. Class I MHC molecules:
    a. Have an MHC encoded alpha chain with 3 domains (a1-3).
    b. Have a non-MHC encoded beta chain (known as beta-2 microglobulin).
    c. The a1 and a2 domains interact with antigen.
    d. Present antigen to CD8-positive T cells leading to cell destruction
    e. Are expressed on most cells except red blood cells.
12. Class II molecules:
    a. Present antigen to CD-4 positive T cells.
    b. Only expressed on dendritic cells, macrophages, and B cells.
    c. IL-2 and interferon gamma (IFN-g) UPREGULATE MHC II expression.

Still with me ?!?!?!?!?!

To reiterate, T cell function is the most important part of rejection, or specifically T cells recognizing foreign (or allo-) antigen. As opposed to the two types of SIGNAL for T cell activation, there are also two PATHWAYS for T cells to recognize alloantigens – DIRECT and INDIRECT.

Direct Pathway

1. T cells recognize allo-MHC on donor cells.
2. This will be important early after transplant as the implantation of the donor graft provides the stimulation for a huge number of T cells and is the mechanism behind acute rejection.

Indirect Pathway

1. T cells recognize alloantigen processed on host-APCs.
2. This is the typical way the immune system works – host-APCs present foreign antigen to T cells.

As Mentioned, There Are Two Types of SIGNAL that Activate T Cells

1. SIGNAL 1 – where the T cell receptor (TCR) interacts with antigen on the antigen-presenting cell (APC).
2. SIGNAL 2 – where there is a costimulatory receptor/ligand interaction on the surface of the T cell and APC.

There are multiple co-stimulatory pathways involving different types of T cells and various cytokines that stimulate and inhibit the signals. This interaction between T cells and the APC is being targeted for new drugs such as belatacept that inhibits the binding in signal 2 (specifically CD28 and B7 ligand interaction) and therefore inhibit T cell function. I doubt this would be asked on the transplant boards.

However, knowing the difference between different types of T cells is important.

T helper cells have two main types: type 1 (Th1) and type 2 (Th2).

Th1 Functions

1. Responsible for acute rejection
2. Produce IL2 and IFN-gamma
3. Induce macrophages, leading to DTH response

Th2 Functions

1. Allograft tolerance involves a switch from Th1 to Th2 cytokine expression
2. Produce IL4, IL5, IL10, IL13
3. Involved in B cell function

After T cells are activated, several enzymatic pathways in the cytoplasm lead to activation of mRNA transcription.

1. Hydrolysis of membrane-bound phosphatidylinositol 4,5-bisphosphate (PIP) to inositol triphosphate (IP3) and diacylglycerol (DAG).
2. IP3 causes release and increase in intracellular calcium.
3. High calcium promotes the formation of calcium--calmodulin complexes that activate several different kinases including the phosphatase calcineurin.
4. Calcineurin dephosphorylates cytoplasmic nuclear factor of activated T cells (NFAT).
5. NFAT is translocated to the nucleus where it binds to the IL-2 promoter sequence and then stimulates transcription of IL-2 mRNA.
6. Tacrolimus and cyclosporine are calcineurin inhibitors but bind to different proteins to form complexes that inhibit the phosphatase activity of calcineurin.
7. Tacrolimus binds to the FK506 binding protein (FKBP).
8. Cyclosporine binds cyclophilin.
9. Sirolimus and everolimus bind to FKBP but work by blocking a p70/S6 kinase that is involved in transducing the IL-2 receptor signal.
10. Nuclear factor kB (NFkB) is activated by several different signals including TNF, IL-1 and lipopolysaccharide (LPS), leading to upregulation of MHC class I, immunoglobulin and IL-2.
11. This pathway is disrupted by corticosteroids.
12. The Janus kinase-signal transducer and activator of transcription (JAK-STAT) pathway is involved in transducing signals provided by interferons and many other cytokines. This works through tyrosine kinase activity providing a target for immunosuppressive drugs.

Allograft Rejection

This involves the mechanisms described above with multiple positive and negative feedback loops. It is very complicated and leads to those amazing cartoon diagrams beloved by immunologists. Important points to remember:

1. There are specific and nonspecific responses.
2. CD4-positive T cells initiate macrophage-mediated DTH.

3. CD4-positive T cells provide help to B cells for alloantibody production.
4. CD8-positive T cells mediate cell-mediated cytotoxicity reactions that lead to cell death and apoptosis.
5. CD8-positive cell-mediated cytotoxicity leads to acute rejection.
6. Chronic rejection is more complicated with upregulation of multiple different T cells and multiple cytokines including IL2, IFNg, IL6, TNF-alpha, nitric oxide synthase, interferon-inducible protein-10 (IP-10, monocyte chemoattractant protein-1 (MCP-1), transforming growth factor (TGF)-beta, platelet-derived growth factor, and endothelin.

Notes

Although immunology seems daunting read through this a few times and at least pick up some of the basics. Rest assured, this will be tested on the boards.

Question 201

Regarding calcineurin inhibitors (CNIs) pharmacokinetics:

A   Tacrolimus absorption is dependent upon bile salts
B   Cyclosporine and tacrolimus do not appear in breast milk
C   CNIs are renally excreted
D   CNIs have high oral bioavailability
E   Tacrolimus half-life is approximately 12 hours

E is the correct answer.

Commentary – CNI Pharmacokinetics

This is important for practical and board reasons.

Cyclosporine and Tacrolimus

1. The absorption and metabolism of CNIs may vary with race and ethnicity.
2. Are absorbed in the small intestine, and peak blood concentrations occur after 1–8 hours and have limited oral bioavailability.
3. Are lipophilic and undergo extensive body distribution.
4. Cross the placenta and appear in breast milk.
5. Are extensively metabolized by cytochrome P-450 CYP3A enzymes in the liver.
6. Are excreted in bile. The elimination half-life varies but is approximately 19 hours for cyclosporine and 12 hours for tacrolimus.
7. Grapefruit contains furanocoumarins that are potent inhibitors of cytochrome P-450 3A4 so can lead to an increase in cyclosporine or tacrolimus levels.

Cyclosporine

1. Has an oral, intravenous, and eye-drop formulation.
2. Nonmodified oral cyclosporine depends upon bile for absorption and has erratic gastrointestinal absorption patterns.
3. Modified cyclosporine is a microemulsion formulation that does not depend upon bile salts for absorption. There is no IV formulation.
4. Should be given at the same time of the day (at 12-hour intervals) and with meals.
5. The absorption of cyclosporine is dependent upon bile salts.
6. Both cyclosporine solutions may adhere to plastic.

Tacrolimus

1. Has an oral, intravenous, and topical formulation.
2. Tacrolimus immediate-release should be given at the same time of the day (at 12-hour intervals) on an empty stomach.

> **Notes**
>
> This is a no-brainer – everyone I have asked after the exam says this came up. Simple stuff to know and remember.

References

https://www.accessdata.fda.gov/drugsatfda_docs/label/2012/050709s031lbl.pdf
https://www.drugs.com/monograph/cyclosporine-systemic.html

Question 202

A 49-year-old female presents with jaundice. She is originally from India and was diagnosed with lymphoma 8 months ago. She has been treated with chemotherapy with good response. She has hypertension controlled on medication and she takes several herbal supplements and drinks 3–4 cups of green tea daily.

Physical examination shows normal vitals, scleral icterus, and a soft, non-tender abdomen

Laboratory studies:

Normal CBC and renal function
ALT 732 U/L
AST 688 U/L
ALP 103 U/L
Tbili 9.8 mg/dL
Anti-HBc IgM positive
AFP 4 ng/mL
US abdomen reveals normal liver contour, mild heterogeneity, normal spleen

▶ Question

Which of the following confers the highest risk of this illness?

A HBsAg negative and taking green tea
B HBsAg positive and received cytotoxic chemotherapy and low dose corticosteroids
C HBsAg negative and received high dose corticosteroids alone
D HBsAg positive and received methotrexate
E HBsAg positive and received rituximab

E is the correct answer.

Commentary – Reactivation of HBV After Chemotherapy

There is another similar question on this topic elsewhere in this book, but it deserves even more attention as it occurs more commonly than it should, and I can almost guarantee there will be a question on the boards.

Reactivation of HBV is a potentially devastating illness so all patients undergoing immunosuppressive therapy should undergo screening for HBV using hepatitis B surface antigen (HBsAg) and HBV core antibody (anti-HBc).

Patients with positive serology for HBV are at risk of reactivation but the risk is increased if the HBsAg is positive (as opposed to just anti-HBc positive) and also depends on the type of immunosuppression, with anti-CD20 therapy conferring a particularly high risk. Once reactivation has occurred (positive HBV DNA) patients should be treated with entecavir or tenofovir as in this case.

The main issue is who should receive prophylactic therapy to prevent reactivation. This is described in the table below. In general, moderate to very high-risk patients should get prophylaxis (so this includes all HBsAg patients) and low or very low risk should be monitored. This is being updated frequently as newer chemotherapy and biological agents are approved.

Drug	HBsAg positive	Anti-HBc positive
Rituximab (or other anti-CD20)	Very high	Moderate
Any regimen with high dose glucocorticoids	High	Low
Cytotoxic chemotherapy	Moderate	Very low
Anti-TNF	Moderate	Very low
Anti-rejection	Moderate	Low (uncertain)
Bone marrow transplant	Very high	Moderate

Notes

You must know this table for clinical practice and I would give even money that this comes up on the boards at least every other year.

Reference

Update on prevention, diagnosis, and treatment of chronic hepatitis B: AASLD 2018 hepatitis B guidance. PMID: 29405329.

Question 203

A 65-year-old male presents with several weeks of vague abdominal pain, dark urine and pruritis. He underwent liver transplant 10 years ago for alcohol related liver disease. He has been taking cyclosporine regularly. His liver and renal function were normal last year.

Laboratory studies:

Tbili 1.8 mg/dL
AST 65 U/L
ALT 93 U/L
ALP 316 U/L
GGT 229 U/L
Ultrasound shows mild ductal dilation. Hepatic artery is patent.
ERCP is performed:

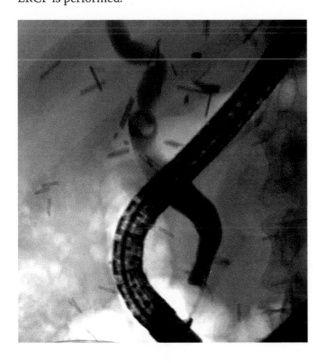

This condition is most likely related to?

A Use of cyclosporine
B Anastomotic stricture
C Bile leak
D Donor BMI
E Prior acute rejection

B is the correct answer.

Commentary – Stone Disease After Orthotopic Liver Transplant

No gallbladder and yet gallstones develop! Magic? Not exactly. I see this quite commonly after transplant and the management can be a bit tricky if there is a stricture as well.

The ERCP image shows a filling defect (likely a gallstone) in the recipient duct just below the duct-to-duct anastomosis. Most gallstones after transplant occur in the setting of strictures. Here the anastomosis was narrow. Type of immunosuppression, leaks, donor BMI, and rejection are not related to stone disease. Remember, this is also likely related to lithogenic bile in the donor and maybe associated with metabolic syndrome in the recipient.

The type of stone can be informative. Cholesterol (yellow) stones are the typical stones seen in the "female, fair, fat, fertile, forty-something" non-transplant patient. Transplant patients can get bile pigment (black) stones or biliary casts if there is ischemic injury (literally sloughing off of the biliary epithelium).

Reference

Endoscopic management of biliary issues in the liver transplant patient. PMID: 30846151.

Question 204

A 44-year-old male underwent a liver transplant 3 weeks ago for acute liver failure. He initially did well but presented with several days of low-grade fever, nausea and abdominal pain. The donor liver was from a 27-year-old female with a BMI of 42 kg/m^2 who died of a drug overdose. The cold ischemia time was 4 hours, and the organ was recovered after cardiac/circulatory death. The left lateral segment was used for an infant.

On exam his temperature is 38.5 °C, HR 108/min, BP 110/60

His abdomen is soft with some upper abdominal tenderness

Laboratory studies:

Tbili 1.1 mg/dL
AST 37 U/L
ALT 43 U/L
ALP 87 U/L
Ultrasound shows no ductal dilation, normal liver parenchyma, patent hepatic artery and some perihepatic fluid collections.
Blood cultures are taken, and he is started on antibiotics and undergoes percutaneous drainage of one of the collections.
ERCP is performed the following day:

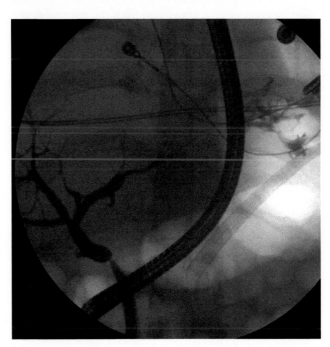

The most likely explanation for this presentation is?

A Donation after cardiac/circulatory death
B High donor BMI
C Donor cause of death
D Split liver allograft
E Acute liver failure

D is the correct answer.

Commentary – Bile Leak Using Split Liver Allograft

The ERCP image shows extravasation of contrast in the right upper corner that corresponds to the area where the left lateral segment would be. This is a surface leak from a small biliary radicle due to the left lateral segment being removed for transplant for the infant.

The duct-to-duct anastomosis looks a little narrow and may have precipitated the leak by increasing the pressure in the intrahepatic bile ducts, explaining the presentation 2–3 weeks after transplant. Placing a stent across the anastomosis should fix the leak.

Bile leaks occur after transplant from the duct-to-duct anastomosis, cystic duct and anywhere there is a cut surface as in this case or in live donor transplant.

The other choices are not associated with bile leaks after transplant.

Reference

Endoscopic management of biliary issues in the liver transplant patient. PMID: 30846151.

Question 205

A 33-year-old male has been in the hospital for 1 week with intermittent fevers to 39 °C, cough, shortness of breath, bloody diarrhea, headache, and oliguria. He underwent a liver transplant 5 years ago for acute liver failure and was doing well prior to admission with normal liver biochemistry and blood count on a stable dose of tacrolimus.

Work up shows negative blood cultures, patent vessels on abdominal ultrasound, and negative CT chest except for minimal pleural effusions and CT abdomen showing a 22 cm spleen. He is treated with antibiotics and undergoes EGD/colonoscopy with negative biopsies and negative CMV serology.

Laboratory studies:

WBC 2.7
Hemoglobin 7.7 g/dL
Platelets 83
Tbili 0.6 mg/dL
AST 37 U/L
ALT 63 U/L
ALP 57 U/L
Creatinine 2.7 mg/dL
Tacrolimus level 2.3 ng/mL
Ferritin 3092 ng/mL (normal 30–400 ng/mL)
Human Herpesvirus 6 DNA 29,400 copies/mL
Human Herpesvirus 8 quant PCR 6,600,000 copies/mL
Soluble IL-2 receptor 32,500 pg/mL (normal <1000)

▶ Question

What is the best management option?

A Treat with ganciclovir
B Increase the tacrolimus dose
C Initiate plasmapheresis
D Perform splenectomy
E Perform bone marrow biopsy and start dexamethasone

E is the correct answer.

Commentary – Hemophagocytic Lymphohistiocytosis (<u>HLH</u>)

This young man has unfortunately developed HLH, likely driven by HHV6 and HHV8 infection due to immunosuppression. HLH is a rare disease of excessive immune activation and can be seen in those with a genetic predisposition and sporadically. It has a poor prognosis. The pathogenesis is thought to be related to over-activated macrophages with failure of NK cells and cytotoxic lymphocytes to eliminate these macrophages leading to elevated levels of circulating cytokines and a cytokine storm. The macrophages ingest red cells (hemophagocytosis). Unfortunately, we have seen several cases in transplant recipients over the years and typically it takes a while to make the diagnosis and the outcome is fatal.

There are several diagnostic criteria including high fever (temperature >38.5°C, splenomegaly, pancytopenia, hemophagocytosis (on smear or bone marrow biopsy), high ferritin, elevated soluble CD25 (IL2 receptor).

There are several potential emerging therapies including dexamethasone, etoposide, and several chemotherapy and immunomodulatory agents.

The diagnosis is usually delayed but fever, splenomegaly, high ferritin, pancytopenia with negative typical infectious work up should raise the alarm for HLH (either pre- or post-transplant).

Reference

Challenges in the diagnosis of HLH: recommendations from the North American Consortium for histiocytosis (NACHO). PMID: 31339233.

Question 206

A 47-year-old male with HIV and HCV-related cirrhosis with a 3 cm HCC is listed for liver transplantation. His HCV was successfully treated, MELD score is 12 with a platelet count of 55. His 42-year-old partner with well-controlled HIV wants to be considered as a potential live donor.

Which of the following statements is TRUE?

A The partner CANNOT be considered as a live donor due to HIV infection

B The partner CAN be considered as a live donor as long as the CD4 count is >200 with a negative HIV viral load for the last 6 months

C The patient is NOT eligible for an HIV-positive, HCV-positive deceased donor allograft

D Live donor transplant in this situation CAN only be performed under a research protocol in a designated center

E The patient is NOT a candidate for transplant unless the HIV viral load is undetectable and CD4 count is >500

D is the correct answer.

Commentary – Liver Transplantation in <u>HIV</u> and the <u>HOPE</u> Act

The HIV Organ Policy Equity (HOPE) Act was passed by the US Congress in 2013 permitting the use of HIV positive organs in HIV positive recipients under a research protocol. Previously the use of these organs was prohibited.

Participation in HIV positive to HIV positive transplant is only permitted if criteria are met in the six categories below:

1. Recipient – has CD4>100 and negative HIV viral load (or in patients intolerant of HIV medications due to severe liver disease, previously documented response).
2. Donor – No opportunistic infection and pre-implantation biopsy. Live donors need to have negative viral load and CD4>500 for at least 6 months. Deceased donors have to have HIV that can be treated with anti-retroviral treatment.
3. Transplant hospital
4. Organ procurement organization (OPO)
5. Protocol to prevent inadvertent transmission of HIV
6. Research – approved study design and outcome measures

In the current case, even though the recipient is HCV negative, he would still be a candidate for an HIV and HCV positive organ as the HCV could be treated after transplant.

Reference

Advancing organ transplantation through HIV-to-HIV transplantation. PMID: 34224501.

Question 207

When using an allograft from a "donation after cardiac/circulatory death (DCD)" for liver transplantation the following outcomes would be expected:

A Less than 70% 3 year graft survival, 20% ischemic cholangiopathy
B Greater than 70% 3 year graft survival, 50% ischemic cholangiopathy
C Less than 70% 3 year graft survival, 50% ischemic cholangiopathy
D Greater than 70% 3 year graft survival, 20% ischemic cholangiopathy
E Greater than 70% 3 year graft survival, 5% ischemic cholangiopathy

E is the correct answer.

Commentary – DCD Organs

With the shortage of deceased donor organs for transplantation, extended criteria donors (ECD) increase the pool of available organs. A DCD organ is not procured until cardiac death is declared in a controlled setting after withdrawal of care. In general, this adds only a few minutes to the time when the organs are recovered compared to conventional procurement after brain death. This increased ischemia time can lead to complications but recent studies using different techniques of hypothermic oxygenated machine perfusion have minimized the main risk – that of ischemic cholangiopathy – to around 5%.

Graft survival should be at least 70% at 3 years. Other factors that used to be considered important for the quality of a DCD organ seem to be less important now. Older donor age and degree of donor steatosis may increase the risk of complications with a DCD organ but is unlikely to be tested in a board exam, as it is controversial. Recent studies suggest older DCD organs and organs with macrosteatosis <30% have comparable outcomes to younger and non-steatotic DCD organs.

Reference

Perioperative and long-term outcomes of utilizing donation after circulatory death liver grafts with macrosteatosis: a multicenter analysis. PMID: 32216008.

Question 208

A 25-year-old male presents to the office with several days of right upper quadrant pain, dark urine, and pruritis. He donated the right lobe of his liver to his 57-year-old father who had cirrhosis and liver cancer, 2 months ago. CT scan shows an enlarged left lobe with mild ductal dilation.

Laboratory studies:

Tbili 3.7 mg/dL
AST 58 U/L
ALT 77 U/L
ALP 464 U/L
INR 1.1
Appropriate imaging is shown below:

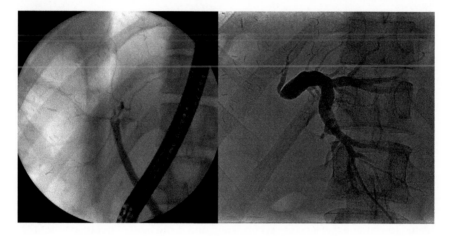

▶ Question

Which statement regarding donor hepatectomy for liver transplantation is TRUE?

A The risk of donor mortality is 0.2–0.4%
B The risk of Clavien grade 1 or 2 complications is 80%
C The risk of Clavien grade 3 or higher complications is 10%
D The complication in this case is Clavien grade 2
E The risk of donor complications decreases with center experience

A is the correct answer.

Commentary – Complications After Donor Hepatectomy

This patient has developed a biliary stricture after right lobe donation. At ERCP (the first image), I could fill the extrahepatic duct but there is essentially non-filling of the intra-hepatics. Percutaneous cholangiogram (the second image) shows a dilated left system but non-filling of the extrahepatic duct. This was due to resection of the right common hepatic duct very close to the bifurcation and slight rotation of the liver during liver regeneration (that typically only takes 1–2 months to get back to >90% of original liver volume) such that the take-off of the left common hepatic duct became stenotic. This required surgery to correct (Roux-en-Y hepaticojejunostomy).

Complications after right lobe hepatectomy for donation can be classified using the Clavien system:

Grade	Definition
I	Any deviation from normal care WITHOUT need for pharmacologic/surgical/endoscopic/radiologic intervention
II	Requiring pharmacologic treatment (except anti-emetics, anti-pyretics) or blood products or parenteral nutrition
IIIA	Requiring pharmacologic/surgical/endoscopic/radiologic intervention WITHOUT general anesthesia
IIIB	Requiring pharmacologic/surgical/endoscopic/radiologic intervention WITH general anesthesia
IVA	Life-threatening requiring ICU, single organ dysfunction
IVB	Life-threatening requiring ICU, multi-organ dysfunction
V	Death

The risk of mortality after right lobe liver donation is 0.2–0.4% (lower for left lobe) and is NOT related to center experience so is consistent and is the figure I quote to potential liver donors. Minor (grade I-II) complications occur in 40% of patients but grade III or more are uncommon (<5%). Hernias and psychological complications can also occur in the long term.

Reference

Complications of living donor hepatic lobectomy – a comprehensive report. PMID: 22335782.

Question 209

A 27-year-old female is 2 years post simultaneous liver and kidney transplant for autoimmune hepatitis. She is doing well and is maintained on tacrolimus 2 mg bid, mycophenolate 500 mg bid, and prednisone 5 mg daily. She has normal liver biochemical tests and renal function. She has recently married and wants to start a family.

What should be the approach to her management?

A She should be advised to adopt a child as pregnancy is unsafe in liver transplant recipients

B The tacrolimus should be replaced by sirolimus

C The mycophenolate should be replaced by azathioprine

D The prednisone dose should be increased as rejection is a risk during pregnancy

E The tacrolimus should be replaced by cyclosporine

C is the correct answer.

Commentary – Mycophenolate and Pregnancy

This is not an uncommon real life clinical scenario and a frequently tested topic on board exams. Knowing which immunosuppressive drugs are safe in pregnancy is important.

Pregnancy is not contra-indicated after liver transplantation and is not associated with an increased risk of rejection. Mycophenolate is category D (associated with increased risk of first trimester loss and congenital malformations) for pregnancy and females of child-bearing age should be counseled on the risks. The drug should be stopped ideally 6 months prior to pregnancy and for the duration. Tacrolimus, cyclosporine, prednisone, azathioprine, and sirolimus can all be used during pregnancy.

In this case, the mycophenolate could be replaced by azathioprine or perhaps stopped and increase the tacrolimus dose depending on liver and renal function.

Clinical Pearls: Pregnancy and LT

1. Pregnancy is not contra-indicated after transplant
2. Mycophenolate is category D in pregnancy- Stop 6 months before pregnancy and for the duration
3. All other immunosuppression drugs are safe

Question 210

A 55-year-old male underwent a simultaneous liver-kidney transplant for HBV-related cirrhosis and HCC six months ago. He was treated with locoregional therapy prior to transplant with normalization of AFP (his AFP had peaked at 800 ng/mL pre transplant). Explant showed multiple treated lesions with microvascular invasion. His post-course has been notable for renal dysfunction with a kidney biopsy 2 months ago showing acute rejection.

He feels well without fever, cough, shortness of breath, abdominal pain, and has not lost weight.

Medications include tacrolimus, mycophenolate, prednisone, and tenofovir. He was CMV donor positive, recipient negative, and is on valganciclovir.

Laboratory studies:

WBC 2.7 (Absolute neutrophil count 0.8)
Hemoglobin 8.9 g/dL
Platelets 124
Tbili 0.5 mg/dL
ALT 28 U/L
ALP 68 U/L
Creatinine 2.4 mg/dL
AFP 2.4 ng/mL
Tacrolimus level 7.3 ng/mL
HBV DNA negative
Routine surveillance CT scan of the chest is shown below:

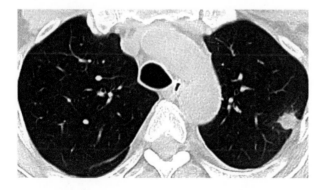

▶ Question

The most likely diagnosis is:

A Metastatic HCC
B *Pneumocystis jirovecii* infection
C Candida albicans infection
D CMV pneumonitis
E *Aspergillus fumigatus*

E is the correct answer.

Commentary – Fungal/Aspergillus Infection After Transplant

This patient has a new lesion in the left lung seen on CT (the circular white lesion on the extreme right of the image) but is asymptomatic. Metastatic HCC would be a consideration, but his AFP is normal and was elevated prior to transplant.

The neutropenia and timing (within the first 6 months after transplant) make fungal infection high on the differential. In addition, his immunosuppression would have been increased recently due to renal rejection, including steroids, increasing the risk of fungal infection even further. Pneumocystis is a common infection in the first 6 months after transplant but typically causes respiratory symptoms without imaging findings. Interestingly, concomitant CMV is associated with pneumocystis. Candida is a common infection after transplant but a rare cause of invasive pulmonary disease. CMV pneumonitis typically presents with bilateral disease affecting the lower lobes. Aspergillus can present as a solitary nodule and can result from primary infection or reactivation of a patient previously colonized. Symptoms can be minimal but invasive disease can occur with necrotizing bronchopneumonia with vascular involvement leading to hemoptysis as well as extra-pulmonary spread.

Other pulmonary infections to consider after transplant include tuberculosis, cryptococcal disease, strongyloides, mucormycosis, and multiple bacteria.

This patient underwent a biopsy that confirmed the diagnosis and was treated with isavuconazole.

Reference

Infection in solid-organ transplant recipients. PMID: 18094380.

Question 211

A 61-year-old male underwent a liver transplant for alcoholic liver disease 3 days ago. He received a 33 year-old allograft from a brain death donor with a BMI of 27 kg/m² and cold ischemia time of 4 hours and warm ischemia time of 33 minutes. Postoperative day 1 ultrasound showed patent vessels. His drain output is bile tinged. Medications include tacrolimus, mycophenolate, and prednisone.

Vital signs T 100.5°F

Laboratory studies:

WBC 13.1
Hemoglobin 7.8 g/dL
Platelets 101
Tbili 3.7 mg/dL (previously 1.8 mg/dL)
ALT 478 U/L (previously 89 U/L)
AST 423 U/L (previously 91 U/L)
ALP 212 U/L (previously 137 U/L)
Creatinine 1.9 mg/dL
Tacrolimus level 5.3 ng/mL

▶ Question

The next step in management should be:

A Increase the tacrolimus dose
B Blood cultures and start antibiotics
C MRI/MRCP
D Doppler ultrasound
E Non-contrast CT scan

D is the correct answer.

Commentary – Hepatic Artery Thrombosis (<u>HAT</u>)

This patient has developed fever, bile-tinged drainage, and a sudden elevation of LFTs early after transplant. Despite the normal ultrasound on day 1, HAT has to be a concern and the Doppler ultrasound should be repeated. If HAT is confirmed or suspected, interventional radiology or operative intervention should be attempted.

In general, early HAT (within 2 weeks) is an indication for relisting as the allograft will not survive long, even if arterial flow is restored and the patient can be listed as status I.

Risk factors for HAT have not been well described except that the incidence of 15–20% in pediatric transplants (compared to 2–5% in adult transplants) suggests smaller vessels, split procedures, and a higher hematocrit are likely important. Other graft characteristics do not appear to be associated with HAT.

For board purposes, a sudden rise in ALT, AST very early after transplant will be HAT.

Reference

Perioperative thrombotic complications in liver transplantation. PMID: 26185371.

Question 212

Which of the following statements regarding sirolimus are TRUE?

A It is approved for use after liver transplantation in the United States

B It binds to sirolimus-binding protein in a similar manner that tacrolimus does to FK-binding protein

C It blocks the transduction signal from the IL-2 receptor, inhibiting T- and B-cell proliferation

D It has renal-protection effects compared to tacrolimus even when given several years after transplant

E Sirolimus monotherapy is recommended after liver transplant in patients with hepatocellular carcinoma

C is the correct answer.

Sirolimus and everolimus are inhibitors of mammalian (mechanistic) target of rapamycin (MTOR). In the United States, everolimus is approved for use in liver transplant recipients (in combination with tacrolimus) but sirolimus is NOT. In fact, sirolimus has a black box warning and is not recommended in liver (or lung) transplant recipients due to excess mortality, graft loss, and hepatic artery thrombosis.

Despite this, sirolimus is used in the liver transplant community. It binds to FK-binding protein, as it is structurally similar to tacrolimus, but does not inhibit calcineurin. It blocks the transduction signal from the IL-2 receptor.

MTOR inhibitors effects on renal sparing are only really seen early before the damage from CNIs becomes irreversible, so typically while the renal function is somewhat preserved in the first few months after transplant. It also has anti-angiogenic properties and so is advantageous in patients with HCC but this is not proven (so should not be on the boards).

Side effects are an easy board question to ask about and they include:

1. Hepatic artery thrombosis (likely dose related) and occurs early
2. Delayed wound healing
3. Hyperlipidemia
4. Bone marrow suppression (particularly anemia with everolimus)
5. Oral ulcers
6. Acne, skin rashes
7. Proteinuria (so urine tests need to be monitored), edema
8. Pneumonia

Notes

Most of the US centers do not use mTORs but they are commonly used in Europe. They received bad press with HAT with sirolimus but this occurred early and was likely related to the dose that was used. In my experience they work quite well but sirolimus causes skin issues like acne and everolimus is associated with anemia.

Reference

https://www.accessdata.fda.gov/drugsatfda_docs/label/2017/021083s059,021110s076lbl.pdf

Question 213

Which of the following statements regarding the prodrugs of mycophenolic acid (MPA) – mycophenolate mofetil (MMF or Cellcept) and mycophenolate sodium (Myfortic) – are TRUE?

A Myfortic is associated with more GI adverse effects, particularly diarrhea
B MMF should be taken with a high fat meal to improve absorption
C Cellcept colitis has a characteristic endoscopic and pathological pattern
D Side effects such as bone marrow suppression are not dose dependent
E MPA inhibits inosine monophosphate dehydrogenase (IMPDH) leading to selective inhibition of B-cell and T-cell proliferation

E is the correct answer.

Commentary – MPA Effects and Formulations

The MPA prodrugs are orally available (as opposed to MPA itself) and undergo renal excretion after glucuronidation. MPA inhibits IMPDH leading to depletion of intracellular guanosine monophosphate (GMP) which prevents cell replication. Most cells have guanine salvage pathways using hypoxanthine-guanine phosphoribosyltransferase, an enzyme that is lacking in lymphocytes.

Both drugs should be taken on an empty stomach (although some advocate taking MMF with food to minimize GI side effects). Myfortic is enteric-coated and delays release until the small intestine leading to less GI side effects. All of the side effects are dose related so if patients develop neutropenia, dose reduction is reasonable. Cellcept colitis describes a variety of different findings seen on colonoscopy and pathology including colitis, discrete ulcers, and even normal looking mucosa.

The MPA prodrugs do not cause some of the troublesome side effects of CNIs such as renal and neuro-toxicity and so are used to decrease CNI and steroid dose in transplant recipients.

Reference

https://www.accessdata.fda.gov/drugsatfda_docs/label/2009/050722s021,050723s019, 050758s019,050759s024lbl.pdf

Question 214

A 45-year-old man presents to the emergency room with abdominal pain, cough, fever, and shortness of breath. He underwent a liver transplant 1 year earlier for end-stage liver disease secondary to HBV and HCC.

He received a 41-year-old allograft with less than 5% steatosis. Both the recipient and donor were CMV positive. His post-operative course was complicated by respiratory failure requiring tracheostomy. He eventually recovered and has been maintained on tacrolimus, mycophenolate mofetil, and tenofovir. He has been taking green tea extract for several months. Liver biopsy 6 months ago after his liver enzymes were elevated demonstrated 25% mixed macro- and micro-vesicular steatosis. There was no evidence of acute cellular rejection.

On exam he has a low-grade fever, scleral icterus but a soft abdomen.

Ultrasound and MRI/MRCP of the abdomen demonstrated a patent hepatic artery and no evidence of biliary ductal dilation.

Laboratory studies:

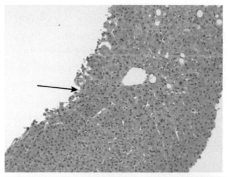
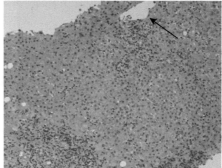

Tbili 17.8 mg/dL
Direct bili 15.1 mg/dL
AST 334 U/L
ALT 357 U/L
ALP 666 U/L
GGT 1252 U/L
Creatinine 1.7 mg/dL
Tacrolimus level 11.7 ng/mL
HBV DNA undetectable
2 months previously his laboratory studies showed normal ALT, AST, bilirubin but ALP of 124 U/L and GGT 389 U/L
A liver biopsy is performed:

▶ Question

The most likely diagnosis is

A Acute rejection
B Chronic ductopenic rejection
C Fibrosing cholestatic hepatitis B
D Drug induced liver injury
E CMV hepatitis

A is the correct answer.

Commentary – Acute Cellular Rejection (ACR)

This patient presents with jaundice and elevated liver enzymes 1 year after transplant. It is reassuring that his imaging shows no biliary obstruction, and his hepatic artery is patent. However, his blood work was essentially normal only a couple of months ago. He has been taking green tea extract which can cause liver injury (typically hepatocellular), his tacrolimus level is a little high and HBV DNA is negative. A liver biopsy is required.

The first image shows marked hepatocytic and canalicular cholestasis (the brownish infiltrate that is arrowed). There is a mixed inflammatory infiltrate in the portal tracts (bottom left of the second image) but also some mild endothelialitis (arrow in second image). Other features that can be seen on high power include bile duct damage and feathery degeneration. The trichrome stain (not shown) demonstrated portal fibrosis with fibrous septa. This is consistent with moderate ACR. Pathological criteria for ACR have been developed and often an RAI (rejection activity index) is given with a score between 1 and 9. In this example, the RAI was 6, consistent with moderate rejection and an indication for treatment.

ACR can occur early after transplant (within 6 weeks) and usually does not adversely affect graft or patient outcomes. However, in this patient, ACR occurred later, and this is often associated with low blood immunosuppression levels and is associated with reduced graft survival. Risk factors for early ACR include lower recipient age, fewer HLA-DR matches, longer cold ischemia time (more than 15 hours), higher donor age (>30 years). Etiology of liver disease may also play a role with lower ACR incidence in viral and alcoholic liver disease, and higher in autoimmune diseases.

The treatment of ACR involves increasing immunosuppression. High dose methyl-prednisolone is usually first line therapy for ACR at a dose of 500–1000 mg given daily for 1–3 days as a bolus. This is effective in 70–80% of cases and can be repeated if necessary. This patient did not improve after two courses of steroids and several options are then available to treat steroid resistant ACR. Drugs that have been used include OKT3 (Muromonab), thymoglobulin, anti-interleukin receptor antibodies, mycophenolate mofetil, sirolimus, and tacrolimus. In this patient, he needed a week of thymoglobulin. Within a month, his liver enzymes and bilirubin almost normalized.

Points to note are that patients who have not been taking their immunosuppression often start taking more when they note jaundice so the level can be high. Fibrosing cholestatic HBV is seen with a very high HBV DNA level. Chronic rejection typically has ductopenia. CMV hepatitis and liver injury from green tea extract do not look like acute rejection on liver biopsy.

Care must be taken in treating patients for ACR since the increased immunosuppression increases susceptibility to infection such as oral candidiasis, cytomegalovirus (CMV), Aspergillus, and *Pneumocystis carinii*. Antimicrobial prophylaxis is usually required.

Notes

Biopsy proven acute rejection is uncommon and this raises the issue that perhaps we are over-immunosuppressing our patients. It used to be thought that a little rejection was not a bad thing but recent studies have suggested that it may not be so benign. Even so, my practice is to keep the immunosuppression on the low side as rejection is easily treated but some of the complications of CNIs are not.

Reference

Acute hepatic allograft rejection: incidence, risk factors, and impact on outcome. PMID: 9731552.

Question 215

A 50-year-old female presents with abnormal liver enzymes. She describes several months of some nonspecific symptoms including fatigue and myalgias but no fever or chills. She has been told she has irritable bowel syndrome with bloating and intermittent diarrhea. Colonoscopy was normal. Her weight is stable. Her past medical history is significant for hypertension controlled on medication. She has also had breast reduction surgery and a hysterectomy.

She denies smoking, alcohol use, intravenous drug use, or cocaine use. She has had no remote blood transfusions.

Her older sister was treated for hepatitis C and has had thyroid problems but there is no other family history.

Exam is unremarkable.

Laboratory studies:

Hb 11.1 g/dL
MCV 73 FL
Tbili 0.8 mg/dL
AST 216 U/L
ALT 401 U/L
ALP 145 U/L
GGT 202 U/L
Albumin 3.7 g/dL
Total protein 8.5 g/dL
Ultrasound abdomen: Normal sized liver but markedly heterogeneous echo pattern. No biliary dilation.
A liver biopsy is performed

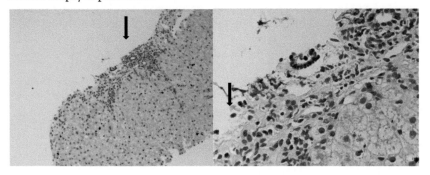

▶ Question

Which statement is TRUE about this condition/patient?

A Interface hepatitis is diagnostic
B Serum IgA and IgM are typically elevated
C ANA is more specific than SMA
D An EGD will be helpful
E Bile ductular reaction is uncommon

D is the correct answer.

Commentary – Autoimmune Hepatitis (AIH)

This patient presents with various symptoms and elevated transaminases. The differential diagnosis includes viral hepatitis (although she has no real risk factors), toxic or drug-induced injury, and autoimmune disease.

The initial work up should include viral hepatitis serology and autoimmune markers including antinuclear antibody (ANA), smooth muscle antibody (SMA), and quantitative immunoglobulins. **SMA is more specific than ANA for AIH.**

AIH is a disease of unknown etiology, much more common in women, with a variable clinical presentation from asymptomatic patients, sometimes debilitating symptoms, and fulminant hepatic failure. Extrahepatic manifestations are common and include hemolytic anemia, idiopathic thrombocytopenic purpura, type 1 diabetes, thyroid disease, celiac disease, and ulcerative colitis.

The incidence of celiac disease is up to 5–10% in some series and the mild microcytic anemia and symptomatology in this case points to that diagnosis so serology and EGD are required.

The liver biopsy findings are **nonspecific** but can confirm the diagnosis. In this case, there is an inflammatory infiltrate in the portal tracts (arrowed) which is made up of lymphocytes and plasma cells (the cells with eccentrically placed nuclei – arrowed in second image). The infiltrate invades the sharply demarcated hepatocyte boundary (limiting plate) surrounding the portal tract and spills into the surrounding lobule (periportal infiltrate) which is termed piecemeal necrosis or interface hepatitis. Bile ductular reaction is very common (in up to 80%). The trichrome stain showed architectural distortion of the hepatic lobule with bridging fibrosis.

The diagnosis of AIH can be difficult and used to be based on a complex scoring system developed by the International Autoimmune Hepatitis Group (IAIHG). This has been simplified for routine clinical practice and involves laboratory studies. Serum IgG is typically elevated, not IgA or IgM. A biopsy is not absolutely essential since a probable diagnosis can be made without histology but a definite diagnosis needs histology. The scoring system is as follows:

Autoantibodies	1 point if the ANA or SMA are 1 : 40
	2 points if the ANA or SMA are ≥1 : 80
IgG	1 point if the IgG is > the upper limit of normal
	2 points if the IgG is >1.10 times the upper limit of normal
Liver histology	1 point if the histological features are compatible with AIH
	2 points if the histological features are typical of AIH
Exclude HCV/HBV	2 points if viral hepatitis has been excluded.

A probable diagnosis of autoimmune hepatitis is made if the total points are 6 while a definite diagnosis is made if the total points are ≥7 (and by definition requires a biopsy).

Reference

Autoimmune hepatitis. PMID: 16394302.

Question 216

The patient in the previous question asks about her management. Which response is TRUE?

A Treatment may be required for several years
B As soon as her LFTs are normal, she can come off medication
C There is a 50% chance she will not respond to treatment
D A repeat liver biopsy will be required prior to withdrawing treatment
E The chance of her needing a liver transplant is less than 1%

A is the correct answer.

Commentary – Treatment of Autoimmune Hepatitis (AIH)

This patient has AIH with symptoms, elevated LFTS, and positive histology findings. In general, treatment is suggested if:

1. ALT >10× ULN
2. IgG >2× ULN if ALT >5× ULN
3. ALT >5× ULN if symptoms, elevated IgG, elevated bilirubin, interface hepatitis on biopsy
4. Bridging necrosis on biopsy
5. Cirrhosis with inflammation

These parameters differ slightly among societies.

AIH is treated with immunosuppression. The American Association for the Study of Liver Disease (AASLD) guidelines suggest:

1. Prednisone in combination with azathioprine or a higher dose of prednisone alone is the appropriate treatment for severe AIH in adults.
2. Prednisone in combination with azathioprine is the preferred initial treatment because of its lower frequency of side effects.
3. All patients treated with prednisone alone or in combination with azathioprine must be monitored for the development of drug-related side effects.

If using azathioprine, thiopurine methyltransferase (TPMT) testing is suggested.

Clinical Pearls: AIH

1. About 65–75% of patients respond by 2 years with normalization of ALT.
2. About 10% do not respond.
3. Withdrawal of treatment can be considered after normal LFTs for 18–24 months.
4. Relapse is common (>50%).
5. Treat again if relapse occurs.
6. Cirrhosis is quite common (at presentation or during follow up) – 20–30%.
7. Ultimately 10–20% need transplant.

Reference

Diagnosis and management of AIH in adults and children: 2019 practice guidelines from the American Association for the Study of Liver Diseases. PMID: 31863477.

Question 217

A 57-year-old male presents with ascites requiring intermittent large volume paracentesis.

He had undergone orthotopic liver transplantation 7 years previously for cirrhosis secondary to chronic hepatitis C. His main complications prior to transplant had been related to portal hypertension including ascites and a right pleural effusion. He received a 19-year-old allograft and developed recurrent hepatitis C that was treated successfully in the first year after transplant. His pretreatment liver biopsy showed minimal fibrosis. He is maintained on tacrolimus-based immunosuppression.

He denied tobacco or alcohol use.

Physical exam demonstrated a healthy-looking male with normal vital signs, BMI 24 kg/m², and no scleral icterus.

Abdomen is soft with moderate ascites. There is no edema.

Laboratory studies:

Tbili 0.5 mg/dL
AST 29 U/L
ALT 22 U/L
ALP 98 U/L
Albumin 4.3 g/dL
INR 1.1
Platelets 171,000
Creatinine 1.1 mg/dL
Ascites fluid analysis SAAG >1.1
HCV RNA negative
Imaging – CT scan and ultrasound showed patent vessels and a normal looking allograft

▶ Question

The most likely diagnosis is:

A De novo NASH cirrhosis
B Allograft cirrhosis from chronic rejection
C Recurrent HCV cirrhosis
D Constrictive pericarditis
E Hepatic venous obstruction

E is the correct answer.

Commentary – Stenosis of Hepatic Vein-Inferior Vena Cava Anastomosis

This is one of my favorite cases. A very interesting case that illustrates the importance of being exhaustive in managing patients after transplant if they do not fit into classic diagnoses.

The differential diagnosis is that of ascites but occurring after transplant in a patient who looks and feels otherwise well. The fluid analysis suggests portal hypertension.

He is unlikely to have cirrhosis given the labs, imaging, and his presentation.

The fact that the imaging and Doppler study did not show any vascular issues was reassuring but the ultimate diagnosis showed that these are unreliable to look for hepatic venous obstruction (as others have documented).

Heart failure, pulmonary hypertension, or constrictive pericarditis could lead to ascites but in general, the patient would be sick with hepatomegaly on exam.

The patient went on to have a transjugular study with a liver biopsy. This showed no evidence of rejection, focal centrilobular congestion, and no significant active hepatitis. Only mild portal fibrosis was noted and no evidence of bridging fibrosis. The hepatic venous pressure gradient was normal. The hepatic veins were determined to be patent. On closer discussion with the radiologist however, the right hepatic vein was not seen. We sent him back for another transjugular study and this time they were able to place a catheter into the right hepatic vein. Right hepatic venogram was performed demonstrating a severe stenosis at the venous anastomosis (first image). Pressure measurements were obtained yielding a hepatic venous pressure of 28 mmHg and a pressure above it of 8 mmHg for a gradient of 20 mmHg. A 10 mm balloon was used to dilate the stenosis (second image) and a repeat venogram (third image) was performed demonstrating better flow through the stenosis. Repeat pressure measurements were obtained yielding a gradient of approximately 4 mmHg. A further dilation was performed using a 12 mm balloon. The patient's ascites resolved.

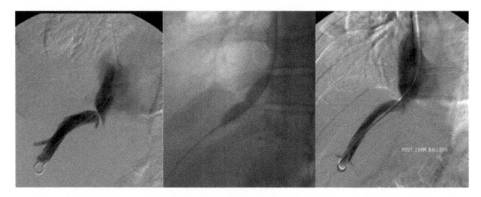

Reference

Outcome of percutaneous transhepatic venoplasty for hepatic venous outflow obstruction after living donor liver transplantation. PMID: 16567488.

Question 218

A 63-year-old female presents with several weeks of nausea, pruritis, weight loss, and jaundice. She has hypertension and diabetes. Medications include metoprolol and insulin.

She underwent total hip replacement 4 months ago and her LFTS were normal at the time.

Examination shows normal vital signs and scleral icterus.

Laboratory studies:

ALT 85 U/L
AST 97 U/L
ALP 578 U/L
Tbili 11.2 mg/dL
INR 1.3
Creatinine 0.5 mg/dL
Ultrasound abdomen – normal liver and biliary tree
HBsAg, anti-Hbc IgM, anti-HAV IgM, anti-HCV all negative
ANA 1 : 40, SMA negative, quantitative immunoglobulins, AMA normal
Anti-HBs positive

▶ Question

Which of the following statements is TRUE?

A Ursodeoxycholic acid will normalize LFTs
B Prednisolone should be started
C A liver biopsy will help to prognosticate
D This is likely DILI from metoprolol
E This is likely AMA-negative primary biliary cholangitis (PBC)

C is the correct answer.

Commentary – DILI causing cholestatic injury with vanishing bile duct syndrome (VBDS)

This patient has a cholestatic liver injury with jaundice. The differential diagnosis is wide but an appropriate work up was performed to exclude the common causes. The clue here is in the history of hip surgery and likely antibiotic use. Viral and autoimmune markers are negative. There is no evidence of biliary disease on imaging and acute cholangitis typically would have more symptomatology. AMA-negative PBC is very uncommon but presents like AMA-positive disease. This patient is very unlikely to have PBC with normal LFTs only 4 months ago.

A liver biopsy is not necessary to make a diagnosis of DILI but characteristic changes can occasionally be seen with certain drugs. In addition, in cases of cholestatic hepatitis, the degree of bile duct loss can prognosticate outcome as it is a harbinger of VBDA that has a poor prognosis without transplant.

Steroids have been used in DILI but there is no good evidence of effectiveness except in cases of drug-induced autoimmune hepatitis.

Metoprolol and beta blockers in general are a very rare cause of DILI.

Many drugs can cause cholestatic hepatitis but typically several antibiotics such as Bactrim, Levaquin, and Augmentin. Augmentin was one of the drugs associated with a VBDS in the DILI Network.

Clinical Pearls: DILI and Cholestasis

1. Cholestatic DILI can lead to bile duct loss
2. Steroids are NOT helpful in cholestatic DILI
3. Antibiotics are a common cause of DILI in general but especially cholestatic

---

Notes

I have been part of the DILI Network in the United States for many years now and most of those we enroll are hospitalized patients with jaundice. Remember that mortality is not insignificant and chronic injury where it persists for more than 6 months occurs in up to 20% of patients.

Reference

Clinical presentations and outcomes of bile duct loss caused by drugs and herbal and dietary supplements. PMID: 27981596.

Question 219

In patients with hepatic amyloidosis

A Hepatomegaly is infrequent
B The degree of hepatomegaly correlates with the amount of amyloid deposition
C It is a common cause of chronic liver disease and portal hypertension
D An elevated ALP is almost universal
E Constitutional symptoms usually reflect significant liver disease

D is the correct answer.

Commentary – Hepatic Amyloidosis

This may come up on board exam as a cause of an elevated ALP, which is seen in nearly all patients. AST can also be elevated. Hepatomegaly is also very common but does not correlate with the degree of amyloid deposition. Both AL and AA amyloid can lead to hepatic involvement. Symptoms are common but usually reflect systemic disease rather than liver disease. It rarely leads to chronic liver disease or portal hypertension although severe cardiac disease or peritoneal disease can lead to ascites. Liver biopsy is usually diagnostic.

Reference

Primary AL hepatic amyloidosis: clinical features and natural history in 98 patients.
   PMID: 14530778.

Question 220

In patients with biliary atresia (BA)

A Jaundice and acholic stools are usually the first sign
B Most infants are low birth weight with failure to thrive
C Liver biopsy is not usually required to make a diagnosis
D ERCP is diagnostic
E A Kasai should be performed once the patient reaches 3 months of age

A is the correct answer.

Commentary – Biliary Atresia

This is fair game, even on the adult board exam as some patients survive to adulthood. BA is rare (1 in 10,000–20,000 live births) but early diagnosis and transfer to a specialized center is imperative. The cause is unknown, but it leads to progressive fibro-obliterative destruction of the biliary tree.

It is the most common cause of neonatal jaundice requiring surgery and the most common indication for liver transplantation in children.

Clinical Pearls: Biliary Atresia

1. Affected infants are usually healthy, full-term, and normal weight.
2. Jaundice and alcoholic stools are the first sign.
3. Ultrasound and HIDA can be performed but usually to exclude other causes of neonatal jaundice.
4. Histology and cholangiogram are very characteristic and required to make a diagnosis.
5. ERCP is technically very challenging and diagnosis can be made in the operating room with direct cholangiogram.
6. Most importantly, Kasai (hepato-porto-enterostomy) should be performed as early as possible – this involves bringing a Roux limb directly to the hilum. The success of the Kasai directly correlates with how early it is performed – ideally before day 30, and definitely before day 90.
7. The vast majority of patients will eventually need transplant for biliary cirrhosis.

Reference

Biliary atresia. PMID: 14562580.

Question 221

All of the following patients would be contraindicated as a live liver donor EXCEPT

A A 17-year-old male with a BMI of 22 kg/m^2

B A 38-year-old female with a BMI of 41 kg/m^2 and prior gastric bypass surgery

C A 23-year-old male with ZZ alpha-1-antitrypsin (A1AT) phenotype and normal LFTs

D A 47-year-old female with a left lobe that is 23% of the total liver volume

E A 45-year-old male with a learning disability

D is the correct answer.

Commentary – Live Liver Donation

Sorry! This was a little bit of a trick question. All of the patients would be contraindicated for a RIGHT lobe donation. The patient in option D could donate the left lobe.

Every center have their own policy on potential donors but for most centers, contraindications for live liver donation include:

1. Age <18 or >60 years
2. Inability to provide informed consent
3. BMI >35 kg/m^2 (some centers will consider higher BMI but make the donor lose weight)
4. Active malignancy
5. Active infection
6. Hypercoagulable disorder
7. ZZ A1AT phenotype
8. Expected left lobe volume <30% of total (for right lobe donation)
9. High suspicion of donor coercion or financial gain

There are several other contraindications but these have become a little controversial including HIV, HBV, and HCV infection in the donor. Some other A1AT phenotypes and some minor coagulation abnormalities can also be considered as donors.

Reference

Selection and postoperative care of the living donor. PMID: 27095648.

Question 222

All of the following are important considerations in the evaluation and potential outcome of live liver donor transplantation EXCEPT

A ABO blood typing on two separate occasions
B Contrast-enhanced cross-sectional imaging of abdomen
C Iron and alpha-1-antitrypsin laboratory studies
D Cardiac testing with echocardiogram and stress test
E Medical, surgical, and psychosocial evaluation of the donor's suitability by the recipient team

E is the correct answer.

Commentary – Evaluation of the Live Liver Donor

All potential live liver donors undergo thorough evaluation including:

1. History and physical
2. Laboratory testing
3. Screening for infectious diseases (this can vary according to geography but definitely includes viral hepatitis, TB, CMV, EBV, HIV, syphilis)
4. Abdominal imaging for anatomy and liver volume
5. Psychosocial assessment
6. Cardiac assessment
7. Age-appropriate cancer screening
8. Independent donor advocate

In the options above, option E would be inappropriate, as the recipient team should not be involved in determining whether the donor is an appropriate candidate for donation. There should be a separate donor team doing the donor evaluation.

Reference

Selection and postoperative care of the living donor. PMID: 27095648.

Question 223

Which of the following combinations would NOT be appropriate for live donor liver transplantation?

Variable	A	B	C	D	E
Recipient weight/kg	100	60	70	90	70
Total donor liver volume/mL	2000	1200	1400	1500	1600
Right lobe liver volume/mL	1300	900	800	900	1000
Left lobe liver volume/mL	700	300	600	600	600

B is the correct answer.

Commentary – Graft to Recipient Weight Ratio (GRWR)

This is an important principle to remember and an easy question for board examiners to ask (hence we have another question in this book that is similar).

Clinical Pearls: GRWR

1. GRWR is the donor graft weight (in kg) (or volume in liters) divided by the recipient weight (kg) (×100).
2. GRWR should be >0.8 ideally and definitely above 0.7 to avoid small for size syndrome where there can be delayed graft function or non-function.
3. Centers have their own policy and can sometimes use otherwise perfect grafts (no steatosis and younger donor) with GRWR of 0.7–0.8 if the MELD is low and there is not a lot of portal hypertension.
4. The volume of the remnant liver needs to be at least 30% of the total volume to prevent a similar small for size syndrome in the donor.
5. The left lobe is generally only a third of the right lobe but can be used in a smaller recipient as long as the GRWR is >0.8. This also equates to a safer donor procedure.
6. The donor vascular and biliary anatomy is not really fair game on the hepatology board exam but generally, two hepatic arteries or two hepatic veins to the right would be contraindications. More than one biliary anastomosis increases the risk of biliary complications but is not a contra-indication.

Notes

If you have a live donor program in your center, I would strongly recommend you attend the live donor conference where the imaging is reviewed. You will learn a lot about liver anatomy from a surgical perspective.

Reference

Liver regeneration after living donor transplantation: adult-to-adult liver transplantation cohort study. PMID: 25065488.

Question 224

The following are true statements regarding the use of anti-thymocyte globulin (ATG) in transplantation EXCEPT

A ATG is a bovine monoclonal immunoglobulin preparation used for induction immunosuppression in renal transplantation

B ATG leads to cell death by complement dependent lysis or Fc receptor mediated lysis and opsonization

C Prophylaxis with antiviral therapy is not necessary prior to ATG use

D ATG is a first line therapy for acute rejection of the liver allograft

E Pretreatment with steroids, antihistamines, and anti-pyretics is rarely necessary prior to ATG infusion.

B is the correct answer.

Commentary – Use of ATG in Transplantation

ATG is prepared by immunizing rabbits or horses with human lymphoid cells derived from the thymus or cultured B cell lines leading to a polyclonal immunoglobulin response to T-cells. ATG acts through complement and the Fc receptor and leads to depletion of T-cells.

ATG is indicated as T-cell depletion therapy for induction and rejection in kidney transplant. Off-label use includes:

1. Induction and rejection in heart transplant
2. Induction and rejection in lung transplant
3. Induction in intestinal and multivisceral transplant
4. Acute rejection in liver transplant (after failure of other therapies)
5. Chronic graft versus host disease

ATG needs to be given with pre-medication as allergic and immune reactions can occur and viral prophylaxis against CMV and HSV is advised. Some centers avoid ATG in patients with leukopenia and thrombocytopenia. I doubt ATG will come up on the boards but it is worth knowing about as it is used perhaps once every couple of years in a big transplant center.

Reference

https://www.fda.gov/media/74641/download

Questions 225–227

A 45-year-old male presents to the emergency room brought in by his family. He has become increasingly jaundiced over the last several days and is mildly confused. His last alcohol was yesterday. He complains of some mild abdominal pain but otherwise denies fever or chills. His past medical history is significant for diabetes and hypertension, but he has been off medication for several months after he lost his job and his medical insurance. He was seen in the ER last month for alcohol intoxication when his renal function was normal and was given furosemide and spironolactone for edema.

Exam demonstrates an obese male, looking older than stated age, with weight 257 pounds, BP 120/80, pulse 104 regular and temperature 100 °F.

He is in no distress but has mild asterixis, scleral icterus with multiple spider nevi and temporal wasting. His heart and lungs are normal, but the abdomen is distended with dilated abdominal veins. His liver is markedly enlarged. Extremities show pitting ankle edema.

Laboratory studies:

Hb 12.6 g/dL
Plts 246,000
WBC 15.3
INR 2.3
Creat 4.3 mg/dL
Tbili 37.5 mg/dL (direct bili 24.3 mg/dL)
AST 210 U/L
ALT 89 U/L
GGTP 456 U/L
ALP 128 U/L
Albumin 2.5 g/dL
Ultrasound of abdomen – hepatomegaly, diffusely echogenic liver, no ductal dilation and moderate ascites.

▶ Question 225

Which of the following is NOT required to make a diagnosis of hepatorenal syndrome?

A Urinalysis
B Intravascular volume expansion
C Ascitic tap
D Renal imaging
E Stopping diuretics

▶ Question 226

The pathogenesis of HRS involves:

Variable	A	B	C	D	E
Cardiac output	Increase	Increase	Decrease	Increase	Decrease
Systemic vascular resistance	Decrease	Increase	Increase	Decrease	Increase
Renal perfusion	Decrease	Increase	Decrease	Increase	Increase
Plasma renin activity	Increase	Increase	Decrease	Increase	Decrease
Urinary sodium excretion	Decrease	Decrease	Increase	Decrease	Increase

▶ Question 227

All of the following can improve renal function in patients with HRS EXCEPT

A Norepinephrine
B Terlipressin
C Midodrine and octreotide
D TIPS
E Dopamine

225 – C is the correct answer.
226 – A is the correct answer.
227 – E is the correct answer.

Commentary – Hepatorenal Syndrome (HRS)

This is one of the more commonly encountered liver complications on the inpatient service at any large transplant program and yet we really have limited effective treatment options. Understanding the physiology is important.

The diagnostic criteria for HRS are strict so it is really a diagnosis of exclusion. Criteria have changed slightly over the last few years. It is essentially an algorithm:

1. Patient with cirrhosis, acute liver failure or portal hypertension with ascites and acute kidney injury (defined as creatinine >0.3 mg/dL in 48 hours or >50% increase in 7 days).
2. Rule out other causes (chronic kidney disease, obstructive kidney disease, hypotension, intravascular depletion, nephrotoxins [mainly drugs], active urine sediment etc.) and treat.
3. Give IV albumin (1 g/kg for 2 days).

If there is no improvement in kidney function then this makes the diagnosis. Analysis of ascites fluid is not required to make a diagnosis of HRS but is important to rule out SBP that can precipitate HRS.

Type 1 HRS is when the serum creatinine increases by at least twofold to a value greater than 2.5 mg/dL during a period of fewer than 2 weeks. If it is less rapidly progressive disease then this is type 2.

Pathophysiology

1. Splanchnic arterial vasodilatation due to portal hypertension is the most important factor.
2. Increased production or activity of vasodilators such as nitric oxide are likely to be involved.
3. Cardiac output rises and systemic vascular resistance falls.
4. There is an increase in renal vascular resistance due to activation of the renin-angiotensin system and sympathetic nervous systems.
5. Reduction in glomerular filtration rate (GFR) and sodium excretion (often to less than 10 mEq/day in advanced cirrhosis).
6. Mean arterial pressure decreases despite renal vasoconstriction.
7. Hence, vasoconstrictors such as vasopressin, terlipressin, and ornipressin; midodrine and octreotide; and norepinephrine can improve HRS by decreasing splanchnic vasodilation and improving the renal hemodynamics.
8. A TIPS will also potentially improve the hemodynamics by reducing portal pressure.

> **Notes**
>
> I would hope by the time this text is published terlipressin would have completed its tortuous journey to FDA approval in the United States. Until then, most of us rely on a study in a handful of patients and continue using octreotide, albumin, and midodrine.

Reference

New developments in Hepatorenal Syndrome. PMID: 28602971.

Questions 228–231

A 58-year-old male presents to the office for routine evaluation with a history of alcoholic liver disease. There is no history of GI bleeding, ascites, or encephalopathy and he has been sober for 2 years, but does continue to smoke. Upper GI endoscopy showed no varices.

Exam is unremarkable

Laboratory studies:

Hb 14.1 g/dL
Plts 84,000
INR 1.2
Tbili 0.7 mg/dL
AST 38 U/L
ALT 20 U/L
ALP 102 U/L
Albumin 3.1 g/dL
Creatinine 0.8 mg/dL
AFP 103 ng/mL
Triple phase MRI scan of a 2.1 cm lesion is shown below:

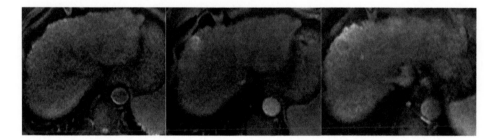

▶ Question 228

Which statement is TRUE?

A A percutaneous liver biopsy is required to make a definitive diagnosis
B He should be considered for a right hepatectomy
C His 5-year survival after liver transplantation is less than 50%
D He will eventually be eligible for a MELD exception
E Locoregional therapy is contraindicated if he meets Milan criteria

▶ Question 229

If resection were to be a consideration, important determinants of outcome include all the following EXCEPT?

A AFP >200 ng/mL
B Tumor >5 cm
C Lymph node metastases
D Positive surgical margin
E Hepatic volumetry

▶ Question 230

All of the following are appropriate management options for this patient EXCEPT?

A Trans-arterial chemoembolization (TACE)
B Yttrium 90 theraspheres
C Radio-frequency ablation (RFA)
D Percutaneous ethanol injection (PEI)
E Stereotactic radiotherapy

▶ Question 231

If he is to undergo liver transplantation (in the United States) all of the following are true EXCEPT?

A His overall 5-year survival after transplant should be at least 75%
B He is immediately eligible for a MELD exception
C He should undergo serial abdominal imaging and a staging CT chest to be eligible for the MELD exception
D His scan shows OPTN class 5B
E Depending on blood type and UNOS region, live donor transplant would be a good option for this patient

228 – D is the correct answer.
229 – A is the correct answer.
230 – E is the correct answer.
231 – B is the correct answer.

Commentary – HCC, Milan Criteria, Loco-Regional Treatment

This patient has developed HCC in the setting of alcoholic liver disease and provides ample opportunity to test your knowledge for examiners. Screening for HCC is discussed elsewhere in this book.

In Terms of Diagnosis

1. HCC can be diagnosed on contrast-enhanced CT, MRI, or US in high-risk patients (such as cirrhosis).
2. LI-RADS is the liver imaging reporting and data system that is used for multiple imaging findings. For liver lesions:
   a. LR1 – definitely benign
   b. LR2 – probably benign
   c. LR-3 – indeterminate probability of malignancy
   d. LR-4 – probably HCC
   e. LR-5 – definite HCC
3. This patient would be considered LR-5 in the LI-RADS for high-risk patients. LR-5 is defined by a lesion on contrast-enhanced CT or MRI that:
   a. Measures >1 cm.
   b. If measures >2 cm should demonstrate at least one of the following three features, and those measuring >1 cm but <2 cm should demonstrate at least two of the three features: non-peripheral washout, enhancing capsule, or growth.
4. There is also an OPTN classification based on the LR-5 lesion as above that is used for the MELD exception. Class 5A and 5B are eligible for the HCC MELD exception (if 5A meet the Milan criteria – see below).

OPTN classification of LR-5 lesions	
Class	Requirement
Class 5A: ≥1 cm and <2 cm measured on late arterial or portal venous phase images	Increased contrast enhancement in late hepatic arterial phase and either washout during later phases of contrast enhancement and peripheral rim enhancement on delayed phase, or biopsy confirmation.
Class 5A-g: same size as OPTN class 5A HCC	Increased contrast enhancement in late hepatic arterial phase and growth by 50% or more documented on serial CT or MR images obtained ≤6 months apart.
Class 5B: maximum diameter ≥2 and ≤5 cm	Increased contrast enhancement in late hepatic arterial phase and either washout during later contrast phases or peripheral rim enhancement (capsule or pseudocapsule) or growth by 50% or more documented on serial CT or MR images obtained ≤6 months apart (OPTN class 5B-g) or biopsy confirmation.
Class 5T: prior regional treatment for HCC	Any class 5A, 5A-g, or 5B lesion that was automatically approved for MELD HCC exception points upon initial request or extension and has been subsequently ablated.
Class 5X: maximum diameter ≥5 cm	Increased contrast enhancement in late hepatic arterial phase and either washout during later contrast phases or peripheral rim enhancement (capsule or pseudocapsule). Not eligible for MELD HCC exception points.

5. The original Milan criteria from 1996 demonstrated that 75% 4 year survival was achievable in patients transplanted for HCC if they had "early HCC": defined as single lesion ≤5 cm, up to three separate lesions, none larger than 3 cm, no evidence of gross vascular invasion, and no regional nodal or distant metastases.

6. To be eligible for the MELD exception the patient needs abdominal and chest imaging to rule out metastatic disease.

7. The MELD exception for HCC is applied if the patient meets Milan criteria AND after 6 months of observation (to weed out tumors with bad biology).

8. Loco-regional treatments for HCC include various embolization and ablation methods and are used as a bridge to transplant. Stereotactic radiotherapy is typically used for large tumors and where the patient is too sick to undergo embolization or ablation.

9. Radiofrequency ablation (RFA) and microwave ablation (MWA) work best in tumors <4 cm. Trans-arterial chemoembolization (TACE) is used most often for the tumors >2 cm. Radioembolization using intra-arterial injection of Yttrium-90 (Y90)-labeled microspheres can be used instead of TACE.

10. There are no head-to-head trials of loco-regional treatments in HCC.

11. Live donor transplant is a reasonable approach for patients that may wait to get transplanted.

12. Surgical resection is usually only an option in 5% of HCC cases.

13. Resection is an option based on the volume and function of residual liver remnant assessed by hepatic volumetry prior to major resection.

14. Significant portal hypertension is a contraindication (presence of varices or platelets <100)

15. Decompensated cirrhosis is a contraindication for resection (High MELD or Childs-Pugh B or C)

16. Since patients undergo comprehensive pre-resection evaluation, outcome after resection is determined by presence of cirrhosis, tumor size, **AFP >1000 ng/mL**, major vascular invasion, positive margins, and metastatic disease.

17. Partial portal vein embolization/ligation can be used prior to resection (ALPPS procedure – associating liver partition and portal vein ligation) to cause hypertrophy of the uninvolved lobe of the liver to allow safer resection of the cancerous lobe.

Reference

Hepatocellular carcinoma. PMID: 29307467.

Question 232

A 33-year-old female presents to the office for persistently elevated liver tests for several months. She complains of fatigue, weakness, and 10-pound weight loss. She denies alcohol or drug use.

Exam shows no distress, BMI 18 kg/m², normal vitals, and temporal wasting. She has difficulty getting up from the examination table.

Laboratory studies:

Hb 12.1 g/dL
Plts 456,000
INR 1.1
Tbili 1.0 mg/dL
AST 598 U/L
ALT 422 U/L
ALP 111 U/L
Creatinine 1.1 mg/dL
Viral hepatitis and autoimmune serology are negative

▶ Question

Which of the following would be most helpful diagnostic test?

A Liver biopsy
B Iron studies
C 24-hour urinary copper
D Brain MRI
E Serum aldolase

E is the correct answer.

Commentary – Other Causes of Elevated LFTs

The clue again here is in the stem. She has weakness and difficulty getting off the examination table. The LFTs are mildly elevated with a hepatocellular pattern. Viral and autoimmune markers are negative. Hemochromatosis could present with these LFTs but not the clinical picture. An eating disorder could also be a cause of this picture. Wilson disease can cause any type of LFT abnormality but characteristically the ALP is very low.

Multiple systemic diseases can cause abnormal LFTs. For board purposes, the following should be remembered:

Hepatocellular LFTs

1. Thyroid disease
2. Muscle disorders – Myositis (as in this case), dermatomyositis – so aldolase and other muscle enzymes are elevated
3. Celiac disease
4. Adrenal insufficiency
5. Anorexia nervosa

Cholestatic LFTs

1. Any infiltrative disease
2. Total parenteral nutrition
3. Sepsis

Notes

This was a case that I remember vividly. She came in and could not get off the examination table without me helping her. Her LFTs normalized after neurology treated her.

Question 233

A 2-year-old male infant is brought into the ER by his parents for fever and cough and is diagnosed with a viral upper respiratory tract infection. On examination, the ER resident notices an enlarged liver. Ultrasound is performed and shows a 6 cm hyperechoic, solid mass in the right lobe of the liver.

Laboratory studies:

Hb 10.2 g/dL
Plts 497,000
INR 1.1
Tbili 0.7 mg/dL
AST 19 U/L
ALT 16 U/L
ALP 76 U/L
AFP 1005 ng/mL

▶ Question

The most likely diagnosis is:

A Fibrolamellar HCC
B HCC
C Angiosarcoma
D Hepatoblastoma
E Epithelioid hemangioendothelioma

D is the correct answer.

Commentary – Hepatoblastoma and Childhood Tumors

If this shows up on the boards, it should be a very straightforward case as shown here. The main differential diagnosis is between HCC and hepatoblastoma. Angiosarcoma occurs in older patients, usually men, with a history of exposure to vinyl chloride and anabolic steroids. Epithelioid hemangioendothelioma affects older women and can be confused with cholangiocarcinoma.

HCC can occur in childhood but rarely before age 5 and occurs in the setting of metabolic and liver diseases such as Alagille's syndrome, hereditary tyrosinemia, progressive familial intrahepatic cholestasis type II, neurofibromatosis, and ataxia-telangiectasia.

For hepatoblastoma, the clinical pearls to know are:

1. Usually before age 2 and almost always before age 5
2. Prematurity is a risk factor
3. Boys are twice as likely to be affected
4. There are several diseases/syndromes that increase the risk
   a. Beckwith Wiedmann
   b. Downs
   c. Von Gierke
   d. Familial adenomatous polyposis.
5. Usually solitary and right lobe
6. AFP is markedly elevated
7. May have sexual precocity due to ectopic gonadotrophin production
8. Embryonal tumor so can mimic other tumor types
9. Liver tests are usually normal
10. AFP usually very elevated
11. Treatment is surgical (resection, transplant)

Notes

There are always a few pediatric questions on the adult transplant hepatology boards. They should be topics that you might see like biliary atresia or where there is some similarity with adult diseases.

Reference

Epidemiology of primary hepatic malignancies in US children. PMID: 12939582.

Question 234

A 53-year-old man undergoes liver transplant for hepatitis B-related cirrhosis and hepatocellular carcinoma. He has a positive HBsAg but undetectable HBV DNA on tenofovir at the time of transplant.

▶ Question

What is the optimal management strategy for control of his HBV after transplant?

A Continue tenofovir indefinitely, hepatitis B immune globulin (HBIG) during anhepatic phase, and then monthly for 10 years.

B Continue tenofovir for 1 year, HBIG during anhepatic phase and then monthly for 1 year with continuation of both tenovofir and HBIG dependent on quantitative anti-HBs titer.

C Continue tenofovir indefinitely, HBIG during anhepatic phase, and then monthly for 3–12 months.

D Continue tenofovir indefinitely, HBIG post-op day 1 and then weekly for 3 months depending on quantitative anti-HBs titer.

E Continue tenofovir indefinitely, HBIG post-op day 1 and then monthly for 12 months.

C is the correct answer.

Commentary – HBIG After Liver Transplant

The use of HBIG dramatically improved the outcome for patients transplanted for HBV related liver disease. HBIG binds to and neutralizes circulating HBsAg and prevents graft infection and also enters the hepatocytes and binds with intracellular HBsAg, decreasing HBsAg secretion. For maximum effectiveness it should be given during the anhepatic phase. It used to be given every month indefinitely after transplant but with the advent of effective antivirals the practice now is to continue antivirals indefinitely and give HBIG during the anhepatic phase and then monthly for up to a year. In our institution, we stop giving it at 3 months as HIBG is quite expensive. Measuring quantitative anti-HBs is possible and a titer of >500 IU/L is thought to be more protective so may be useful in patients with a higher risk of reinfection (such as those with HCC).

Reference

Liver transplantation in European patients with the hepatitis B surface antigen. PMID: 8247035.

Question 235

Which of the following recipient/donor combinations would NOT be currently appropriate for liver transplantation?

	A	B	C	D	E
Recipient	HCV RNA+	HCV RNA+	HBsAg+	HCV RNA+	HCV RNA−
Donor	HBsAg+	HCV RNA+	Anti-HBc+	Anti-HBc+	HCV RNA+

A is the correct answer.

Commentary – HBV/HCV Positive Donors

The lack of donor organs coupled with effective antiviral treatments for HCV and HBV means that donors with positive serology for viral hepatitis are appropriate candidates for donation to the right recipient. The HOPE Act allows HIV positive donors to donate to HIV positive recipients, but for HBV and HCV, the decisions are center specific and may change in the future depending on even more effective antivirals, particularly if there is a "cure" for HBV.

In General

1. Anti-HBc positive donors are appropriate for all recipients but oral antiviral prophylaxis should be given indefinitely.
2. HCV RNA positive recipients can receive HCV RNA positive donors and should be treated with antivirals after transplant.
3. HCV RNA negative recipients can receive HCV RNA positive donors if they consent and need to be treated with antivirals shortly after transplant.
4. HBsAg positive donors should only be used in HBsAg positive recipients.

Reference

Expanding the donor pool: Hepatitis C, hepatitis B, and human immunodeficiency virus-positive donors in liver transplantation. PMID: 31885421.

Question 236

A 68-year-old female underwent a liver transplant 3 weeks ago for cryptogenic cirrhosis. She has had an uneventful recovery. She presents to your clinic now with fever, headache, abdominal pain, and some confusion. Medications include tacrolimus, mycophenolate mofetil, prednisone, trimethoprim-sulfamethoxazole, and valganciclovir.

Laboratory studies:

Tbili 1.4 mg/dL
AST 25 U/L
ALT 41 U/L
ALP 117 U/L
Hb 8.7 g/dL
WCC 6.5
Plt 177
Creat 2.8 mg/dL
Tacrolimus level 23 ng/mL
She is started on broad spectrum antibiotics but develops worsening dyspnea and mental status requiring intubation. CT head is negative. Respiratory syncytial virus is positive in sputum. Yeast species are identified in blood cultures on day 3. A lumbar puncture is performed with an opening pressure of 36 cm.

▶ Question

Which statement is TRUE?

A Serial lumbar puncture should be performed until the pressure is below 20 cm
B Cryptococcal antigen in the CSF is specific but has poor sensitivity
C Cryptococcal culture from CSF will take 3–4 weeks to result
D 1 week of induction therapy with fluconazole 200 mg followed by 6 weeks of maintenance therapy at 100 mg daily cures infection in 90%
E The prognosis is poor with 50% 1-year survival

A is the correct answer.

Commentary – Cryptococcal Meningitis After Liver Transplant

This patient has developed fever shortly after transplant with respiratory symptoms but then starts growing yeast in blood cultures with worsening mental status. Cryptococcus neoformans infection is a concern with both disseminated disease and meningo-encephalitis.

Clinical Pearls: Cryptococcal Meningitis and LT

1. Consider Cryptococcal meningitis in a post-transplant patient with fever and neurological symptoms.
2. Occurs in a 2–3% of patients after transplant.
3. It can occur early but generally occurs in first 1–2 years (median time to onset is 21 months).
4. Acquired through inhalation and then spreads to CNS where CSF is a favorable growth medium.
5. Presents with fever and usually neurological symptoms.
6. Diagnosis is with India ink stain (for encapsulated yeast forms), cryptococcal antigen (sensitive and specific), and culture (takes 3–5 days).
7. Treatment is with induction with amphotericin B and flucytosine for at least 2 weeks and then consolidation with high dose fluconazole (400–800 mg) for 8 weeks and then maintenance fluconazole (200 mg) for at least a year (or more).
8. Therapeutic lumbar puncture to reduce intracranial pressure is helpful in patients with neurological symptoms.
9. Prognosis in transplant recipients is generally good.

Notes

This is another disease that you need to look out for, particularly in older patients as it responds well to treatment. Patients can be in a coma and be back to normal in a few months.

Reference

Clinical practice guidelines for the management of cryptococcal disease: 2010 update by the IDSA. PMID: 20047480.

Questions 237–243 (Infections and Prophylaxis)

▶ Question 237

Regarding testing and management of tuberculosis (TB) in potential liver transplant patients, which of the following statements is TRUE?

A The tuberculin skin test (TST) and interferon-gamma release assay (IGRA) (Quantiferon) are equally sensitive tests for latent TB in patients with end-stage liver disease.

B The IGRA is unreliable in patients who received BCG vaccination at an early age.

C If a patient has close contact with someone with active TB, a negative IGRA is sufficient to prevent the need for treatment of latent TB.

D Patients with latent TB can be treated after liver transplantation.

E The dose of calcineurin inhibitor needs to be increased when isoniazid is used to treat latent TB after transplant.

D is the correct answer.

Commentary – TB and Transplant

This is an easy arena to garner questions from and examiners have loved TB since the dawn of exams.

All potential liver transplant candidates need to be tested for latent TB.

Clinical Pearls: TB and LT

1. The TST is an unreliable test and has been superseded by the IGRA (Quantiferon)
2. IGRA is not affected by prior BCG and is more sensitive in patients with end-stage liver disease.
3. However, even the IGRA is not perfect so in patients with an indeterminate test, it should be repeated.

Candidates for Treatment of Latent TB Include

1. Positive TST or positive IGRA
2. History of untreated latent TB
3. History of close contact with active TB (irrespective of IGRA or TST result)
4. Donor with positive TST/IGRA or untreated latent TB

Treatment for latent TB can wait until after transplant, particularly in patients with advanced liver disease given the potential hepatotoxicity of anti-TB medications. Rifampin is the drug that induces cytochrome p450 so decreases CNI levels. Treatment of latent TB is for at least 4 months using rifampin containing regimens and longer when isoniazid is used. Local resistance patterns and infectious diseases specialist will determine length of treatment. Liver tests need to be closely monitored during treatment and oral pyridoxine should be given.

Reference

Mycobacterium tuberculosis infections in solid organ transplantation: Guidelines from the infectious diseases community practice of the AST. PMID: 30817030.

▶ Question 238

Which of the following vaccines are recommended for ALL adult liver transplant recipients?

Vaccine	A	B	C	D	E
Seasonal influenza	+	+	−	+	+
Pneumococcus	+	-	+	−	+
HAV/HBV	+	+	+	−	+
Recombinant zoster	−	−	+	+	+
Meningococcus	−	+	−	+	−
Human papillomavirus	−	−	+	−	+
Tetanus/diphtheria/pertussis	+	−	−	+	+
COVID 19	+	−	+	−	+

▶ Question 239

Which of the following vaccines is contraindicated AFTER liver transplantation?

A Hepatitis B
B Pneumococcal conjugate (PCV13)
C Pneumococcal polysaccharide (PPSV23)
D Shingrix (zoster)
E Varicella

238 – A is the correct answer.
239 – E is the correct answer.

Commentary – Vaccines in Liver Transplant Recipients

This is important to remember for practical purposes as I get asked several times a month by transplant recipients: "Is this vaccine ok to take?"

Essentially, live attenuated vaccines are contraindicated after transplant (so if they are needed give before and ensure transplant is at least several weeks after).

Live vaccines include: live attenuated influenza (intranasal), oral polio, measles/mumps/rubella, rotavirus, varicella, yellow fever, live zoster (not available in US).

Recommended vaccines for transplant patients are as listed in choice A in the previous question.

There are two types of pneumococcal vaccine – PCV and PPSV – and PPSV – and both are indicated in solid organ transplant recipients. Recombinant zoster is indicated in adults over age 50. Remember, the varicella-zoster vaccine (Zostavax) is live and so is contraindicated. Shingrix is a recombinant vaccine so ok after transplant. Meningococcal and hemophilus influenzae vaccines are indicated if there is an additional risk factor such as asplenia (or stem cell transplant for hemophilus). HPV vaccine is not generally indicated after age 26. COVID 19 should be given to all transplant recipients and preferably prior to transplant as the response is diminished in patients on immunosuppression.

Reference

https://www.cdc.gov/vaccines/hcp/acip-recs/general-recs/immunocompetence.html

▶ Question 240

Which of the following is the most appropriate *immediate pre and peri*-transplantation infection prophylaxis regimen in liver transplant recipients?

Regimen	A	B	C	D	E
Empiric antibiotics to cover gram negative organisms	+	–	–	+	–
Antibiotics based on institutional protocol	–	+	+	–	+
Empiric antifungals	+	–	–	+	+
Targeted antifungals based on risk factors for fungal infection	–	+	+	–	–
Empiric antivirals	+	–	+	–	–
Antivirals in CMV negative recipients	–	–	–	+	

▶ Question 241

Targeted antifungal prophylaxis should be considered in all the following patients undergoing liver transplantation EXCEPT

A Retransplantation
B Prolonged total parenteral nutrition (TPN)
C Massive transfusion requirement
D Prior splenectomy
E Intraoperative bile leak

▶ Question 242

Which statement regarding antifungal drugs used in transplant recipients is TRUE?

A The dose of tacrolimus needs to be increased with fluconazole due to induction of cytochrome P450.
B Patients should be monitored for arrhythmias due to QT prolongation with caspofungin.
C Voriconazole can cause dose-related hepatotoxicity.
D Amphotericin B is useful for invasive Aspergillosis as the dose does not need to be adjusted in renal failure.
E Patients on micafungin need a reduction in tacrolimus dose as it inhibits cytochrome P450.

▶ Question 243

A 58-year-old male with hepatocellular carcinoma underwent liver transplantation yesterday. He received a deceased donor allograft from a 37-year-old donor who was CMV

IgG positive. The recipient is CMV IgG negative. He has been started on tacrolimus, mycophenolate, and prednisone.

Which of the following statements regarding CMV infection in this patient is TRUE?

A He should be continued on life-long CMV prophylaxis with valganciclovir

B CMV prophylaxis will reduce the risk of bacteremia, fungal infection, and acute rejection

C Pre-emptive therapy (treating when evidence of viremia) is not recommended as the outcomes are worse compared to prophylaxis

D Valganciclovir is preferred over ganciclovir as it is FDA approved in liver transplant recipients

E Ganciclovir is preferred over valganciclovir as is has activity against HSV and VZV

240 – B is the correct answer.

This is a bit of a trick question. For the immediate peri-operative period in liver transplantation, all patients receive antibiotic prophylaxis according to institutional protocols based on organisms, susceptibility, and patient factors. Antifungals are used in certain patients depending on risk factors for fungal infection and again will vary by center. Antivirals are not used in the peri-operative period, but prophylaxis starts in the post-operative phase.

241 – D is the correct answer.

As with all issues regarding infection prophylaxis, each center develops their own protocol based on incidence and specifics of fungal infection seen in transplant recipients. However, the following are considered appropriate criteria for fungal prophylaxis:

1. Retransplantation
2. Massive blood requirements
3. Bile leak
4. Renal failure
5. Known fungal colonization prior to transplant
6. Prolonged antibiotic use prior to transplant
7. Prolonged TPN

242 – C is the correct answer.

There are three types of antifungals and none are perfect. The important points to remember for the boards are listed below.

The Azoles

1. Inhibit cytochrome P450 so INCREASE tacrolimus/cyclosporine levels.
2. Are hepatotoxic, especially voriconazole.
3. Cause prolonged QT interval.

Amphotericin B is nephrotoxic and is ineffective at low dose for invasive infection (especially Aspergillus).

Echinocandins such as caspofungin and micafungin do not affect cytochrome P450 but can cause elevated LFTs.

243 – B is the correct answer.

Commentary – CMV Prophylaxis

CMV is a common issue after liver transplantation so a very appropriate topic for a board exam. CMV infection refers to the presence of virus (blood, tissue, etc.), while CMV disease is infection with signs and symptoms.

CMV prophylaxis is pretty much universally recommended by most transplant programs, but the strategy differs. Universal prophylaxis is recommended for everyone for several months (usually 3–6 months) after transplant depending on center preference. A CMV positive donor to a CMV negative recipient has the highest risk and so is usually treated for longer. Pre-emptive therapy has been shown to be equally effective.

The two drugs that are used are valganciclovir (oral) and ganciclovir (IV in US). They are both effective against HSV and VZV but only ganciclovir is FDA approved for prophylaxis in liver transplant recipients.

CMV prophylaxis has the added benefit of reducing the risk of other bacterial and fungal infections and reducing the risk of acute rejection.

Reference

The third international consensus guidelines on the management of cytomegalovirus in solid organ transplantation. PMID: 29596116.

Question 244

A 28-year-old female presents with a 3-day history of abdominal pain, nausea, vomiting, diarrhea, shortness of breath and fevers to 103 °F.

She underwent a liver transplant 4 months ago for acute liver failure due to acetaminophen overdose. She is on tacrolimus, mycophenolate and prednisone. Trimethoprim-sulfamethoxazole, fluconazole, and valganciclovir were stopped a month ago. There was no recent travel or sick contacts and no history of recent alcohol or drugs.

Physical Examination

Dyspnea, mild icterus, no oral mucocutaneous lesions, no stigmata of chronic liver disease.
No hepatosplenomegaly or ascites. Alert and oriented without asterixis.

Laboratory studies:

Total bilirubin 3.9 mg/dL
AST 4,500 U/L
ALT 3,900 U/L
ALP 127 U/L
INR 3.4
Tacrolimus level 6.7 ng/mL
WBC 13.2 (25% bands)
Liver biopsy is performed:

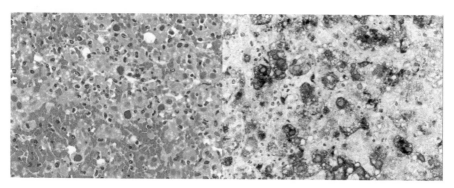

▶ Question

Which of the following statements is TRUE?

A The tacrolimus should be increased
B Fluconazole should be restarted
C She is likely taking high doses of acetaminophen again
D She should be started on broad spectrum antibiotics
E She should be started on acyclovir

E is the correct answer.

Commentary – HSV Infection After Transplant

Unfortunately, this lady has developed HSV hepatitis, a disease with high fatality. The clues are the high fever, high LFTS, and the recent cessation of prophylaxis. The biopsy shows intranuclear inclusions in the middle of the first image (the larger purple lesions) and a positive immunostain for HSV in the second image (the darker brown staining).

Clinical Pearls: Post-transplant HSV Hepatitis

1. CMV prophylaxis is protective against reactivation of HSV after transplant.
2. Some of the typical symptoms of HSV hepatitis may be absent in post-transplant patients such as high fever.
3. Treatment with IV acyclovir is the same as in immunocompetent patients.
4. It can be associated with lung and GI involvement.

Reference

HSV hepatitis after solid organ transplantation in adults. PMID: 1850439.

Questions 245 and 246

You are visited by a smartly dressed rep from a new technology company that has a "novel" blood test (CA 20-2) that they claim will revolutionize the diagnosis of cholangiocarcinoma (CCA) in patients with PSC.

She shows you a brochure that shows data from an international multicenter study of 100 patients who underwent surgery for suspected CCA, 69 had pathological evidence of CCA and 31 had benign disease with inflammatory pseudotumor.

The blood test CA20-2 has a normal range of 6–35 U/L. In the 69 patients with CCA, the CA20-2 was >35 U/L in 57 patients. In the 31 patients without CCA, the CA20-2 was >35 U/L in 10 patients.

▶ Question 245

What are the sensitivity and specificity of the CA20-2 test in diagnosing CCA?

	A	B	C	D	E
Sensitivity	83%	57%	83%	85%	83%
Specificity	30%	10%	68%	64%	90%

▶ Question 246

What are the positive and negative predictive values of the CA20-2 test in this population?

	A	B	C	D	E
Positive predictive value (PPV)	83%	57%	83%	85%	83%
Negative predictive value (NPV)	30%	10%	68%	64%	90%

245 – C is the correct answer.
246 – D is the correct answer.

Commentary – Sensitivity/Specificity/PPV/NPV

There will almost certainly be a statistics question on every single medical board exam. This is very straightforward if you draw your 2×2 table with disease on one side and test on the other.

	CCA (+ disease)	No CCA (− disease)	
CA20-2 >35 U/L (+ test)	57 (TP)	10 (FP)	67
Normal CA20-2 (− test)	12 (FN)	21 (TN)	33
	69	31	

Sensitivity is the proportion of patients who tested positive out of all patients with CCA. So 57 patients were truly positive (TP) and 12 patients were falsely negative (FN) out of the 69 patients who had CCA at surgery. So sensitivity is $57/69 = 83\%$.

Specificity is the proportion of patients who tested negative out of all patients who did not have CCA. So 21 patients were truly negative (TN) and 10 patients were falsely positive (FP) out of the 31 patients who had benign disease at surgery. So specificity is $21/31 = 68\%$.

Positive predictive value determines, out of all of the positive results on the test, how many patients had CCA. So PPV is $TP/TP + FP$, in this case, $57/57 + 10 = 85\%$. Negative predictive value determines, out of all of the negative results on the test, how many patients did NOT have CCA. So NPV is $TN/TN + FN$, in this case, $21/21 + 12 = 64\%$.

The population being tested in this example were patients who were already suspected of having CCA so the CA20-2 is a diagnostic test as opposed to a screening test.

Remember, disease prevalence in a population affects PPV and NPV but not sensitivity. So for a screening test, when a disease is highly prevalent, the test is better at "ruling in" the disease and worse at "ruling it out."

Question 247

A 23-year-old female presents to the office for a routine visit. She underwent liver transplantation 10 years ago for fulminant liver failure of indeterminate etiology. She has been prescribed tacrolimus and has been getting regular bloodwork that shows normal liver and renal function. She is working and feels well. However, a call from the specialty pharmacy reveals that she has not taken her immunosuppression for over a year.

Laboratory studies:

ALT 23 U/L
ALP 89 U/L
Total bilirubin 0.7 mg/dL
Creatinine 0.6 mg/dL
Tacrolimus level undetectable

▶ Question

Which of the following statements is TRUE?

A Operational tolerance can be expected in up to a third of pediatric liver transplant recipients.
B If rejection occurs after withdrawal of immunosuppression, there is a high rate of graft failure.
C This patient will likely have normal liver histology on biopsy.
D The development of de novo donor specific antibodies after withdrawal of immunosuppression is associated with operational tolerance.
E She will likely need to go back on immunosuppression in the near future.

A is the correct answer.

Commentary – Withdrawal of Immunosuppression and Operational Tolerance

This is an interesting area of research that is still evolving so will be unlikely on a board exam, but several points are worth noting. Several immunosuppression withdrawal after liver transplantation trials have been performed or are still ongoing and use frequent liver biopsies to assess outcome since there are no reliable biomarkers for rejection.

Clinical Pearls: Operational Tolerance

1. Operational tolerance refers to indefinite allograft acceptance after withdrawal of immunosuppression.
2. In pediatric patients, up to a third can develop operational tolerance.
3. Patients with normal LFTS can often have biopsy findings of inflammation/rejection.
4. If operational tolerance occurs, it is usually robust and maintained.
5. The development of de novo donor specific antibodies after withdrawal of immunosuppression is associated with acute rejection, not operational tolerance.

Notes

It is surprisingly common for patients not to take immunosuppression as prescribed. Through the years I have had many patients eventually admit to taking the tacrolimus only once a day or once a week with the classic excuses: "I forgot," "they run out otherwise," or my favorite "I like to take it before I go to church."

Reference

Efficacy and safety of immunosuppression withdrawal in pediatric liver transplant recipients: moving toward personalized management. PMID: 32786149.

Questions 248 and 249

A 55-year-old male presents for EGD. He has a history of NASH cirrhosis and diabetes. He denies ascites, GI bleeding, or encephalopathy. Contrast imaging last month showed cirrhosis but no HCC.

On exam he is alert in no distress without scleral icterus. BP 130/80, pulse 78.

Laboratory studies:

Hb 12.9 g/dL
Tbili 1.3 mg/dL
INR 1.2
Plt 128
Creatinine 1.7 mg/dL
EGD shows grade I (small) esophageal varices with red wale signs, no gastric varices and mild portal hypertensive gastropathy.

▶ Question 248

Which statement is TRUE?

A Use of a nonselective beta-blocker will reduce the risk of a first variceal hemorrhage but does not affect progression to larger esophageal varices.
B If the patient is started on nadolol, the starting dose needs to be adjusted due to the renal insufficiency.
C The patient's risk of esophageal variceal bleeding is reduced by 5–10% with a nonselective beta-blocker.
D A distal splenorenal shunt can be considered if he is intolerant of beta-blockers.
E A TIPS can be considered if he is intolerant of beta-blockers.

He presents a year later for repeat EGD and denies any GI bleeding. The esophageal varices are now large with red wale signs and there are several 1–2 cm varices in the fundus. BP is 100/60 and pulse is 56.

Laboratory studies:

Hb 12.1 g/dL
Tbili 1.7 mg/dL
INR 1.3
Plt 103
Creatinine 1.8 mg/dL

▶ Question 249

What is the most appropriate management option?

A The gastric varices should be injected with cyanoacrylate.
B A TIPS should be placed
C The esophageal varices should be sclerosed with ethanolamine
D The esophageal varices should be banded
E The nadolol should be replaced with propranolol

248 – B is the correct answer.
249 – D is the correct answer.

Commentary – Primary Prophylaxis of Variceal Hemorrhage

This is of practical significance as well as board testing material. There are some caveats but there have been several randomized clinical trials in this area so guidelines have some good evidence.

Clinical Pearls: Primary Prophylaxis for Variceal Hemorrhage

1. Pre-primary prophylaxis – beta-blockers (timolol) do not prevent formation of varices in patients that do not have varices.
2. Patients with cirrhosis should undergo EGD to look for varices. There is some evidence that a platelet count >150 and liver stiffness of <20 kPa in patients with cirrhosis from HCV are very unlikely to have varices.
3. Primary prophylaxis reduces the risk of a first variceal bleed and the risk of bleeding-related death.
4. Screen with EGD- if no varices and compensated cirrhosis, repeat in 2–3 years. If decompensated cirrhosis, repeat annually.
5. If varices are detected, the size and therapy will determine timing/need for repeat.
6. Varices are graded as small or large (the grades I–IV are no longer used).
7. Small EV without red wale and Child's A cirrhosis can be observed and repeat EGD in 1–2 years.
8. Small EV with red wale or if Child's B or C, or large EV, should be treated.
9. Nonselective beta-blockers (NSBB) should be used for primary prophylaxis and started at low dose and titrated up to target heart rate of 55–60 as long as BP and side effects not problematic.
10. Nadolol is renally excreted so dose needs to be adjusted.
11. NSBB reduce the progression of small EV to large EV.
12. NSBB (nadolol, propranolol, carvedilol) reduce the risk of EV bleeding from about 20% (controls) to 10% in treated patients.
13. Number needed to treat is about 11 (to prevent one bleed).
14. Nitrates do not work as primary prophylaxis.
15. Endoscopic variceal ligation (EVL) is an alternative to NSBB for large varices, if varices enlarge despite NSBB and if patients are intolerant of NSBB or where NSBB are contra-indicated. EVL should be performed by experienced providers.
16. Surgical shunts, TIPS, and sclerotherapy are not recommended for primary prophylaxis.
17. For gastric varices, NSBB are recommended but cyanoacrylate injection is not for primary prophylaxis. Remember that cyanoacrylate is used for acute GV bleeding but is not approved in the US for endoscopic use.

Reference

Portal hypertensive bleeding in cirrhosis: Risk stratification, diagnosis and management. PMID: 27786365.

Questions 250 and 251

A 42-year-old female is in the intensive care unit of a local hospital after a catastrophic intracranial bleed. Her living will and her family are hoping she can become an organ donor.

▶ Question 250

Based on current organ allocation policy (since December 2018), what is the sequence that this organ will be offered to compatible wait-listed patients (assuming NOT a DCD donation and the local hospital is in the contiguous USA).

Potential recipient	A	B	C	D	E
Status 1A 600 nautical miles away	5	3	2	3	4
MELD 38 240 nautical miles away	2	1	3	1	3
MELD 15 120 nautical miles away	4	5	5	4	5
MELD 30 60 miles away	3	4	4	5	1
Status 1A 400 miles away	1	2	1	2	2

▶ Question 251

Assuming the same 42-year-old female patient as in the previous question is offered as a deceased donor but now it is a DCD organ, what is the sequence that this organ will be offered to compatible wait-listed patients (assuming the local hospital is in the contiguous USA).

Potential recipient	A	B	C	D	E
Status 1A 100 nautical miles away	1	2	1	1	2
MELD 25 240 nautical miles away	4	4	4	3	3
MELD 15 120 nautical miles away	5	5	3	4	5
MELD 30 60 miles away	3	3	2	5	1
MELD 38 400 miles away	2	1	5	2	4

250 – A is the correct answer.
251 – C is the correct answer.

Commentary – Deceased Donor Liver Allocation

This is a bit of a moving target but the current organ allocation for deceased donor livers takes into account how sick patients are AND eliminates the arbitrary geographical boundaries based on the original 11 UNOS regions and the donation service areas. This came into effect in December 2018.

Essentially, once an organ is available, the sequence for allocation is status 1A or 1B patients within 500 nautical miles of the donor get priority. After that, it is based on donor age and whether the organ is a DCD since older organs and DCD organs should have a shorter preservation time to improve outcomes.

For an organ under 70 years and not a DCD, the sequence is:

1. MELD or PELD score of 37 or higher within 150 nautical miles from the donor, then 250 nautical miles, then 500 nautical miles.
2. MELD or PELD scores from 33 to 36 within 150 nautical miles from the donor, then 250 nautical miles, then 500 nautical miles.
3. MELD or PELD scores from 29 to 32 within 150 nautical miles from the donor, then 250 nautical miles, then 500 nautical miles.
4. MELD or PELD scores from 15 to 28 within 150 nautical miles from the donor, then 250 nautical miles, then 500 nautical miles.

For an organ 70 years or older and/or a DCD, the sequence is:

1. MELD or PELD of 15 or higher within 150 nautical miles, then 250 nautical miles, then 500 nautical miles.

Note how the MELD score is almost irrelevant for the older, DCD organ.

For pediatric donors (under age 18), the allocation is to all pediatric patients within the 500 nautical mile radius first. For donors from outside of the contiguous USA (Hawaii and Puerto Rico), blood type O donors are offered to all local candidates first.

Reference

https://unos.org/policy/liver-distribution

Question 252

A 27-year-old female is referred to your office for possible liver transplantation. After several years of multiple emergency room visits for severe abdominal pain without an obvious etiology, she was diagnosed with acute intermittent porphyria. She continues to have frequent attacks despite treatment. She has evidence of some peripheral neuropathy but no motor weakness. Her laboratory studies are normal except for mildly elevated ALT and AST.

She is very anxious and asks you multiple questions about porphyria and liver disease and the role of liver transplantation.

Which of the following statements is TRUE?

A   She is still at risk of progression of neurological symptoms after liver transplantation.
B   Her liver can be used for a domino transplant without risk of neurovisceral symptoms in the recipient.
C   The prognosis after transplant is 50% 5 year-survival.
D   Without transplant she is at risk for hepatocellular carcinoma.
E   Live donor transplant from her sister is possible as this is an autosomal recessive condition.

D is the correct answer.

Commentary – Liver Transplantation for Acute Intermittent Porphyria (AIP)

This is not a common condition but comes up occasionally in a busy transplant program so fair game for the boards.

The porphyrias are a group of disorders caused by defects in enzymes involved in heme production. They present with neuro-visceral symptoms and in some patients, photosensitivity. Heme synthesis occurs mainly in the bone marrow but also in the liver where there are several regulatory pathways involving delta-aminolevulinic acid synthase. Treatment of porphyria relies on pain medication and infusion of heme during an attack. Liver transplantation has been reported as a treatment for AIP that does not respond well to medical management.

Clinical Pearls: Deceased Donor Liver Allocation

1. AIP is autosomal dominant but with low penetrance due to partial deficiency of porphobilinogen deaminase.
2. The presentation is variable and affected by several exacerbating factors.
3. Abdominal pain, peripheral neuropathy, and progressive autonomic and central nervous system involvement can occur.
4. Liver tests are usually normal or mildly elevated.
5. There is a significant risk of HCC, particularly after age 50 (so screen).
6. Renal dysfunction is common as the disease progresses.
7. Liver transplantation has excellent prognosis (80–90% 5-year survival).
8. Progression of neurological disease is halted by transplant (and occasionally can improve).
9. Domino transplant is possible but there is a risk of neuro-visceral symptoms in the recipient after a few years (so can use for domino in select cases after careful discussion).
10. Liver transplantation has also been performed for other porphyrias, particularly erythropoietic protoporphyria that can lead to cirrhosis, gallstones, and biliary disease.

Notes

I used to think this was just for textbooks until I helped take care of a young woman who was miserable with AIP and on long-term narcotics. She had a MELD of 6 and we eventually were able to get her transplanted and she was a completely different person.

Reference

Liver transplantation for acute intermittent porphyria. PMID: 33259654.

Question 253

A 10-year-old Caucasian female presents with abnormal liver tests. Her mother states that she has always been a "sick" child with multiple visits to the pediatrician for GI symptoms, skin rashes, nail infections, and occasionally seizures. She was recently diagnosed with diabetes and has been started on insulin.

Exam reveals a small child in no distress. There are several small patches of hair loss on the back of her scalp. Her nails are disfigured.

Laboratory studies:

ALT 118 U/L
AST 97 U/L
Tbili 1.4 mg/dL
ALP 67 U/L
ANA negative
SMA negative
Immunoglobulins normal
A liver biopsy shows a mild lymphoplasmacytic portal infiltrate and mild fibrosis.

▶ Question

Which of the following statements is TRUE?

A IL-17 deficiency can lead to this syndrome
B She is at risk for invasive candida infection
C Laboratory studies are likely to show hypercalcemia and hypermagnesemia
D Steroids and azathioprine should not be used to treat her hepatitis
E Genetic testing may show deficiency of the autoimmune regular (AIRE) gene on chromosome 21

E is the correct answer.

Commentary – AIRE and Autoimmune Polyendocrinopathy-Candidiasis-Ectodermal Dystrophy (APECED)

Don't blame me for this question! This topic has turned up on prior board exams and I have seen a couple of cases.

The clue is in the stem. The disfigured nails are due to fungal and/or staphylococcal infections, she has diabetes and alopecia (autoimmune conditions), a history of seizures (maybe due to low calcium or magnesium due to hypoparathyroidism), and an autoimmune hepatitis like presentation and biopsy with negative autoimmune markers.

Chronic mucocutaneous candidiasis is seen in several conditions but classically with autoimmunity involving the endocrine system. There is no invasive candidiasis. There are several genetic associations, mainly due to variants in the AIRE gene and signal transducer and activator of transcription 1 gene (STAT1). The AIRE gene is located on chromosome 21, so not part of the HLA genes that are on chromosome 6.

Clinical Pearls: LT for AIP

1. APECED is associated with a classic triad of candidiasis, hypoparathyroidism, and adrenal failure but there are multiple other autoimmune conditions that are seen.
2. AIH type liver disease is an increasingly recognized association.
3. AIH markers are usually negative.
4. It can be treated with steroids and azathioprine.
5. Multiple mutations in IL-17 genes leading to IL-17 deficiency have been identified that are associated with mucocutaneous candidiasis and staphylococcal infections but NOT with APECED.

Reference

APECED-associated hepatitis: clinical, biochemical, histological and treatment data from a large, predominantly American cohort. PMID: 32557834.

Question 254

For the following drugs used for infection prophylaxis after liver transplant, several adverse effects/pharmacokinetics are listed. Four of the choices are accurate. Which drug does not have the correct adverse effect listed?

A	Trimethoprim-sulfamethoxazole	Hyperkalemia	Pancytopenia	Hypoglycemia	Hyponatremia	Hepatotoxicity
B	Valganciclovir	Pancytopenia	Risk of seizure with imipenem	Decreased sperm count	Acute kidney injury	Tremor
C	Fluconazole	Prolonged QT	Stevens-Johnson	CNI interaction	Pregnancy category D	Hepatotoxicity
D	Pentamidine	Pancreatitis	Bronchospasm	Pancytopenia	Hepatotoxicity	Hypocalcemia
E	Atovaquone	Diarrhea	Cholestatic hepatitis	Interaction with rifampin	Take with high fat meal	Vomiting

D is the correct answer.

Commentary – Side Effects of Commonly Used Drugs for Infection Prophylaxis

This is must-know stuff, although some of the drugs are used less often, you are the prescriber so you should know the adverse effects.

Remember that pancytopenia can occur with Bactrim, valcyte, and pentamidine.

The risk of seizure with imipenem is increased when using valcyte (so do not combine them!) and the decreased sperm count is a good board question.

You must know the prolonged QT interval with fluconazole and the interaction with CNIs.

Pancreatitis with pentamidine is a well-known adverse event, as is bronchospasm but the other 3 adverse events are false.

Patients do not like taking atovaquone because of the GI side effects (a bit like mycophenolate).

Notes
This is pretty much guaranteed board material and important clinically

Question 255

A 72-year-old female presents to the hospital with complaints of shortness of breath for one day. She has a past medical history of atrial fibrillation, CAD, and ischemic cardiomyopathy (EF 25%). On arrival to the emergency room, the patient is complaining of feeling light-headed and is somnolent. Her systolic BP 68/34, HR 110, saturation is 82%. Outpatient mediations include coumadin. She denies acetaminophen.

WBC 14, Hb 8.9, platelets 222
Na 133, Cr 2.1
TBili 1.1, AST 11,054, ALT 10,009, ALP 129
Albumin 2.9; INR 2.4
LDH 2450

RUQ US reveals mild hepatomegaly, no ascites or lesions, patent vessels but a dilated IVC and flattening of the doppler waveform in the hepatic veins.

The patient is admitted to the cardiac care unit and is intubated. She is started on inotropes and hemodynamics improve significantly over the next 8 hours: HR 74, systolic BP 110, saturation 96%.

Anti-HAV IgM, HBsAg, HCV RNA all negative.

Cardiology consults you on day 3 for increasing bilirubin.

Laboratory studies on hospital day 3 reveal a TBili 3.4, AST 2400, ALT 1900, ALP 112; Cr 1.6

The most likely cause of the patient's liver injury is:

A Hepatic blood-flow is critically insufficient for hepatocyte survival
B Hepatic glutathione pathway is overwhelmed by NAPQI
C An intense immune reaction against host liver antigens
D Activation of CD8+T cells
E Direct damage to lipid bilayers and disturbance of lysosomal and mitochondrial function

A is the correct answer.

Clinical Pearls: Ischemic Hepatitis

1. Also known as hypoxic hepatitis; we would recommend against using the term "shock liver"
2. Present in 1–2.5% of ICU admissions. Should be on the differential of any ICU patient with marked elevation in LFTs
3. The mean age in large case series is >65 years
4. Injury occurs as a result where hepatic blood-flow is critically insufficient for hepatocyte survival
   a. Two hit hypothesis: (i) a predisposing low flow state (typically right sided heart failure); (ii) 2nd hit during acute cardiac, circulatory, or respiratory failure
5. Characterized by marked exclusive elevation in transaminases (that occur within 24–48 hours of the ischemic event) and that rapidly improve as hemodynamics and oxygenation improve; labs typically normalize within 7–10 days
   a. AST and ALT are typically in the 1000s with normal ALP and only very mild elevation in TBili (upon presentation TBili is almost never above 3); bilirubin can lag however as liver enzymes improve, especially in patients with underlying liver disease.
   b. Concomitant AKI is common
   c. Check LDH! Usually markedly elevated (many times in the 1000s)
6. The diagnosis is one of exclusion
   a. Other causes of liver injury should be excluded
      i. The pre-requisite ultrasound should be done with dopplers to ensure no evidence of thrombus. Clues on RUQ US may include dilated IVC and hepatic veins, flattening of doppler waveform in hepatic veins, and "to-and-fro" motion in hepatic veins and IVC
   b. Biopsy is almost never required but can confirm the diagnosis by showing prominent centrilobular hepatocyte necrosis in the absence of other abnormalities; injury is to zone 3 hepatocytes
7. Passive hepatic congestion (especially elevated right-sided pressures) is almost always a precondition for ischemic hepatitis. >75% of patients will have a predisposing acute cardiac event.
   a. Documented hypotension seen in ~50% of cases
   b. Sepsis ~25% of cases
   c. Exacerbated chronic respiratory failure as the underlying condition is likely under-recognized and can account of up to 10% of cases
8. Can cause an ALF like picture (with coagulopathy and mental status changes) especially in patients with underlying chronic liver disease and those with underlying heart failure
9. In-hospital mortality associated with ischemic hepatitis is about 50%
10. Treatment is directed at the underlying hemodynamic disturbances (as opposed to any specific therapy for the liver injury)

Notes

Cards always calls us on day 3 of "shock" (their words, not mine) liver. The increasing TBili is usually what prompts the consult. Reassure them and they will reward you by giving you a consult on a different patient for "cardiac ascites". AST and ALT >10,000? Can only be two things: acetaminophen or ischemia. If you have seen a case debunking this claim, I am more than happy to hear you out, but make sure your case isn't clouded by a concomitant ischemic event. In particular, exacerbation of chronic respiratory failure probably goes under-recognized. Fellows, I want to know the LDH level when you present a case of suspected ischemic hepatitis!

Reference

Current concepts in ischemic hepatitis. PMID: 28346236.

Question 256

A 17-year-old Caucasian female presents to your outpatient office after a recent admission for variceal bleeding. EGD in the hospital noted large esophageal varices that were banded. Her past medical history is significant for cystic fibrosis (CF) and she follows with the pediatric CF team and has been started on a new CFTR modulator drug.

Examination reveals a thin, pale individual with no distress. Vital signs are normal, BMI 17 kg/m^2

There is no scleral icterus. There is a 5 cm liver edge and a palpable spleen tip.

Laboratory studies:

Hb 11.7
Plt 105
Tbili 1.0 mg/dL
ALT 89 U/L
ALP 303 U/L
INR 1.6
Creat 1.1 mg/dL
Ultrasound shows a smooth, enlarged liver with increased echogenicity. The gallbladder is not well seen.

▶ Question

Which of the following is TRUE?

A Being a Caucasian female increases her risk of disease progression and need for liver transplant
B Percutaneous liver biopsy should be considered to look for cirrhosis
C She is at increased risk of gallbladder cancer
D Nutritional supplementation with a low carbohydrate, high fat diet is recommended
E If she needs transplant, lung-liver is her only option

D is the correct answer.

Commentary – Cystic Fibrosis Related Liver Disease (CFLD)

The increased life expectancy of CF patients means that adult hepatologists will see CFLD and therefore is a reasonable board exam topic.

Biliary cirrhosis is the common reason for CF patients to undergo liver transplantation but there is a whole spectrum of liver (and biliary) abnormalities associated with CF. Clinical CFLD is thought to occur in almost 50% of CF patients.

The CF transmembrane conductance regulator (CFTR) is located on the biliary epithelium and promotes bile flow by regulating chloride and bicarbonate secretion. In CF, genetic mutations of the CFTR leads to bicarbonate-poor bile with increased viscosity leading to biliary obstruction, fibrosis and cirrhosis.

The other incorrect options in the question are discussed in detail below. Her sex and race are favorable in terms of outcome and liver biopsy if performed, should be trans-jugular as non-cirrhotic portal hypertension is common. Gallbladder cancer is not a feature of CFLD but a small, contracted gallbladder is seen. The need for high fat diet and fat/fat-soluble vitamin supplementation is strongly recommended.

Clinical Pearls: CF-related Liver Disease

1. Abnormal LFTs, hepatomegaly, and radiographic and histologic abnormalities historically defined CFLD.
2. Abnormal LFTs can be found in up to 50–90% of CF patients (intermittent, transient, or persistent).
3. Ultrasound abnormalities can be found in 20% of patients.
4. The most common pathologic finding is steatosis but does not correlate with the risk of fibrosis. Fibrosis is usually patchy.
5. Older autopsy studies in adults suggest biliary cirrhosis/advanced fibrosis in most CF patients.
6. Registry studies suggest 10% of CF patients develop biliary cirrhosis. Usually there is well-preserved synthetic function and jaundice is rare. Malnutrition is very common due to fat malabsorption and many patients also have pancreatic insufficiency.
7. Portal hypertension can be related to biliary cirrhosis or non-cirrhotic portal hypertension (NCPH) and is associated with worse outcome.
8. In patients with NCPH, NRH can occur.
9. Risk factors for more advanced disease and poor outcome include:
   a. *F508del* variant of the CFTR gene
   b. Male sex
   c. Hispanics
   d. Concomitant PiZ A1AT (heterozygosity)
10. Management should concentrate on nutritional optimization. Nutritional supplementation with fats rather than carbohydrates and high dose fat soluble vitamins is recommended.

11. Ursodeoxycholic acid use is common but unproven (so should not come up on the boards).
12. The new CFTR modulator drugs are used on patients with eligible mutations of the CFTR gene. They can cause elevated LFTs and routine LFT monitoring is recommended. They also have CYP P450 3A4 interactions.
13. Liver transplantation is appropriate for decompensated disease. Lung-liver transplant has been performed but is uncommon. Survival is similar for liver alone or lung-liver transplant.
14. Five-year survival after liver transplantation is reported at 75%
15. Biliary disease includes cholelithiasis, cholecystitis, micro-gallbladder, and a sclerosing cholangitis subtype that can lead to a recurrent pyogenic cholangitis- type presentation with hepaticolithiasis and biliary strictures.

Notes

We see CFLD a few times a year and we have transplanted a handful of patients. The portal HTN is often much more pronounced than the degree of liver synthetic dysfunction would suggest, emphasizing the role NCPH plays. Surprisingly, I have only seen one case of the sclerosing cholangitis type, although it is well-described.

Reference

Features of severe liver disease with portal hypertension in patients with cystic fibrosis. PMID: 27062904.

Question 257

A 58-year-old male is referred to your clinic for clearance for cardiac transplantation. He has a history of ischemic cardiomyopathy with New York Heart Association class IV heart failure. In addition to dyspnea he complains of abdominal distension and edema. During a recent admission, he underwent paracentesis with a SAAG of 1.2 mg/dL.

On examination his O_2 saturation is 92% on room air, pulse 88, BP 110/60

He has jugular venous distension, a 4/6 pansystolic murmur at the right sternal edge, pulsatile tender hepatomegaly, and moderate ascites.

Laboratory studies:

Hb 10.3 g/dL
Plt 134
Tbili 2.7 mg/dL, direct 0.8 mg/dL
ALT 46 U/L
ALP 273 U/L
Albumin 3.5
INR 1.7
Creat 1.0 mg/dL
Viral and autoimmune markers negative
Ultrasound abdomen – heterogeneous enlarged liver, dilated hepatic veins

▶ Question

Which of the following statements is TRUE?

A His ascites fluid protein level will likely be <1 mg/dL
B A transjugular liver biopsy will show an elevated hepatic venous pressure gradient
C Liver histology will likely show bridging fibrosis between adjacent hepatic veins with sparing around portal areas
D A nutmeg liver refers to the reddish cirrhotic nodules seen on gross examination in this condition
E If biopsy confirms cirrhosis, he should be declined for heart transplant and needs combined heart-liver transplant

C is the correct answer.

Commentary – Congestive Hepatopathy/Cardiac "Cirrhosis"

Liver disease in patients with heart disease/failure is commonly seen at large tertiary centers and the above example is discussed a few times a year in our recipient review conference. In general, it is rare that a heart transplant would be contra-indicated because of liver disease.

In this patient, the presentation and physical findings indicate high right-sided pressures with tricuspid regurgitation explaining the pulsatile hepatomegaly and dilated hepatic veins seen on imaging. The pearls below go into more depth, but ascites fluid protein should be elevated, the HVPG will be normal (no gradient), nutmeg liver refers to the gross appearance (and an imaging equivalent) with reddish central areas of congestion and bleeding into the dilated sinusoids and the paler spared areas. Even with "cirrhosis," heart transplant alone is usually sufficient.

Clinical Pearls: Congestive Hepatopathy/Cardiac Cirrhosis

1. Laboratory abnormalities typically include elevated indirect bilirubin (that correlates with the degree of right-sided pressure) but jaundice is uncommon. The ALP is usually elevated, and the transaminases may be slightly elevated.
2. Imaging usually shows an enlarged heterogeneous liver due to stagnant blood flow and dilated hepatic veins and IVC.
3. The SAAG should be >1.1 mg/dL and the ascitic fluid protein is elevated to >2.5 mg/dL as there is preserved liver synthetic function and presumed increased leakage from hepatic lymphatics that are protein rich.
4. A trans-jugular biopsy will show elevated free and wedged hepatic vein pressures, with a normal gradient. Example: Wedge 26 mmHg, Free 23, IVC 23, RAP 22.
5. Liver biopsy will show congestion with dilated sinusoids, variable zone 3 hemorrhage and necrosis, variable cholestasis.

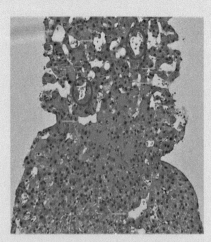

Yellow arrows highlighting dilated sinusoids, blue circles highlighting areas of hemorrhage.

6. In well-established disease, fibrosis occurs in zone 3 and extends out from the central vein. It can link to the portal areas (cardiac sclerosis) or bridge between adjacent hepatic veins and spare the portal areas (cardiac fibrosis or "cirrhosis").
7. HCC can rarely occur.
8. Treatment is to treat the underlying heart failure.
9. Cardiac "cirrhosis" is not *necessarily* a contraindication to a heart transplant.
10. Between 1988 and 2015 only 192 combined heart-liver transplants were performed in the United States (on average less than 10 per year). The most common indications for combined heart-liver transplant are familial transthyretin amyloid and hemochromatosis and less frequently heart failure with "cardiac" cirrhosis.

Notes

For the boards, the ascitic fluid analysis and HVPG findings are easily testable. In clinical practice, this is not a difficult diagnosis to make, and a liver biopsy is not usually necessary unless the cardiologists demand it. As the "stakes" with transplants are so high, it is understood that these patients should be evaluated at large experienced centers. Decisions regarding single or combined transplantation should be made in a multi-disciplinary fashion involving both the transplant hepatology and transplant cardiology teams.

Reference

Assessment of advanced liver fibrosis and the risk for hepatic decompensation in patients with congestive hepatopathy. PMID: 29672883.

Index

The numbers in the right indicate question numbers.

Hepatology and Transplant Hepatology Board Review, First Edition. Jawad Ahmad and Shahid M. Malik.
© 2023 John Wiley & Sons Ltd. Published 2023 by John Wiley & Sons Ltd.